The Geography of Disease

Scientific Editor: *Sir Richard Doll*

Professor Sir Richard Doll chaired the committee, which included Professor E D Acheson, Mrs Paula Cook-Mozaffari and Professor G A Rose, that planned this number of *British Medical Bulletin*. We are grateful to them for their help, and particularly to Professor Doll who acted as Scientific Editor for the number.

British Medical Bulletin is published by Churchill Livingstone
British Council, 10 Spring Gardens, London SW1A 2BN.

* As the pagination is continuous throughout the four numbers of Volume 40, the first page in this number is 307 and not 1.

British Medical Bulletin (1984) Vol. 40, No. 4, p. 307

INTRODUCTION

RICHARD DOLL DM FRCP FRS

Imperial Cancer Research Fund
Cancer Epidemiology and Clinical Trials Research Unit
University of Oxford

The paths that lead to the discovery of the causes of disease are often long and tortuous, including along the way clinical impression, vital statistics, and a wide range of epidemiological and laboratory investigations. They may begin in physiological experiments, theoretical deductions, or serendipity, but they have often also started from a simple count of patients and a description of where, when, and how they lived. Such studies of the geography of disease, or geographical pathology as it tended to be called on the continent of Europe, were one of the principal means by which clues to aetiology were obtained in the last century, and led to the discovery of the causes of many parasitic and infectious diseases, of vitamin and trace element deficiencies, of chronic intoxications like ergotism, and of cancers of the buccal cavity in SE Asia, and of the skin of the abdomen in Nepal. Now, however, with the development of such refined and powerful tools as the electron microscope, the mass spectrometer, and DNA probes, we turn naturally to laboratory investigation as our method of choice and the value of simple observational studies tends to be overlooked. This, I believe, is a mistake. The world has not yet become a uniform unit; culture, standards of living, and external environments vary greatly; and knowledge of the geographical distribution of disease is still far from complete.

If anyone doubts the wealth of clues that remain to be followed up and explained from such studies, he will certainly not do so after reading the series of articles in this issue of the Bulletin. The topics that have been chosen for review include only a small fraction of those that might have been covered, varying from every type of common cancer to diseases like Balkan nephropathy and Japanese Itai-Itai disease that occur only in strictly localized areas. Two of the topics illustrate methodologies that are relevant to the study of the geography of disease wherever it may occur: a technique for separating purely geographical factors from the socio-economic ones with which they may be confounded, and the use of migrants as a means for distinguishing genetic and environmental factors. The others mostly examine single diseases or groups of diseases that are major contributors to mortality or show particularly striking variations in incidence which challenge research workers for an explanation. Two have been selected for other reasons: Paget's disease, to show how diseases that might seem to be poor candidates for geographical investigation may pay unexpected dividends, and mental disease, because of its increasing importance in the world and the paucity of clues to the causes of its various components.

Like all branches of medicine, the study of the geography of disease has developed its own special techniques, which sometimes involve complex statistical analysis. This, however, seldom intrudes into these papers and many of them require no more specialist knowledge than an understanding of the standardized mortality ratio or SMR, which is now generally understood to mean the number of deaths observed in a given population expressed as a percentage of the number that would have occurred, if the population under study had experienced the same sex- and age-specific mortality rats as some larger standard population.

The new and encouraging feature of many of the studies reported is the close collaboration that has developed between epidemiologists and laboratory workers, to the enrichment of the work of both. This is particularly evident in the study of cancer of the liver, where the discovery of the carcinogenic potency of aflatoxin led to surveys of its presence in samples of food; and the persistent evidence of an association between cancer and hepatic fibrosis in high-incidence areas led to a search for the presence of hepatitis B antigen in livers in which cancer had developed. The extent to which both factors need to be present to produce the disease is still unclear. It is of great interest to the understanding of the mechanisms of carcinogenesis, and may prove to be important in practice for, as Cook-Mozaffari and van Rensburg suggest, it may be possible to get a quicker effect by reducing the amount of aflatoxin in food before the viral carrier states can be eliminated by immunization at or soon after birth. Similar cooperative research is now promising to explain how the reproductive factors that have long been associated with the production of cancer of the breast, may actually modify the incidence of the disease, although in this case an understanding of the mechanism by which it is produced may still leave us a long way from being able to prescribe a practical means of prevention.

Some of the studies reported in this issue are close to, if they have not already achieved, fruition. Others, like those of cancer of the oesophagus and stomach, and of hypertension and other cardiovascular disease, provide clues that could hardly be clearer but yet are exasperatingly difficult to follow up. All, however, have the common feature that they demonstrate that the diseases with which they are concerned vary greatly in incidence, independently of genetic susceptibility, and are therefore in principle capable of being avoided. As these diseases are amongst the commonest causes of morbidity and mortality throughout the world, the study of their geographical distribution strengthens the belief that preventive medicine will have even more opportunities for improving health in the future than it has already.

Another Munksgaard Journal

LIVER

AN INTERNATIONAL JOURNAL

Editors
HEMMING POULSEN, Copenhagen, Denmark
PER CHRISTOFFERSEN, Copenhagen, Denmark

Associate Editors
VALEER DESMET, Leuven, Belgium
JOHAN FEVERY, Leuven, Belgium
JENS O. NIELSEN, Copenhagen, Denmark
SHEILA SHERLOCK, London, U.K.

This journal, international in scope, is intended for pathologists, clinicians, immunologists and others concerned with all aspects of liver function and diseases.
The general aim of LIVER is to promote and maintain communication in the fields of basic and clinically applied liver morphology.

Subscription
As of 1983, LIVER is extended from 4 to 6 issues of about 64 pages. LIVER is published bimonthly. Subscription price 1984: D.kr. 634.00 including postage (£ 48.00, DM 188.00). USA and Canada: US$ 76.00 including postage and air freight, payable in advance. Prices are subject to exchange-rate fluctuations.

Please order from the Publisher at the address below – or through any bookseller.

MUNKSGAARD
International Publishers Ltd.

35 NÖRRE SÖGADE P.O. BOX 2148 DK-1016 COPENHAGEN K DENMARK

British Medical Bulletin (1984) Vol. 40, No. 4, pp. 309–314

APPROACHES TO STUDYING THE EFFECT OF SOCIO-ECONOMIC CIRCUMSTANCES ON GEOGRAPHIC DIFFERENCES IN MORTALITY IN ENGLAND AND WALES*

A J FOX BSc DIC PhD

D R JONES BA MSc PhD

Social Statistics Research Unit
The City University
London

P O GOLDBLATT BSc MSc PhD

Medical Statistics Division
Office of Population Censuses and Surveys
London

1   Methods
    a OPCS Longitudinal Survey
    b Mortality differentials
    c Area classification
2   Results
    a Mortality 1971–81 by socio-economic ward clusters
    b Socio-economic structure of four selected clusters
    c Mortality by socio-economic characteristics within
       selected clusters
3   Discussion
4   Conclusions
    References

Since the first Annual Report[1] of the Registrar General, analysis of geographic mortality differentials has formed a central part of annual reports and of more detailed decennial supplements, the most recent of which[2] covers the period 1969–73.

These statistics are used by two main groups of people. The first, health and other public administrators, are primarily interested in differences between areas, such as health regions and districts, which reflect the administrative organization of services. Their interests may arise from responsibility for the provision and distribution of resources and desire to relate expenditures to 'need'[3] for services, or a wish to compare performances between areas. Measures of need based on mortality use it as a proxy for morbidity and therefore as a measure of demand; measures of performance use mortality as a proxy for output from the health services.

Comparisons using geographic differences in mortality to measure performance are often based on the assumption that health services have an important contribution to make to the avoidance of early death. However, most investigations of 'avoidable deaths' focus on a small proportion of total deaths.[4] For most deaths it is difficult to identify which could have been avoided or delayed by improved medical care. More generally, use of geographic mortality statistics as indicators of 'need' and of output are based on untested assumptions.

The second large group of users of geographic mortality statistics comprises epidemiologists and other researchers studying individual diseases. For these, geographic patterns provide an important source of clues about the causes of the diseases in question. The main body of papers presented in this publication reflects this interest. The units of area used in studies of disease causation will in future become less dependent on administrative boundaries than has been the case to date; since 1981, post-coding of death and census populations (i.e. the use of the postal code of the address) has provided the potential for more studies to use geographic areas which reflect the distribution of the factors under study more directly.

The range of such studies includes those concerned with local variations in socio-economic circumstances,[5] distribution of industry[6] and local environment.[7] At a broader level, international comparisons[8] may examine mortality in relation to stage of socio-economic development, dietary differences and the differences in culture and behaviour. The main emphasis of all these studies has been on improving understanding of factors causing a particular disease by noting geographic correlations.

Thus far, we have referred to the characteristics of geographic areas. These characteristics must, however, be considered as distinct from those of individuals living in these areas. Geographic correlation studies provide a weak basis for making inferences about the relationships between the health of individuals and their life style, socio-economic circumstance, and their personal exposure to environmental hazards, at least when the units of area used are large. Difficulties arise because in more affluent areas there are poor people and in less affluent areas there are people who are well-off, in areas with a high proportion of smokers there are many non-smokers, etc. This type of difficulty is often termed the ecological fallacy.[9]

In most developed countries, routine mortality statistics are derived by counting the number of deaths with particular characteristics, as recorded at death registration, and then relating this to an estimate of the mid-year population of the locality under study, with the particular characteristics. In this way, geographic analyses are based on 'usual residence at the time of death'. Every 10 years in the UK, use is also made of information provided at death registration about 'the last occupation of the deceased'. One such application is the allocation of individuals to social classes. This enables analyses to be performed by social class *within* each area to measure the degree to which geographic differences reflect the socio-economic variation between areas.[10]

In recent years the Office of Population Censuses and Surveys (OPCS) has been assembling longitudinal data on a 1% sample of the population of England and Wales.[11] This study, the OPCS Longitudinal Study (LS), provides a unique source for examining many of the points made above. In so doing, it demonstrates how an understanding of these issues is relevant to both the health service administrators and planners concerned about administrative areas, and to researchers and epidemiologists with their emphasis on the aetiology of particular diseases.

The first major report from this source[11] described mortality differences in 1971–75 between administrative areas, such as regions, and showed how it was possible to look at individuals' characteristics, such as their migration histories, to see how these influenced the geographic gradients. Our paper now presents some early results of a project using the full decade of deaths between 1971 and 1981 Censuses to investigate geographic mortality differentials further. Here we describe differences in mortality between areas of the country defined in terms of the socio-demographic characteristics of people living in them. For four selected socio-demographic areas we look at the degree to which differences in mortality between the areas are explained by the housing tenure, social class, and the economic position of the *individual* people living in those areas. In this paper social class refers to the Registrar General's grouping of individual occupations into broad categories such as professional, administrative, junior non-manual, skilled manual, semiskilled manual, and unskilled manual occupations. We also include a preliminary investigation of the extent to which differences in area characteristics explain differences in mortality by housing tenure, social class, etc. These results will be incorporated in our main project in an analysis of the impact of socio-economic circumstances on individual and area differences between administrative and geographic areas.

1 Methods

a *OPCS Longitudinal Study*

Since the early 1970s OPCS has been bringing together Census and vital events records for 1% of the population of England and Wales. The sample, all people born on one of four birth dates in each year, was initially selected from the 1971 Census. Subsequent additions of new births occurring on these dates and of immigrants with these birth dates who register with the NHS have been made so that the sample should continue to represent about 1% of the population. Subsequent censuses will supplement this operation. Demographic, social and economic characteristics of the sample in 1971 were obtained by reference to their 1971 Census schedules, which include information about the sample member and other people in the same household.

For each person in the sample, vital events occurring in the period 1971–1981 are being incorporated into the data set. The events covered include (i) live and still births to men and women in the sample; (ii) deaths under one year of age of these children; (iii) immigration and emigration; (iv) death of a spouse; (v) cancer registration; and (vi) death. OPCS are currently incorporating information about the sample from the 1981 Census (this includes information for people added to the sample between the censuses). Once again, this information will relate to the individual sample member *and* to other people in the same household.

b *Mortality Differentials*

The methods used to analyse mortality differentials in this paper are described in detail in the first report from the Longitudinal Study.[11] In summary, deaths and person-years-at-risk of the sample population between the Censuses are separated by sex, age at death (5-year age-groups) and then further sub-divided by characteristics recorded in the 1971 Census. Deaths in a sub-group are then compared with the number expected, obtained by multiplying the person-years-at-risk by age-specific death rates for a standard group, usually the total Longitudinal Study population of the same sex. In this way mortality can be analysed by characteristics derived from Census questions on economic activity, household composition, marital and family status, housing, marriage and fertility history (for women under 60 years of age only), education, area of residence, migration history from 1966 to 1971 and country of birth of the individual and of their parents. For the present paper we concentrate on area of usual residence (see below), economic position (i.e. whether or not the sample member was working the week before the Census), social class, and housing tenure.

c *Area Classification*

The geographic framework used in the 1971 Census permits analysis by groupings based on enumeration districts (of which there were 110000 in 1971). Such groupings include standard regions, conurbations, counties, London boroughs and county boroughs, wards, parliamentary constituencies etc.[12]

During the 1970s, OPCS sponsored a series of analyses which aimed to group areas according to their socio-economic composition.[13] In this paper we compare mortality in 36 geographic clusters derived by grouping Census wards on the basis of 40 census variables.[14] The titles given to these clusters and families are:

FAMILY 1: Areas of young and growing population
1 New towns
2 Planned developments, smaller town
3 Very new council housing
4 Modern, low-cost, owner-occupier housing
5 Not-owner-occupied housing in areas of growth
6 Modern high-status housing, young families
7 Military bases
FAMILY 2: Areas of older settlement
8 Edwardian development
9 Older industrial settlements with low stress
10 Market town
11 Inner areas with low-quality older housing
12 Poor-quality housing in areas of economic decline
FAMILY 3: Rural areas
13 Villages with some non-agricultural employment
14 Rural areas with large land holdings
15 Rural areas with small land holdings
FAMILY 4: Urban council estates
16 Overspill estates
17 Local-authority housing in Scotland and North East
18 Urban local authority estates with good job opportunities
19 Mining areas
20 Inter-war local authority housing
21 Inner-city council estates
22 Areas of local authority housing with single people
FAMILY 5: Areas in Scotland suffering from acute social disadvantage
23 Clydeside peripheral estates
24 Clydeside inner areas
FAMILY 6: Areas of multi-occupancy students and immigrants
25 Inner London
26 Multi-occupied inner London
27 Multi-occupied and immigrant areas
28 Student areas and high-status Central London
29 High-status rooming-house areas
FAMILY 7: Areas of established high status and resorts
30 Modern high-status areas
31 Mock-Tudor areas
32 Established high-status suburban areas
33 Rural established high-status areas
34 Very-high-status areas
35 Residential retirement
36 Seaside and retirement

We have chosen to concentrate on areas defined in terms of characteristics, rather than administrative areas, and to measure the degree of within-area variation by socio-economic characteristics because others have suggested the use of these area measures as alternatives to measures based on the circumstances of individuals.[15,16] Restrictions on space and time have forced us to concentrate on four clusters and to look only at male mortality to illustrate the approach. A fuller analysis, including analyses by administrative areas, will be covered in our main report of this project.

The relative importance of cluster and individual measures of social class, tenure or economic position has been assessed in part by fitting nested regression models to the data, using a log link function and Poisson error structure[17] to describe numbers of observed deaths in terms of expected deaths alone (the 'null' model) or in combination with socio-economic variables.

The object of these initial analyses is to obtain an indication of the extent to which the socio-economic characteristics explain the cluster differences or the cluster differences explain the socio-economic differences.

2 Results

a *Mortality 1971–81 by Socio-economic Ward Clusters*

The overall differences in mortality between the 36 individual clusters of areas are summarized in Table I and Fig. 1. These 36 areas were grouped by continuing the clustering process into seven 'families' as indicated by Table I and Fig. 1. The reader should, however, recognize the limitations of these titles and refer to the original analysis which describes the characteristics of people in each cluster.[14]

The first point that is clear from the table is that, because the Longitudinal Study is confined to people usually resident in England and Wales in 1971, not surprisingly we have few people in Family 5 (areas in Scotland suffering from acute social disadvantages). In the original cluster analysis,[14] this family comprised mainly, but not exclusively, Scottish areas. Consequently, clusters

23 and 24 in this family, are excluded from the comments below. This family title provides an extreme example of the need for caution in interpreting the titles given to individual clusters and to families of clusters.

Even though more than 1000 men in our sample were usually resident in even the smallest of the remaining 34 clusters in 1971, the final column of Table I shows that the confidence limits around individual cluster SMRs are still fairly broad.

The cluster with the most significantly raised SMR (based on the maximum of 34 chi values, see Reference 12, p. 15) is Cluster 11 (inner areas with low-quality, older housing). Other clusters with significantly raised SMRs include Cluster 16 (overspill estates), Cluster 18 (urban local-authority estates with good job opportunities), Cluster 19 (mining areas), Cluster 21 (inner-city council estates) and Cluster 27 (multi-occupied and immigrant inner areas).

Those clusters with significantly lowered SMRs include Cluster 30 (modern high-status areas), Cluster 32 (established high-status surburban areas), Cluster 35 (residential retirement areas), Cluster 33 (rural established high-status areas), Cluster 34 (very-high-status areas), Cluster 6 (modern high-status housing, young families) and Cluster 29 (high-status rooming-house areas). These areas are found by Webber[20] (see for example p. 54) to be

TABLE I. Mortality in 1971–1981 of males, by socio-economic area cluster of residence in 1971

Cluster	Number of men in 1971	Deaths in 1971–81			Approximate 95% confidence limits
		Observed	Expected	SMR	
Family 1					
1	8 106	698	703.1	99	92–107
2	4 800	494	479.3	103	94–113
3	4 721	315	285.5	110	98–123
4	12 664	1270	1 173.0	108	102–114
5	13 119	1299	1 344.8	97	91–102
6	8 017	551	631.1	87	80–95
7	1 473	57	78.1	73	55–94
Family 2					
8	13 105	1687	1 628.4	104	99–109
9	13 392	1853	1 769.0	105	100–110
10	12 821	1809	1 817.0	100	95–104
11	5 695	763	589.0	130	120–139
12	12 248	1885	1 649.9	114	109–120
Family 3					
13	8 278	1057	1 150.1	92	86–98
14	3 904	506	559.4	90	83–99
15	3 034	389	465.6	84	75–92
Family 4					
16	8 168	917	725.7	126	118–135
17	2 761	282	245.6	115	102–129
18	12 337	1474	1 295.5	114	108–120
19	9 774	1274	1 111.6	115	108–121
20	3 100	397	410.8	97	87–107
21	2 961	375	303.8	123	111–137
22	1 635	250	226.8	110	97–125
Family 5					
23	455	30	33.0	91	61–127
24	76	5	3.1	161	49–338
Family 6					
25	7 537	955	907.3	105	99–112
26	2 601	279	268.5	104	92–117
27	6 183	707	628.8	112	104–121
28	3 545	426	452.5	94	85–103
29	7 866	917	1 013.3	90	85–97
Family 7					
30	13 364	1308	1 517.5	86	81–91
31	13 393	1505	1 635.4	92	87–97
32	10 599	1239	1 425.9	87	82–92
33	4 620	558	673.5	83	76–90
34	4 551	513	603.7	85	78–93
35	6 510	1250	1 430.0	87	83–91
36	2 751	595	644.0	92	85–100

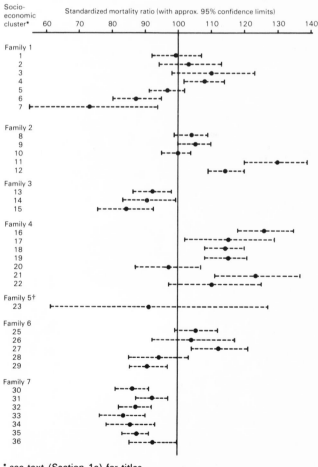

FIG. 1. Male mortality in 1971–1981 by socio-economic area

* see text (Section 1c) for titles
† Cluster 24 95% confidence interval (49—338)

311

areas with a high proportion of two-car households, professional people and owner-occupiers with large accommodation.

The main conclusion from this table and figure is a pattern of low mortality in 'high-status' clusters and high mortality in 'low-status' clusters.

At the broader level of families of areas, the results are not as homogeneous. Only in Family 3 (rural areas) and Family 7 (areas of established high status and resorts) is there a high degree of homogeneity; all clusters in both families have significantly lowered SMRs. Both Family 6 (areas of multi-occupancy student and immigrants) and Family 1 (areas of young and growing population) contain clusters with mortality significantly above average and clusters with mortality significantly below average.

b *Socio-economic Structure of Four Selected Clusters*

In the following sections we focus on four relatively large clusters with contrasting socio-demographic structures and mortality levels to see if differences in mortality may be associated with their socio-economic structure. We consider Cluster 35 (residential retirement areas) which has low mortality; Cluster 1 (new towns) and Cluster 9 (older industrial settlements with less stress) which have mortality near to the average; and Cluster 11 (inner areas with low-quality older housing) which has high mortality.

Table II summarizes, in terms of housing tenure, social class and economic position, the socio-economic structure of these clusters.

Comparing these four clusters, the low mortality areas, Cluster 35, contain the highest proportion of owner-occupiers and the lowest of local-authority tenants; the highest proportion of men in Social Classes I and II (broadly professional, managerial and administrative) and the lowest in Social Classes IV and V (semi-skilled and unskilled manual); and the highest proportion retired and the lowest proportion employed.

In contrast, Cluster 1 contains the highest proportion of men in local-authority housing, a fairly high proportion of men in non-manual occupations and a high economic activity rate, with very few retired men and a large proportion of dependent children.

Clusters 9 and 11 are clearly of 'lower status' but differ in

interesting ways. The proportion of men in owner-occupied housing in Cluster 9 is nearly as high as in Cluster 35, whereas in Cluster 11 the largest proportion of men live in privately rented accommodation. Cluster 11 has the lowest proportion of men in Social Classes I and II and highest proportion 'sick'.

c *Mortality by Socio-economic Characteristics Within Selected Clusters*

Tables III–V give the observed and expected male deaths in 1971–1981 in the same four clusters by housing tenure, by social class and by economic position within the four selected clusters. Table VI shows the fit of a series of regression models to the data in these tables.

We shall consider first the analysis by housing tenure (Table III). Within each tenure category, men in Cluster 11 had the highest SMRs and men in Clusters 35 and 1 has the lowest SMRs. This suggests that cluster differences persist within tenure groups. However, it is interesting to compare Cluster 35 and Cluster 1. As has already been noted, the former comprises mainly owner-occupiers whereas the largest group in the latter are local-authority tenants. Overall, the SMR for Cluster 35 is 87 (95% confidence

TABLE II. Distributions of males in selected area clusters by housing tenure, by social class and by economic position

| | Socio-economic area cluster | | | | | | | |
| | 35: Residential retirement areas | | 1: New towns | | 9: Older industrial settlements with low stress | | 11: Inner areas with low-quality, older housing | |
	No.	%	No.	%	No.	%	No.	%
Tenure								
Owner Occupier	4545	69.8	2760	34.0	8126	60.7	1996	35.0
Local Authority	782	12.0	4751	58.6	3369	25.2	1206	21.2
Privately Rented	903	13.9	488	6.0	1775	13.3	2289	40.2
Other	280	4.3	107	1.3	122	0.9	204	3.6
Total	6510	100.0	8106	100.0	13392	100.0	5695	100.0
Social class								
I + II	1608	24.7	1021	12.6	1547	11.6	259	4.5
III N & M	2101	32.3	2837	35.0	5271	39.4	1888	33.2
IV & V	957	14.7	1446	17.8	2624	19.6	1573	27.6
Other	1844	28.3	2802	34.6	3950	29.5	1975	34.7
Total	6510	100.0	8106	100.0	13392	100.0	5695	100.0
Economic position								
Employed	3310	50.8	4895	60.4	7991	59.7	2996	52.6
'Sick'	115	1.8	105	1.3	245	1.8	175	3.1
Retired	1419	21.8	393	4.8	1401	10.5	471	8.3
Other	1666	25.6	2713	33.5	3755	28.0	2053	36.0
Total	6510	100.0	8106	100.0	13392	100.0	5695	100.0

TABLE III. Mortality in 1971–1981 of males in selected clusters in 1971, by housing tenure in 1971

| Cluster* | Housing tenure | | | | | |
| | Owner occupied | | Privately rented | | Local authority | |
	Deaths: Observed Expected†	SMR	Deaths: Observed Expected†	SMR	Deaths: Observed Expected†	SMR
35: Residential retirement areas	916 1097.1	83	182 188.1	97	92 88.1	104
1: New towns	188 239.9	78	52 67.0	78	429 383.2	112
9: Older industrial settlements with low stress	1000 1060.1	94	322 279.7	115	488 409.9	119
11: Inner areas with low-quality, older housing	208 186.0	112	357 261.1	137	164 122.8	134

* Craig-Weber, see Table I
† Expected on the basis of death rates in 1971–1981 in 5-year age groups for all males in the LS 1971 Census sample

TABLE IV. Mortality in 1971–1981 of males in selected clusters in 1971, by social class in 1971

| Cluster* | Social class | | | | | |
| | I & II | | III N & M | | IV & V | |
	Deaths: Observed Expected†	SMR	Deaths: Observed Expected†	SMR	Deaths: Observed Expected†	SMR
35: Residential retirement areas	395 494.2	80	446 524.4	85	246 265.1	93
1: New towns	68 103.1	66	292 300.0	97	238 213.9	111
9: Older industrial settlements with low stress	233 253.1	92	827 811.1	102	552 534.9	103
11: Inner areas with low-quality, older housing	42 34.3	122	300 239.7	125	299 234.9	127

* Craig-Weber, see Table I
† Expected on the basis of death rates in 1971–1981 in 5-year age groups for all males in the LS 1971 Census sample

TABLE V. Mortality in 1971–1981 of males in selected clusters in 1971, by economic position the week before the 1971 census

Cluster*	Economic position					
	Employed		Retired		'Sick'	
	Deaths: Observed Expected†	SMR	Deaths: Observed Expected†	SMR	Deaths: Observed Expected†	SMR
35: Residential retirement areas	341 447.9	76	819 920.7	89	65 21.3	305
1: New towns	383 429.8	89	260 232.1	112	35 15.0	233
9: Older industrial settlements with low stress	792 821.1	96	890 862.2	103	114 42.3	270
11: Inner areas with low-quality, older housing	313 268.2	117	336 263.0	128	73 23.6	309

* Craig-Weber, see Table I
† Expected on the basis of death rates in 1971–1981 in 5-year age groups for all males in the LS 1971 Census sample

TABLE VI. Scaled deviances of regression models for observed deaths by cluster and tenure (Table III), social class (Table IV) or economic position (Table V)

Model	Scaled deviance	Degrees of freedom
Cluster by tenure (Table III)		
Null model	123.2	11
Cluster alone	54.1	8
Tenure alone	50.3	9
Cluster and tenure	6.5	6
Cluster by social class (Table IV)		
Null model	84.6	11
Cluster alone	21.7	8
Social class alone	54.2	9
Cluster and social class	9.1	6
Cluster by economic position (Table V)		
Null model	300.1	11
Cluster alone	232.1	8
Economic position alone	68.0	9
Cluster and economic position	9.4	6

limit 83–91) and that for Cluster 1 is 99 (95% confidence limit 92–107). Within housing-tenure groups there is no systematic difference between these two clusters.

While this analysis by geographic cluster within tenure category suggests that tenure might explain some, but not all, of the geographic cluster differences, we need to look at tenure differences within geographic clusters to see whether the converse may be happening. Within each geographic cluster, owner-occupiers have substantially lower SMRs than local-authority tenants. Men in privately rented accommodation in Clusters 35, 9 and 11 have similar mortality rates to local-authority tenants. Only in Cluster 1 (for which this is a small group) is the SMR for men in privately rented accommodation similar to that for owner occupiers.

This picture is broadly confirmed by the regression approach outlined earlier. As Table VI shows, inclusion of a cluster term alone or of a tenure term alone in the regression model explained a substantial proportion of the variation in Table III. The two terms combined yield a model which fits the data well, the scaled deviance of this model being similar to its degrees of freedom.[17] There is no evidence that a cluster–tenure interaction term is

needed; within each cluster category the relationship with tenure is similar and within each tenure category the relationship with cluster is similar.

The analysis of mortality by social class within geographic clusters (Table IV) indicates that both social class and cluster contributes to observed differences, a broadly similar conclusion to the analysis by tenure within clusters. Cluster 11 has the highest SMR within each social class grouping; Clusters 35 and 1 generally have the lowest. This suggests an area component which is independent of the social classes of the men in these types of area. Also, within each geographic cluster, men in Social Classes I and II had lower mortality than men in Social Classes IV and V, with those in Social Class III in between.

This is again confirmed by the regression analysis (Table VI) which indicates that inclusion of a cluster term alone reduces the deviance considerably; inclusion of a social-class term alone leads to a smaller reduction. However, neither on its own provides a satisfactory fit to the data. This is obtained by fitting both, without a cluster–social-class interaction, again suggesting a similar relationship with social class in each cluster and vice versa.

It is worth noting that the differences in SMRs by housing tenure within geographic clusters are wider than those by social class, within clusters. In Table III tenure gave a better fit than cluster, whereas in Table IV cluster gave a better fit than social class (Table VI). This was despite the distributional differences noted in Table II which shows that the population of men in owner-occupied housing was much larger than the proportion in social classes I and II.

Table V considers men in each cluster separated by economic position. The two major groups of interest are the employed and the retired, but the table also includes the 'sick' (i.e. those who, in the week before the 1971 Census, were temporarily out of work but intending to seek work and those who were permanently sick). Although the 'sick' make up a small proportion of each area, they are a group with exceedingly high mortality.

Within each geographic cluster, the employed have low mortality and the retired have higher mortality. Within the employed and the retired, Cluster 11 has high SMRs and Cluster 35 has low SMRs. The only SMR which appears out of place is the relatively high SMR for retired people in New Towns (Cluster 1). The size of sampling variations for men who were 'sick' in 1971 means that the power to detect a geographic cluster pattern within this category is small. The SMR for Cluster 35 is as high as that for Cluster 11, but those for Cluster 1 and Cluster 9 suggest that some differences within the category of 'sick' men remain. This is reflected in the goodness of fit of a regression model including only an economic-position variable. This explains a good deal of the variation in Table V, whereas a model with just a cluster term fits much less well. Once again, the model including both terms, in this case cluster and economic position, without an interaction term provides a satisfactory fit.

3   Discussion

It has not been our intention here to present the final results of an analysis of housing tenure, the effects of social class or employment on geographic differences, but rather to illustrate one approach we are taking. We have concentrated our analysis here on geographic areas clustered according to the socio-demographic characteristics of people in these areas. Marked differences between clusters were found, with areas identified by Webber as high-status areas having low mortality and those identified as low-status areas having high mortality. We then proceeded to investigate whether the differences in mortality between four of these clusters could be explained by the pattern within different housing tenure groups, social classes and economic position categories. In most instances, only a part of the geographic cluster differences could be explained by differences in the distribution of people by socio-economic characteristics. Within each geographic cluster, socio-economic differences in mortality were found by housing tenure, by social class and by economic position. In view of the emphasis of the titles of the geographic clusters on the housing characteristics of the areas, and the number of housing variables included in the clustering process (14 out of 40), it is perhaps striking that parallel tenure differences were observed within clusters.

As was indicated above in the introduction, the original review of regional differences in 1971–75 looked at mortality of migrants and assessed the contribution of migration to differences between administrative areas. Relationships between migration and health will also need to be considered when we extend the present analysis to look at the contribution of cluster and individual socio-demographic differences to differences in mortality between administrative areas.

A further extension of this paper will be to repeat the analyses for females and to look at all clusters to see whether these findings are confirmed. We would also wish to examine more conventional geographic differences between the north and west regions and those in the south and east. We could then investigate the extent to which conventional region differences can be explained by the socio-economic characteristics of areas within these regions as distinct from the socio-economic characteristics of individuals within these areas.

4 Conclusions

While it would be difficult to draw firm conclusions from the data presented here, one or two comments may be made. Differences in mortality between clusters are observed. However, when clusters are either aggregated to 'families' or disaggregated according to the characteristics of individuals, little homogeneity is retained. This preliminary analysis would suggest that when it is possible to record the circumstances of an individual, such as their housing tenure, this provides a considerably better measure of their risk of mortality than surrogate measures derived from a knowledge of the area in which they live, the interpretation of which is subject to the ecological fallacy.

ACKNOWLEDGEMENTS

We gratefully acknowledge the contribution of many members of OPCS staff and the Medical Research Council who are supporting a programme of mortality analysis at The City University.

REFERENCES

1 Registrar General. First annual report of the Registrar General of births, deaths and marriages in England [1837–1838]. London: HMSO, 1839

2 Office of Population Censuses and Surveys. Area mortality 1969–73. (Series DS no 4) London: HMSO, 1981

3 Department of Health and Social Security. Sharing resources for health in England and Wales. London: HMSO, 1976

4 Charlton JRH, Hartley RM, Silver R, Holland WW. Geographical variations in mortality from conditions amenable to medical intervention in England and Wales. Lancet 1983; 1: 691–696

5 Kitagawa EM, Hauser PM. Differential mortality in the United States: a study in socio-economic epidemiology. Cambridge MA: Harvard University Press, 1984

6 Blot WJ, Fraumeni JF Jr. Geographic patterns of lung cancer: industrial correlations. Am J. Epidemiol 1976; 103: 539–550

7 Gardner MJ. Using the environment to explain and predict mortality. J R Stat Soc A 1973; 136: 421–440

8 Doll R, Peto R. The causes of cancer. Quantitative estimates of avoidable risks of cancer in the United States today. J Natl Cancer Inst 1981; 66: 1191–1308

9 Goodman LA. Ecological regressions and behavior of individuals. Am Sociol Rev 1953; 18: 663–664

10 Office of Population Censuses and Surveys. Occupational mortality 1970–72. (Series DS no 1) London: HMSO, 1978; 179

11 Fox AJ, Goldblatt PO. Socio-demographic mortality differentials from the OPCS Longitudinal Study 1971–75. (Series LS no 1) London: HMSO, 1980

12 Denham C. The geography of the Census 1971 and 1981. Popul Trends 1980; 19: 6–12

13 Webber R, Craig J. Which local authorities are alike? Popul Trends 1976; 5: 13–19

14 Webber R. The classification of residential neighbourhoods: an introduction to the classification of wards and parishes. (PRAG Technical Report TP23) London: Centre for Environmental Studies, 1977

15 Morgan M. Measuring social inequality: occupational classifications and their alternatives. Community Med 1983; 5: 116–124

16 Morgan M, Chinn S. ACORN group, social class and child health. J Epidemiol Community Health 1983; 37: 196–203

17 McCullagh P, Nelder JA. General linear models. London: Chapman and Hall, 1983

British Medical Bulletin (1984) Vol. 40, No. 4, pp. 315–319

MIGRANT STUDIES IN BRITAIN*

A M ADELSTEIN MD FRCP FFCM

M G MARMOT MB MPH PhD

Department of Medical Statistics and Epidemiology
London School of Hygiene and Tropical Medicine
London

L BULUSU MA FSS

Medical Statistics Division
Office of Population Censuses and Surveys
London

The main part of this paper is a review of our analysis of causes of death of immigrants in England and Wales during 1970–78.[1] Additional mortality figures come from OPCS publications on perinatal and infant mortality, and we review relevant morbidity studies in the UK. Finally, we refer to a number of studies of immigrants in other countries, which include emigrants from the UK or include immigrants born in countries which also sent immigrants to the UK.

Uses of studies of disease in immigrants. Studies of mortality (or morbidity) of immigrants in various countries have been shown to be useful for investigating causes of disease, validating differences between countries and identifying problems of immigrants. They show that rates of diseases in immigrants are often broadly similar to rates in their country of origin, and that these may change within the first or later generations towards the risk of the host population. This would point to influence of the environment.

1   Mortality of Immigrants in England and Wales in 1970–78

An analysis of mortality of immigrants in England and Wales followed the introduction in 1969 of a statement of place of birth on registration of death. From a similar statement on the 1971 Census the numbers of persons born in each country outside England and Wales were available as denominators for calculation of the standardized mortality ratios (SMRs)† in 1970–72. Furthermore, deaths of immigrants in the period 1970–1978 were analysed by

proportional mortality rates (PMRs): that is, ratios for which the denominator is not population but deaths. For this purpose, immigrants were regarded as persons born outside England and Wales; it included people born in Scotland or Ireland, although these are not usually thought of as immigrants in the UK. This definition is not always equatable to ethnic origin, especially when referring to people born in the Indian sub-continent, Africa, or the Caribbean. A measure of ethnicity was available for the first two by classifying names of the deceased; thus among the deaths of persons born in the Indian sub-continent, British could be distinguished from Indian, and both could be distinguished from Africans among immigrants born in Africa. These subsidiary ethnic analyses are based on PMRs, there being no corresponding population denominators. Using deaths in England and Wales as a standard, ratios of each cause of death were compared between England and Wales, each specific immigrant group, and its respective home country (if figures were available). A weakness of the study is the absence of a date of entry into England and Wales of each deceased person.

Table I shows mortality ratios (SMR or PMR) for selected causes in some countries and in their respective immigrants in England and Wales for the period 1970–72. SMRs (or PMRs) are based on rates in England and Wales in 5-year age groups, separately for each sex. Immigrants' SMRs refer to ages '20 and over', and PMRs to ages 20–69 while for home countries SMRs refer to ages 15–74. The text which follows includes discussion of data not shown in the Table.

a   *Mortality From 'All Causes'*

SMRs of immigrants are mostly lower than in their old countries, although they correlate with them, suggesting that immigrants are healthier than the population from which they come. Male immigrants born in Ireland are an exception; for them SMRs are higher than in both their old and new countries.

Selection and adaptation. The lower mortality of immigrants compared to their respective old countries, apparently due to 'selection', appears in ratios for many causes of death in this study and has been noted in other studies including those of emigrants *from* the UK and from Ireland.[2] In the course of time, the immediate effect of selection may wear off, and the 'underlying' trend become manifest. However, the rate may be further influenced by the new environment, especially if immigrants adopt new ways. Examples of selection and late adaptation will be cited in respect of cardiovascular disease and of various cancers in emigrants *from* the UK. The high mortality of Irish immigrants may reflect both 'selection' of disadvantaged immigrants and adverse social conditions in the host country.

Social class. A gradient of mortality between social classes, as observed in the UK and in other industrialized countries, was not observed in migrants except those from Ireland (figures for social class of migrants from Scotland were not available). Apparently the processes of selection and adaptation have so varied between classes as to eliminate differences which are presumed to be present in industrialized countries of origin. In countries with little industry categories of class, based as they are on occupations in industrialized countries, probably have different meanings.

b   *Specific Diseases*

Infections: tuberculosis. The general picture of high SMRs for immigrants and their respective home countries (when known) shown in Table I is familiar. The highest SMR, over 1000, is for women from the Indian sub-continent. Throughout this work, SMRs are based on figures of each sex separately and are not

TABLE I. Examples of SMRs in country of birth and corresponding migrant group (England and Wales = 100)

| | | Ireland | | France | | Italy | | Caribbean | | Indian sub-continent | | | |
| | | | | | | | | | | All ethnic groups | | Indians* (PMR) | |
		M	F	M	F	M	F	M	F	M	F	M	F
All causes	Home	99	117	96	84	91	92	119	171	–	–	–	–
	Migrant	114	109	88	88	77	84	94	117	98	106	–	–
	Migrant deaths	16742	13506	419	961	756	668	1545	1163	4352	98	–	–
All cancers	Home	83	103	100	80	95	85	45	8	–	–	–	–
	Migrant	109	106	102	87	77	87	79	86	69	90	46	46
	Migrant deaths	3759	2982	99	167	162	179	316	262	722	656	190	88
Intestine	Home	116	133	99	78	84	71	77	51	–	–	–	–
	Migrant	118	99	145	74	27	70	65	47	55	80	38	23
	Migrant deaths	266	284	10	17	4	13	17	11	38	58	10	3
Trachea, bronchus and lung	Home	57	90	43	25	56	35	15	19	–	–	–	–
	Migrant	111	159	78	54	68	67	40	33	53	86	25	32
	Migrant deaths	1537	475	28	10	52	14	61	10	218	65	39	6
Breast	Home	–	88	–	64	–	67	–	55	–	–	–	–
	Migrant	–	88	–	79	–	85	–	73	–	80	–	37
	Migrant deaths	–	552	–	29	–	44	–	60	–	131	–	21
Ovary	Home	–	–	–	–	–	–	–	–	–	–	–	–
	Migrant	–	86	–	110	–	71	–	37	–	104	–	53
	Migrant deaths	–	181	–	13	–	12	–	10	–	57	–	9
Diabetes	Home	146	151	169	149	239	293	1081	1310	–	–	–	–
	Migrant	82	69	66	97	109	102	321	436	188	146	243	330
	Migrant deaths	77	95	2	12	7	9	36	46	55	52	28	18
Hypertensive disease	Home	111	133	53	62	101	163	357	690	–	–	–	–
	Migrant	135	108	85	75	111	80	343	430	128	79	168	103
	Migrant deaths	302	244	6	16	16	11	84	63	85	45	41	6
Ischaemic heart disease	Home	96	118	30	31	43	52	70	120	–	–	–	–
	Migrant	104	109	85	89	74	79	51	89	115	115	119	119
	Migrant deaths	4669	2796	115	218	209	117	257	113	1533	739	606	53
Motor vehicle accidents	Home	144	133	206	179	218	135	138	101	–	–	–	–
	Migrant	166	134	215	245	119	87	97	96	110	139	107	83
	Migrant deaths	390	134	14	17	31	8	61	19	134	45	93	16
Immigrant population (in thousands)		399.3	427.0	9.7	23.4	22.0	22.7	121.4	118.0	213.7	150.7	–	–

* Indian refers to all persons born in the Indian sub-continent who have ethnicity of the countries in the Indian sub-continent

directly comparable between sexes. This high ratio in immigrants from the Indian sub-continent is confined to ethnic Indians; people of British background born in the Indian sub-continent have ratios only marginally raised. High mortality ratios are attributed to tuberculosis also in immigrants from Ireland, the Caribbean, Africa and to a lesser extent from Scotland. Countries of origin with high SMRs include Poland, Italy, France and Spain; but migrants from these countries have lower ratios, mostly between ratios of the old and new countries. The high mortality ratios especially among immigrants from the Indian sub-continent have been consistently noted in morbidity studies.[3]

Malignant neoplasms. SMRs for cancers of all sites together are generally low among immigrants and in their home countries (where figures are available); there are large differences in mortality between countries and also between immigrant groups. For example, immigrants from the Indian sub-continent, especially when of Indian background, have very low mortality ratios for a number of cancers; e.g. for stomach, intestine, rectum, 'trachea, bronchus and lung', breast, ovary, cervix, and skin. High ratios were found in both ethnic communities born in the Indian sub-continent for primary liver cancer; and elevated ratios were also found for cancers of the buccal cavity and pharynx and for lymphomas in females.

Mortality ratios from many types of cancers in immigrants born in the Indian sub-continent with British names were between ratios for England and Wales and for immigrants with Indian names. This suggests that British people born in the Indian sub-continent acquired some protection from that environment.

High ratios for liver cancer were found in immigrants from the Caribbean and from Africa in addition to those mentioned above in immigrants born in the Indian sub-continent. Also low ratios for colon cancer were found in immigrants from the Caribbean and from Italy and Spain. As expected, ratios for cancer of the lung were low in all immigrant groups born outside of the British Isles as also in their old countries.

In contrast with American findings,[4] rates for cancers of the intestine, breast, and prostate do not appear to have changed in the first generation. Cancers thought to be caused by a combination of smoking and drinking alcohol—i.e. cancers of the mouth and larynx—were highly in excess in France, Spain and Italy, where the consumption of alcohol is high. Cancer of the oesophagus has a high ratio in France. For these three sites, large differences between countries are confined to males, and immigrants have much lower ratios than in their old countries.

Cigarettes. Smoking is probably the only relevant environmental hazard for which there are available estimates of exposure for individuals. Surveys of cigarette smoking by OPCS[5] show that immigrants from the Indian sub-continent, the Caribbean, and Africa smoke much less than the rest of the UK population. Although immigrants from Europe currently seem to smoke about the same as the indigenous population, figures from their old countries suggest that the amount may have been increased later in life.

The nervous system. The main finding is the very low mortality attributed to multiple sclerosis in immigrants born in the Caribbean, in Africa, and in the Indian sub-continent, particularly in those of Indian origin. Mortality ratios for motor neurone disease, looked at as a 'control' for possible selection against nerve diseases, are more or less as in England and Wales. These figures supplement studies of hospital admissions by Dean *et al*, and are in accord with a hypothesis that in poor countries, early infection protects against subsequent development of paralysis.[6]

Diseases of the cardiovascular system and diabetes. In general, immigrants have mortality ratios between those of their old countries and of England and Wales. Low ratios are noted in immigrants from France, Italy and Spain, and high ratios in immigrants from the Indian sub-continent, more pronounced among ethnic Indians, who have the highest mortality from ischaemic heart disease. In this respect it is notable that ethnic Indian immigrants have a very low ratio for cancer of the intestine, unlike the usual pattern among countries where rates for these diseases are correlated.[7] Very high mortality ratios for hypertension and stroke and low ratios for ischaemic heart disease occur in immigrants from the Caribbean and from Africa.

Mortality from diabetes is very high in immigrants from the Caribbean and from the Indian sub-continent—the latter high ratio being confined to ethnic Indians among whom there are numerous reports of high mortality from diabetes in the Indian sub-continent and in Indian immigrants in other countries.[8]

Diseases of the respiratory system. Mortality from obstructive lung disease is generally low in countries of birth of immigrants born outside of the British Isles; the only two exceptions (with sufficient numbers) are for women in the Caribbean and for both sexes in South Africa.

Immigrants retain the low ratio of their countries of origin. The two ethnic groups of immigrants born in the Indian sub-continent are affected about equally. Studies of British migrants in other countries—Australia, USA, South Africa—show that they retain the high ratio of mortality from bronchitis.[9] These observations of migrants both into and away from the UK are in accord with research findings which link exposure to hazards—e.g. air pollution, respiratory infections in childhood, smoking—with later chronic respiratory disease.

Disease of the digestive system. All the countries of origin whose figures were available showed high ratios for this group of diseases made up mostly from peptic ulcer and liver cirrhosis. In most countries outside the British Isles there are high ratios for liver cirrhosis, and generally immigrants have lower ratios than are reported in their country of origin. Immigrants born in Scotland or Ireland, however, retain high ratios. There are high ratios for cirrhosis in immigrants from the Indian sub-continent, the Caribbean, and Africa.

Diseases of the genito-urinary system. Considering genito-urinary diseases together (mainly nephritis and nephrosis), the principal features are the high ratios in immigrants from the Caribbean, Africa, and the Indian sub-continent, with the last confined to ethnic Indians. These are groups who have high mortality ratios attributed to hypertensive disease, not surprisingly since the two diseases may be related.

Maternal mortality (complications of pregnancy, childbirth and puerperium). Even after standardizing for the number of births, mortality ratios were very high in women who were born in the Caribbean, in Africa, and to a lesser extent in the Indian sub-continent.

Accidents, poisoning and violence (including suicide). Immigrants, with the exception of the Italian-born, have somewhat high mortality ratios, reflecting rates in their home countries, and determined largely by motor vehicle accidents. Deaths due to falls, probably at work, are frequent in immigrants born in Ireland, as also are deaths due to fire. High mortality ratios from suicide were found in immigrants from Poland, Germany and the USSR.

2 Perinatal and Infant Mortality

From records of stillbirths and by linking each record of death within the first week of life with its corresponding record of birth, OPCS produces analyses of perinatal death rates which among other variables include country of birth.[10] The latest published, for 1978 and 1979, shows that perinatal and neonatal death rates are relatively high in children of mothers born in the Indian sub-continent, the Caribbean, or Africa.

3 Morbidity

a *General*

Although mortality rates of specific diseases are often a reasonable index of underlying morbidity, they do not reflect the frequency of some types of illness; for example, mental disorder or rheumatic afflictions. Many research papers on the morbidity of immigrants have been published, and we review here very briefly only those which appear to indicate important issues not already observed in mortality studies.

b *General Practice*

Morbidity statistics from general practice 1970–1971 (socio-economic analysis)[11] are derived from volunteer members of Royal College of General Practitioners who recorded each contact with a patient. Country of birth analysis is included, but the sample of patients was too small for reliable statistics among immigrants from any but the most frequent conditions. This shows that persons born in the Indian sub-continent consult more often than average. Illnesses with high ratios are spread throughout the various chapters of the International Classification of Diseases. Among the few with low ratios are 'mental disorders' and neoplasms in persons born in Pakistan. The first may reflect doctors' perceptions of neurosis; but, as pointed out later, other research confirms these low rates. A low rate for neoplasms agrees with mortality statistics in persons born in Pakistan.

c *Cardiovascular Disease*

Studies of hospital records confirm in general the differences observed in mortality: for example, Beevers and Cruikshank[12] showed that, in their hospital in Birmingham, proportional rates of admission for heart attacks were half as common in West Indians and slightly above normal in persons born in the Indian sub-continent, and that admissions for stroke were much commoner in West Indians.

Cruikshank and Allyne[13] showed that in diabetics, myocardial infarction was more common in blacks although peripheral vascular disease was not. Cataracts were much more frequent in black patients and retinopathy slightly more. The best known study of morbidity for coronary heart attacks in England and Wales in a defined population which included immigrants was by Tunstall Pedoe *et al.*[14] in Tower Hamlets (the east end of London) between April 1970 and December 1972. All cases below age 65 were registered and followed up for 1 year. Immigrants from Asia had above the average and those from the Caribbean only one tenth of the average attack rate.

d *Rickets and Osteomalacia*

Asian immigrants have been known to develop higher rates of rickets or osteomalacia than the indigenous population[15] and it has been shown that a high proportion have evidence of vitamin D deficiency.

Rashid *et al.*[16] showed that Asians in Pakistan had a normal range of serum 25-hydroxycholecalciferol whereas their relatives in England had a considerably lower range. They consider that the evidence for vitamin D deficiency of some Asians in the UK points to an environmental factor. They suggest that in Pakistan the high levels of sunshine compensate for the low intake of vitamin D in the diet, which is reduced by the high intake of fibre, which in turn reduces the half-life of the vitamin.[17] In the UK, the amount of sunshine is insufficient to compensate for the dietary lack. They support the addition of vitamin D to the diet, which has been shown to be effective.

That diet has an effect is further supported by the observation that the incidence of osteomalacia has not changed, while that of rickets in children has decreased considerably, presumably as a result of the second generation of immigrants taking a diet closer to that of the UK[18] (i.e. less fibre, more animal protein). Deficiency of vitamin D was apparently implicated in 10 cases of cochlear deafness reported by Brookes:[19] 4 cases were Asian.

e *Mental Illness*

Cochrane[20] analysed statistics of the Mental Health Enquiry, a national system of hospital records, in 1971. The age-standardized admission rate, irrespective of diagnosis, showed very high rates for people born in the Irish Republic and moderately high rates for female West Indians. Dean *et al.*[21] analysed records of first admissions in South-East England in 1976: immigrants from the Indian sub-continent had fewer admissions for all diagnoses grouped together than expected from the rates for the whole population.

High rates of first admissions, for all diagnoses combined, were registered in immigrants who were born in Ireland, the Caribbean, or Africa. Irish immigrants had a rate of admission between that for England and the higher rates in Ireland. Rates were especially high for alcohol-related disorders and schizophrenia.

In both studies, schizophrenia is diagnosed greatly in excess of expected numbers in all immigrant groups. This raises the possibility that paranoid delusions are being incorrectly recorded as present in some immigrant patients through a lack of familiarity with their culture.[22] There seems to be no agreement whether there is a real excess of schizophrenia or whether the apparent excess is due to a combination of special ways of referring and diagnosing immigrants as a result of both the preconceptions of clinicians and the different customary behaviour of immigrants. Cochrane and Stopes-Roe, declaring that hospitalization[23] rates are an insensitive index of psychological disturbance, carried out a survey using standardized measures of psychopathology among samples of immigrants born in Pakistan and of the native community in and around Manchester. They found that the average level of symptoms was similar in the two populations. This, they conclude, supported the findings that hospital admissions for mental illness as a whole are low in immigrants from Pakistan and that the diagnosis of schizophrenia, particularly the paranoid type, seems to be related to circumstances surrounding the way diagnoses are made.

4 Various Studies of Immigrants from a Common Country of Origin

The interpretation of studies of disease ratios in immigrants may be taken further by comparing findings between countries that have immigrants from a common source, such as the USA,[2,4] Australia, and the UK, each of which has received immigrants from the 'same' countries, e.g. Italy. In Italian-born immigrants in each of these analyses only one major site of cancer (that is, the stomach) has a mortality ratio that is higher than for any of the respective host countries. Furthermore, when Italian and British immigrants in Australia are compared, these results are supported, as Italian-born immigrants have a higher cancer rate than British-born only for cancer of the stomach. An important point is revealed when stomach cancer figures for immigrants from England and Wales are sub-divided; immigrants from Wales have higher rates than those from England and this reflects the national rates within the UK.

These comparisons between studies in different countries increase our confidence in international and immigrant mortality figures. Earlier studies[24] had strengthened the view that cancer of the 'trachea, lung and bronchus' was truly an epidemic of the British Isles; it had been found that British migrants to South Africa, Australia, New Zealand and the USA had a much higher mortality from respiratory cancer than the populations in the receiving countries. This relatively high mortality in Britain is confirmed by the low mortality of all immigrant groups from outside of the British Isles to England and Wales, and by high rates of British migrants compared with those of other migrants in Australia.

Another interesting comparison between studies relates to oesophageal cancer. Analyses in the USA showed that many immigrant groups, especially males, had higher rates of mortality from oesophageal cancer than the populations both of the USA and of their respective countries of origin. A similar picture is shown by immigrants from Ireland in England and Wales, and by immigrants from Ireland and female immigrants from England and Wales in Australia. It would seem to follow either that these immigrants include people who drink and smoke more than average, or, alternatively, that the process of immigration leads to these habits. Selection of immigrants as healthier than the population from which they come is discussed in the Australian report. It is pointed out that mortality ratios for some cancers rise shortly after immigration, presumably as a result of loss of the selective effect, and that subsequently the rate moves towards that of Australia—presumably as a result of developing a new life style in the new environment.

ACKNOWLEDGEMENT

Dr Adelstein undertook this work with the support of a fellowship of the Cancer Research Campaign.

REFERENCES

1 Marmot MG, Adelstein AM, Bulusu L. Mortality by cause in immigrants in England and Wales 1970–1978. OPCS. London: HMSO, 1984 (Studies on population and medical subjects; no 47) in press
2 Armstrong BK, Woodings TL, Stenhouse NS, McCall MG. Mortality from cancer in migrants to Australia 1962–1971. University of Western Australia, 1983
3 Medical Research Council: Tuberculosis and Chest Diseases Unit. National survey of tuberculosis notifications in England and Wales 1978–9. Br Med J 1980; 281: 895–898

4 Haenszel W. Variation in incidence of and mortality from stomach cancer, with particular reference to the United States. J Natl Cancer Inst 1958; 21: 213–262
5 Office of Population Censuses and Surveys. General Household Survey. Social Survey Division, Series GHS. Unpublished tables, 1975, 1976, 1978
6 Dean G, Brady R, McLoughlin H, Elian M, Adelstein AM. Motor neurone disease and multiple sclerosis among immigrants to Britain. Br J Prev Soc Med 1977; 31: 141–147

7 Doll WRS, Peto R. The causes of cancer: quantitative estimates of the avoidable risks of cancer in the United States today. Oxford: Oxford University Press, 1981

8 Jackson WPU. Racial and geographic factors in diabetes. Lancet 1971; 1: 601–602

9 Reid DD. The future of migrant studies. Isr J Med Sci 1971; 17: 1592–1596

10 Office of Population Censuses and Surveys. Mortality statistics, perinatal and infant: social and biological factors. Review of the Registrar General on deaths in England and Wales 1978 and 1979. London: HMSO, 1982 (Series DH3 no 7)

11 Royal College of General Practitioners, Office of Population Censuses and Surveys and Department of Health and Social Security. Morbidity statistics from general practice 1970–1. Socio-economic analyses. London: HMSO, 1982. (Studies on medical and population subjects no 46)

12 Beevers DG, Cruickshank JK. Age, sex, ethnic origin and hospital admission for heart attack and stroke. Postgrad Med J 1981; 57: 763–765

13 Cruickshank JK, Alleyne SA. Vascular disease in West Indian and white diabetics in Britain and Jamaica. Postgrad Med J 1981; 57: 766–768

14 Tunstall Pedoe H, Clayton D, Morris JN, Brigden W, McDonald L. Coronary heart attacks in East London. Lancet 1975; 2: 833–838

15 Department of Health and Social Security. Rickets and osteomalacia. Report of the Working Party on Fortification of Food with Vitamin D. London: HMSO, 1980. (Reports on Health and Social Subjects no 19)

16 Rashid A, Mohammed T, Stephens WP, Warrington S, Berry JL, Mawer EB. Vitamin D state of Asians living in Pakistan. Br Med J 1983; 286: 182–184

17 Batchelor AJ, Compston JE. Reduced plasma half-life of radio-labelled 25-hydroxyvitamin D3 in subjects receiving a high fibre diet. Br J Nutr 1983; 49: 213

18 Dunnigan MG, Robertson I. Residence in Britain as a risk factor for Asian rickets and osteomalacia. Lancet 1980; 1: 770

19 Brookes GB. Vitamin D deficiency—a new cause of cochlear deafness. J Laryngol Otol 1983; 97: 405–420

20 Cochrane R. Mental illness in immigrants to England and Wales: an analysis of mental hospital admissions. Soc Psychiatry 1977; 12: 25–35

21 Dean G, Downing H, Shelley E. First admissions to psychiatric hospitals in south-east England in 1976 among immigrants from Ireland. Br Med J 1981; 282: 1831–1833

22 Paranoia and immigrants [Editorial]. Br Med J 1980; 281: 1513–1514

23 Cochrane, R, Stopes-Roe M. A survey of psychological morbidity in Pakistani immigrants to England. Paper read at the Royal College of Psychiatrists. London, 1981

24 Reid DD. Studies of disease among migrants and native populations in Great Britain, Norway, and the United States. I. Background and design. In: Haenszel W. ed. Epidemiological approaches to the study of cancer and chronic diseases. Bethesda, Maryland: US Department of Health, Education and Welfare. Public Health Service 1966. (National Cancer Institute Monograph 19)

British Medical Bulletin (1984) Vol. 40, No. 4, pp. 320–328

MAPPING CANCER MORTALITY IN ENGLAND AND WALES

M J GARDNER BSc DipMathStat PhD

Medical Research Council's Environmental Epidemiology Unit
Southampton General Hospital

The geography of cancer within countries has become a subject of increased activity in recent years with the aim of detecting causes of the disease. This paper reviews the developments in England and Wales in cancer mapping and related studies.

1 History of Cancer Mapping

There has been an interest in the geographical distribution of cancer in England and Wales since the middle of the last century.[1] The first Decennial Supplement on Area Mortality was published 120 years ago,[2] and the first cancer map—which was based on deaths in women during the years 1851–60—was produced on a county scale by Haviland.[3] Little more attention was paid to the geography of cancer over the next 50 years. Stocks[4] commenting on this lack of investigation, in a way which suggested that it would not have been a very fruitful exercise anyway, said '... during the period when both the accuracy of diagnosis and the completeness of death certification of cancer was improving year by year ... it was natural to suppose that the more rapid progress in these directions around London and certain hospital centres might be the chief factor in producing such local differences as appeared to exist ...'. However, in a pioneer effort produced in three parts, Stocks presented maps based on the years 1921–30 on a county basis for 17 different types of cancer.[4–6] These three papers also described the geographical distributions of the various cancers taking account of the age and sex composition and the degree of

urbanization of each county. Regions of high and low mortality were pointed out, and Stocks proposed some tentative explanations of these differences in relation to climate, geology, diet, occupation and other factors. Cruickshank demonstrated that in the maps which Stocks had produced there was strong evidence of a geographical pattern for the majority of cancer sites.[7]

In 1963 an atlas of mortality for a selection of causes of death was prepared by a committee formed by the Royal Geographical Society,[8] containing mortality data for the years 1954–58. These maps were supplemented by others based on deaths during the years 1959–63 in a later edition.[9] Smaller areas than counties were used for these atlases—such as county and metropolitan boroughs and aggregated urban and rural districts within counties—but only four cancers (lung, stomach, breast and uterus) were included. Howe has experimented with non-standard presentation of maps—such as demographic base maps where an area is represented proportionally to its population size rather than geographical area.[9,10] A recent collection of maps at a regional level was based on 5 years' mortality data around the 1971 census,[11] including a large number of sites of cancer. These maps have been particularly helpful for depicting the geographical patterns of the different cancers on a large area scale.[12]

Using deaths which occurred during the years 1968–78 in England and Wales, an atlas of cancer maps in colour has been produced for a smaller scale of area.[13] The areas used were the boundaries of the 1366 local authorities as constituted prior to reorganization in 1974—namely, the county, London and municipal boroughs and the urban and rural districts. In this volume, 23 maps were presented on this scale for the most important cancers numerically, with a further 44 maps for other types of cancer being provided on a county scale. By using these finer geographical divisions, the marked regional patterns of earlier maps can be dissected into their smaller components.

2 Interpreting the Maps

In the following sections some of the findings from these geographical studies are discussed, as well as other aspects of the variations of cancer mortality around England and Wales. One of the main interests in studying the distribution of cancer in the country is to look for clues to aetiology in any emergent patterns. The desirability for new knowledge in this field is obvious for a cause of death to which some 120 000 deaths (20% of the total) are registered annually. It is interesting to reflect in this connection upon the long duration of time which elapsed between the period when Stocks produced his maps and the more recent versions. As Doll[14] conjectured, this may be due, in part at least, to the strong belief in the mid-years of this century that laboratory-based experimental work would soon discover the causes of cancer and lead to its irradication. Also, the annual number of cancer deaths in England and Wales during 1921–30—a figure of about 52 000 deaths per year[4]—was less than half the current level.

a *Quality of Diagnosis and Certification*

The theme of the quotation from Stocks[4] above, although almost half a century ago, is still an issue of some concern. Over the years a series of papers has raised the problems of inaccurate diagnosis and certification of the cause of death, three of the more recent being by Cameron and McGoogan,[15] Cochrane and Moore[16] and Alderson *et al.*[17] However, these difficulties appear to be less severe for cancer than for some other causes of death—and less severe for some cancer sites than others. Also, the degree of

PLATE I

MAPPING CANCER MORTALITY IN ENGLAND AND WALES   *M J Gardner*

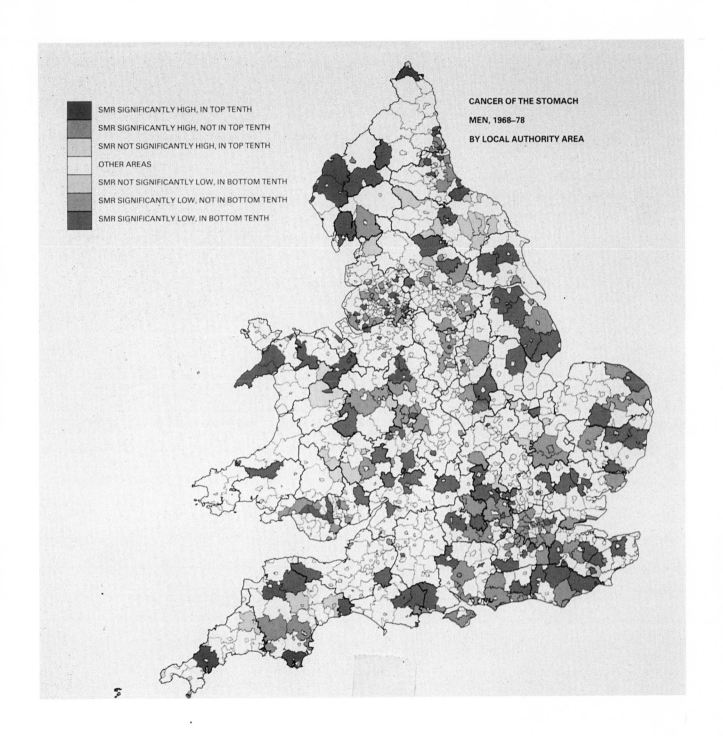

SMR SIGNIFICANTLY HIGH, IN TOP TENTH

SMR SIGNIFICANTLY HIGH, NOT IN TOP TENTH

SMR NOT SIGNIFICANTLY HIGH, IN TOP TENTH

OTHER AREAS

SMR NOT SIGNIFICANTLY LOW, IN BOTTOM TENTH

SMR SIGNIFICANTLY LOW, NOT IN BOTTOM TENTH

SMR SIGNIFICANTLY LOW, IN BOTTOM TENTH

CANCER OF THE STOMACH

MEN, 1968–78

BY LOCAL AUTHORITY AREA

PLATE II

MAPPING CANCER MORTALITY IN ENGLAND AND WALES *M J Gardner*

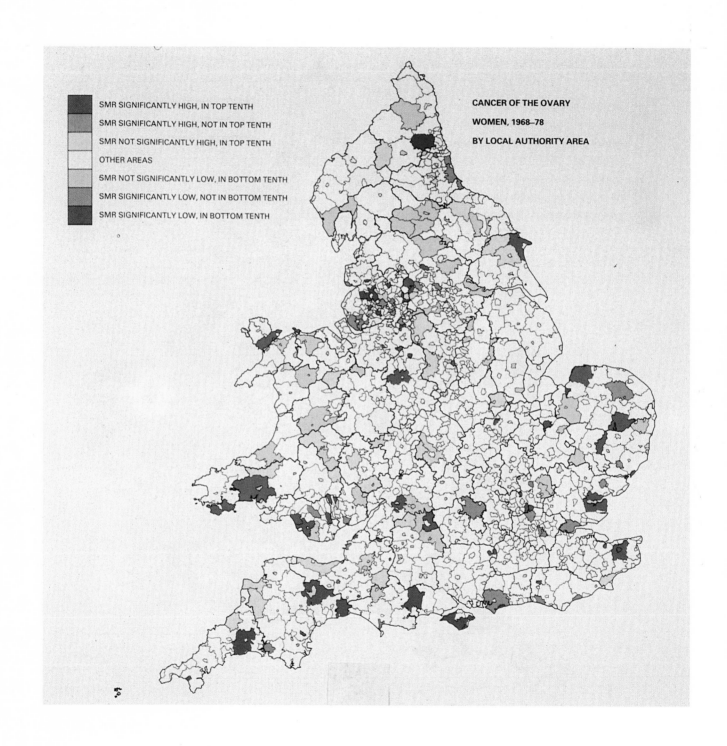

SMR SIGNIFICANTLY HIGH, IN TOP TENTH

SMR SIGNIFICANTLY HIGH, NOT IN TOP TENTH

SMR NOT SIGNIFICANTLY HIGH, IN TOP TENTH

OTHER AREAS

SMR NOT SIGNIFICANTLY LOW, IN BOTTOM TENTH

SMR SIGNIFICANTLY LOW, NOT IN BOTTOM TENTH

SMR SIGNIFICANTLY LOW, IN BOTTOM TENTH

CANCER OF THE OVARY

WOMEN, 1968–78

BY LOCAL AUTHORITY AREA

PLATE III

MAPPING CANCER MORTALITY IN ENGLAND AND WALES   *M J Gardner*

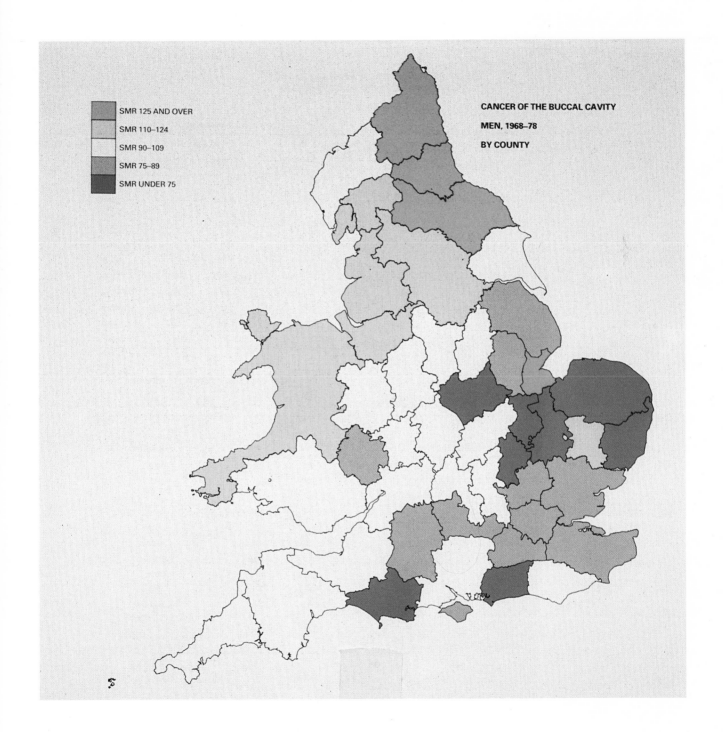

SMR 125 AND OVER
SMR 110–124
SMR 90–109
SMR 75–89
SMR UNDER 75

CANCER OF THE BUCCAL CAVITY

MEN, 1968–78

BY COUNTY

PLATE IV

MAPPING CANCER MORTALITY IN ENGLAND AND WALES   *M J Gardner*

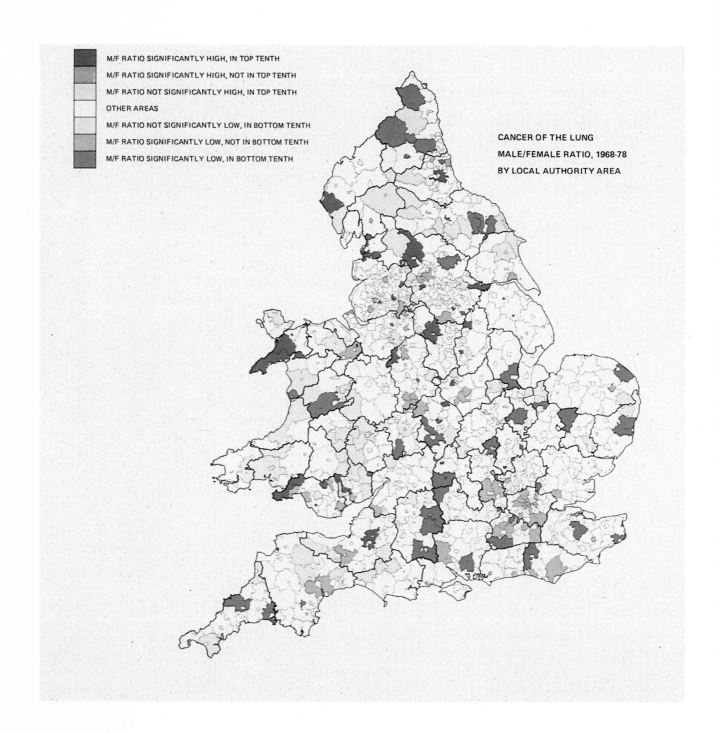

M/F RATIO SIGNIFICANTLY HIGH, IN TOP TENTH

M/F RATIO SIGNIFICANTLY HIGH, NOT IN TOP TENTH

M/F RATIO NOT SIGNIFICANTLY HIGH, IN TOP TENTH

OTHER AREAS

M/F RATIO NOT SIGNIFICANTLY LOW, IN BOTTOM TENTH

M/F RATIO SIGNIFICANTLY LOW, NOT IN BOTTOM TENTH

M/F RATIO SIGNIFICANTLY LOW, IN BOTTOM TENTH

CANCER OF THE LUNG

MALE/FEMALE RATIO, 1968-78

BY LOCAL AUTHORITY AREA

inaccuracy is usually not serious in the context of the epidemiological uses of death certificates.[18] It seems most unlikely that the present level of inaccuracy is associated with producing a distorted picture of the geographical distribution of cancer. Rather, if the errors are of a random nature, they will act to diminish any real geographical differences in mortality. At the present time there is little hard evidence on this point, although what is available does not support the presence of bias.[19] Nevertheless, since only some 20–30% of deaths come to autopsy in England and Wales,[20] it would be a wise precaution to check with other sources of information, such as pathology records and local diagnostic and registration practices, before accepting that a local area death rate is either particularly low or high.[21]

b *Mortality or Morbidity Data?*

A strong theoretical argument could be made in favour of using morbidity data rather than mortality statistics for the description of the relative frequency of cancer in different subgroups of the population. In this way a measure of the incidence of the disease, rather than the death rate, would be provided. For some cancers, particularly those for which treatment is more successful, mortality is clearly an understatement of occurrence and so morbidity would be more suitable. Although survival after diagnosis varies from one type of cancer to another, there are no suggestions of any major differences in outcome between regions of England and Wales.[22] Thus mortality figures, although underestimating the full cancer burden, are unlikely to provide a distorted view of the geographical distribution. On the other hand collection of morbidity information, in the form of Cancer Registries, is a much more recent development than death certification. Cancer registration, having been set up on a national scale only in 1962,[23] post-dates death certification which commenced in 1839 by over 100 years. Also, in contrast to the legal requirement that every death be registered, the notification of patients diagnosed with cancer to the appropriate regional Cancer Registry is a voluntary scheme, dependent for its quality on the cooperation of the patients' doctors and hospitals. For these reasons, similar to Stocks' earlier doubts about the suitability of death certification data, it seems premature to use cancer morbidity data for geographical comparisons.[24]

c *Migration*

Another consideration which must always be borne in mind when interpreting geographical data of this nature is that people, to some extent, are mobile creatures and do not all come to life, live and die in the same place. Statistics of cancer mortality (and morbidity) assign individual cases to their area of home residence at the time of death (or onset), except in some particular instances mentioned below. These areas, of course, are not necessarily the ones where they spent a large portion of their lives, or where they might have been exposed to the experiences which led to them developing cancer. However, there is little to suggest that migration between large areas is of a sufficient level to influence greatly the true mortality patterns,[25] either by diminishing geographical differences to such an extent that they become blurred, or by creating impressive but misleading differences through biased movement of the susceptible/unsusceptible or sick/healthy. This is not to say that the early experiences of migrants are not important in their future mortality, as is well exemplified by the excess death rates from lung cancer among English migrants and both lung and stomach cancer among Welsh migrants to Australia. This excess mortality over their Australian-born contemporaries diminishes as their duration of residence in Australia increases.[26]

d *Coding of Area of Residence*

There can be difficulties with the assignment of area of residence when an individual dies in an institution.[27] For acute general hospitals the death will usually be coded to the person's home address; but for some long-stay institutions the death can be coded to the area in which the institution lies, regardless of how long the patient was there or from where they came. In the small-area scale cancer atlas referred to earlier[13] there was one rural district which appeared to have high mortality on 19 out of 23 cancer maps for men and women. It turned out that this was an artefact due to the presence of a terminal care hospital for cancer patients of all ages in the district (Stone Rural District), which itself had a relatively small population. Since many patients were admitted from the large neighbouring areas of Stoke-on-Trent County Borough and Newcastle under Lyme Municipal Borough, the apparent cancer death rates in Stone were all grossly inflated. On the other hand, mortality from non-cancer causes of death in Stone was not exceptional.[86] In general, the problems of migration and coding of area of residence are more critical as the size of the area studied becomes smaller, and more care should be taken in interpretation to ensure that these are not important influences.

There are other potential difficulties—for example, the appropriateness of the population base used for the calculation of rates—which must also be considered. Some are described in papers by Davies[28] and Davies and Chilvers.[29]

3 Geographical Distribution of Cancer Mortality

The colour plate shows, as examples, three maps reproduced form the cancer atlas for 1968–78.[13]

a *Maps on a Small-Area Scale*

Plates I and II show two cancers mapped on the small local authority area scale—namely, stomach cancer in men and cancer of the ovary in women respectively. The green shaded areas are those which experienced low mortality rates compared to the national average, while the red areas had high rates. Different densities of colour shading are used according to the statistical significance (at the 5% level) of the local standardized mortality ratio* (SMR) compared to the national average value of 100, and according to whether or not areas have SMRs in the extreme tenths of the distribution of cancer mortality among the 1366 local authority areas. The first criterion was used to reduce the attention given to low or high rates based on small numbers of deaths in areas of limited population size, and the second criterion to indicate particularly the areas with the numerically lowest and highest SMRs.

For cancer of the stomach in men, low rates are concentrated in East Anglia, central south England and the south-west. By contrast, areas with high rates are found mainly in Wales, Staffordshire, south Lancashire, parts of Cumberland and the West Riding of Yorkshire, Durham and Tyneside. As far as London is concerned there is a cluster of boroughs in the east with high rates compared with the low rates of the western boroughs. For ovarian cancer in women, the main areas with low rates are in the north and west of the country, particularly in many districts of Lancashire and south Wales. Areas with high rates are predominantly in the south and east.

---

* See Introduction (p. 307) for definition.

b *Maps at County Level*

Plate III shows mortality from cancer of the buccal cavity for men on a county level, with the Welsh counties being grouped into two standard regions and Rutland combined with Leicestershire because of their relatively small populations. On this map, areas have been classified into groups simply on the basis of the numerical value of the SMR from cancer of the buccal cavity, with lower rates being shown in blue and higher rates in orange. There is clearly a distinctive pattern with generally lower rates in the south of the country compared to the north.

4 Patterns of Cancer Mortality, 1968–78

Among other maps in the atlas, not all cancers show such clear patterns as those illustrated here. However, in general terms it can be said that mortality from cancers of the pharynx, rectum, cervix and kidney tended to be lower in the south than in the north. On the other hand, cancers of the breast, brain, melanoma and non-Hodgkin's lymphoma were distributed in the reverse direction. High rates from lung cancer occurred mainly in some of the conurbations and from cancer of the oesophagus in Lancashire and among women in Wales. In the case of death from cancer where the primary site was not specified on the death certificate, it is interesting to note that rates were highest in many of the London boroughs and in Birmingham. These deaths are mainly recorded as carcinomatosis, and it is unlikely that any medical significance can be attached to this distribution.

a *Comparisons with Earlier Years*

Figure 1 reproduces the map of ovarian cancer mortality in women during 1921–30 in England and Wales from the report of Stocks.[4] Mortality is shown on a similar percentage scale as the modern SMR, but a further correction for degree of urbanization as well as age is incorporated into the comparison between counties. However, this extra factor is unlikely to have modified the geographical pattern as the urban and rural rates for cancer of the ovary are comparable (see Table I). The map in Fig. 1 shows a similar picture to that of Plate II, and indicates that over a period of some 50 years the areas of low and high mortality have remained much the same. The similarity of the geographical distributions in the 1921–30 and 1968–78 maps is also apparent for a number of further cancers, such as stomach, breast and prostate, but not for others where changes have occurred, such as cancers of the lung and bladder.

b *High and Low Areas*

Earlier in this paper it was mentioned that one area, Stone Rural District, appeared on 19 out of 23 maps (for 21 sex- and site-specific cancers and all cancers combined in each sex) due to an artefact in area coding. Table II shows other areas which appeared most frequently on the cancer maps according to the joint criteria of having a statistically raised SMR which was above the top decile of the distribution. It is clear how exceptional Stone Rural District is in this respect, since the next highest area, Kirkby Urban District, is on only 10 as compared to 19 maps. After Kirkby Urban District, the number of areas occurring with any given frequency increases. This does not, of course, exclude the area coding difficulties with regard to deaths in institutions (or different problems) having affected areas other than Stone Rural District, but it has not occurred elsewhere in such an extreme manner. Table III shows, by contrast, the local authority areas which are most frequently 'low' in terms of their cancer mortality. It is

Fig. 1. Cancer of the ovary by area in England and Wales during 1921–30 in women aged 25 and over

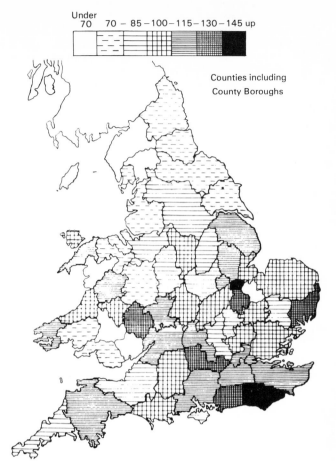

Under 70   70 – 85 – 100 – 115 – 130 – 145 up

Counties including County Boroughs

Shows actual mortality per cent of that expected from the distribution of female population by age and class of district

noticeable that, generally speaking, the areas with low and high death rates are geographically separated, spreading from the south to the north. Also there is a predominence of rural districts among the low mortality areas, with urban districts being more common at the high levels.

c *Urban/Rural Ratios*

This difference in urban/rural mortality experience, which is, incidentally, even more marked for non-cancer mortality, has been known and examined for many decades.[4,30,31] Table I shows urban/rural mortality ratios for each sex, with the sites being ranked from high to low in terms of the ratio for men, except for single-sex cancers which are ranked separately at the bottom of the table. The ratios have been produced by amalgamating the county, London and municipal boroughs together with the urban districts and comparing these with all rural districts combined. A common standard poulation—that of the combined male and female population of England and Wales by age-groups—has been used to calculate directly standardized death rates by sex for each type of area, and hence their ratios. From the table it can be seen that the urban/rural mortality ratio is greater than unity for the majority of cancers, indicating higher mortality in the towns than in the

TABLE I. Urban/rural and male/female ratios for cancer mortality during 1968–78 ranked by decreasing urban/rural ratio among men

Cancer	Urban/Rural		Male/Female		Urban/Rural* male/female
	Male	Female	Urban	Rural	
Pleural mesothelioma	2.04	1.47	4.16	2.99	6.11
Liver (primary)	1.37	1.13	2.37	1.95	2.67
Larynx	1.36	1.11	6.41	5.22	7.11
Trachea, bronchus and lung	1.32	1.24	5.81	5.44	7.19
Pharynx	1.23	1.00	2.08	1.69	2.08
Bladder	1.22	1.17	3.75	3.58	4.38
Stomach	1.20	1.17	2.11	2.05	2.46
Nose	1.20	1.10	1.83	1.67	2.01
Unspecified site	1.19	1.09	1.36	1.24	1.48
Gall bladder	1.14	0.98	0.90	0.78	0.89
Kidney	1.14	1.09	2.20	2.10	2.40
Buccal cavity	1.10	1.06	2.56	2.47	2.72
Bone	1.10	1.09	1.68	1.67	1.83
Pancreas	1.08	1.03	1.65	1.56	1.69
Rectum	1.07	1.06	1.75	1.75	1.86
Oesophagus	1.04	0.98	1.93	1.81	1.89
Large intestine	1.03	1.02	1.07	1.06	1.09
Non-Hodgkin's lymphoma	1.02	1.01	1.55	1.53	1.56
Hodgkin's disease	1.02	0.96	1.85	1.75	1.78
Acute myeloid leukaemia	1.02	1.09	1.35	1.45	1.48
Multiple myeloma	0.99	0.96	1.37	1.32	1.31
Chronic lymphatic leukaemia	0.99	1.05	2.17	2.29	2.27
Connective tissue	0.98	0.92	1.28	1.20	1.18
Other skin	0.97	0.99	1.78	1.82	1.76
Chronic myeloid leukaemia	0.97	0.94	1.42	1.38	1.34
Melanoma	0.96	0.91	0.94	0.89	0.85
Brain	0.96	1.01	1.56	1.64	1.57
Thyroid gland	0.96	1.04	0.54	0.59	0.56
Acute lymphatic leukaemia	0.96	0.85	1.68	1.49	1.43
Prostate	0.99	–	–	–	–
Testis	0.93	–	–	–	–
Cervix uteri	–	1.14	–	–	–
Breast	–	1.01	–	–	–
Ovary	–	0.98	–	–	–
Other uterus	–	0.95	–	–	–
Vulva and vagina	–	0.92	–	–	–
All cancers	1.18	1.05	1.71	1.54	1.81

* The figure in this column is the square root of the product of the figures in the first four columns

TABLE II. Areas with SMRs from 23 various cancers* in both sexes most frequently significantly high and in the top tenth of the distribution among the 1366 local authority areas

Area	Number of 'high' rates
Stone Rural District, Staffordshire	19
Kirkby Urban District, Lancashire	10
Huyton-with-Roby Urban District, Lancashire	8
Jarrow Municipal Borough, Durham	8
Widnes Municipal Borough, Lancashire	8
Barking London Borough, Greater London	7
Longbenton Urban District, Northumberland	7

* All cancer, oesophagus, stomach, large intestine, rectum, pancreas, lung, breast, cervix, other uterus, ovary, bladder, prostate, pleural mesothelioma

country. However, there are some cancers with ratios which show up to 15% lower death rates in urban compared to rural areas. In general the ratios for men are higher than those for women, indicating a higher relative risk of cancer among men living in towns compared to the country than among women. Some particularly high urban/rural ratios for both sexes are from pleural mesothelioma and from cancers of the lung, bladder, and stomach. There is an interesting clustering of related sites in parts of the ranking. Thus, respiratory cancers are largely high, followed by a collection of gastrointestinal cancers, and then the lymphomas, leukaemias, and skin cancers with low urban/rural ratios.

TABLE III. Areas with SMRs from 21 various cancers* in both sexes most frequently significantly low and in the bottom tenth of the distribution among the 1366 local authority areas

Area	Number of 'low' rates
Carmathen Rural District, Carmathenshire	6
Northallerton Rural District, Yorkshire North Riding	6
Billesdon Rural District, Leicestershire	5
Blandford Rural District, Dorset	5
Caistor Rural District, Lincolnshire (Lindsey)	5
Chorleywood Urban District, Hertfordshire	5
Deben Rural District, East Suffolk	5
Kettering Rural District, Northamptonshire	5
Llandeilo Rural District, Carmathenshire	5
Ripon and Pateley Bridge Rural District, Yorkshire West Riding	5
Scalby Urban District, Yorkshire North Riding	5
Yeovil Rural District, Somerset	5

* As for Table I, excluding pleural mesothelioma

d *Male/Female Ratios by Cancer Site and Area*

Table I also shows the male/female mortality ratios within urban and rural areas, calculated as indicated in the previous paragraph. There is a tendency for these male/female ratios to be ranked in a similar order to the urban/rural ratios, although this is not consistent. The numerical magnitudes of the two sets of ratios are quite different, however, with both some very large sex ratios (for cancers of the larynx, lung and bladder, and pleural mesothelioma) and one very small ratio (for cancer of the thyroid gland). In keeping with the urban/rural ratios being higher in men than women, the male/female cancer mortality ratios are nearly all higher in urban than rural areas. The exceptions—namely, acute myeloid leukaemia, chronic lymphatic leukaemia, and cancers of the skin (other than melanoma), brain and thyroid gland—all have low urban/rural mortality ratios and are generally among the lowest in terms of the male/female ratios also.

The final column of Table I shows the mortality ratios for urban men compared to rural women—which is, for the majority of cancers, the widest contrast. It can be seen that the numerical values are extremely high for cancers of the lung and larynx and pleural mesothelioma with mortality over six times higher in urban men than rural women, followed by bladder cancer. A number of other cancers have more than double the death rate among urban men than rural women. At the other extreme, rural women fare worse than urban men for only melanoma of the skin and cancers of the gall bladder and thyroid gland. In the last case the relative excess among rural women is highest—by a factor of 1.79 times (= 1/0.56).

An extension to looking at male/female ratios in the totality of urban and of rural districts as in Table I, is to study the variation of the ratio between Local Authority areas geographically. Plate IV shows, in a similar manner to the SMRs in Plates I and II, the pattern of the ratios of male/female lung cancer mortality in the local authority areas of England and Wales. An area is coloured in a shade of green or magenta if its male/female mortality ratio is low or high in relation to the national ratio of 5.72, in terms again of statistical significance and position in the distribution among the 1366 areas. There is seen to be a tendency for the ratio to be lower in the south and south-east, including Greater London and its surrounds, and higher in Wales, the Midlands and parts of Lancashire and the West Riding of Yorkshire. The geographical picture shown in Plate IV is independent of the absolute numerical levels of the mortality rates in men and women, and depicts only the spread of their relative magnitudes. This is, in fact, different to the geographical patterns of the high SMRs from lung cancer themselves which are concentrated in the conurbations, including London, for both men and women.

c *Clusters of High or Low Rates*

One interest in studying the maps is to search for clusters of adjoining areas with similarly low or high values. This could lead to the identification in these locations of either the absence or presence of potential causes. One such example is seen in Plate IV for the 'Black Country', where there are six contiguous areas with high male/female ratios for lung cancer. For each of the six, the SMR for men is in the top tenth of the distribution, with values ranging from 113 to 130 each based on over 1000 deaths. The rates among women, on the contrary, are relatively low with five of the six SMRs being in the lower half of the female distribution with values of between 69 and 83—the remaining SMR is 105. Other clusters are also apparent in the various maps, such as oesophageal cancer in North Wales and in south Kent, and kidney cancer in the north-west.

As well as clusters of areas with unusually high rates, there can also be particular interest in isolated localities with raised mortality. An example of such an instance is the excess death rate from nasal cancer among both men and women in the London borough of Tower Hamlets.[32] These high rates spread, at slightly lower levels, into some neighbouring boroughs. As a consequence of this observation a case-control study is under way in east London to attempt to elicit the reason for these increases, in collaboration with the local hospitals. A similar approach is being adopted to look at raised bladder cancer in east London (P J Baxter, in preparation) and Weymouth (M J Gardner *et al*, in preparation).

5 Reasons for Geographical Variation

The real test of whether drawing maps—and looking at the geography of cancer—is productive depends upon the success or otherwise of gaining useful information from them directly or from the outcome of associated studies. In particular, their value eventually relates to whether advances can be made as a result through the modification of factors found to cause the disease.

a *Pleural Mesothelioma*

Considering first a cancer with one of highest urban/rural and male/female mortality ratios, pleural mesothelioma, this is a case where, in regard to its extreme position, it might be thought that its aetiology should be easier to determine. The main, if not the only, cause in this country is well known to be asbestos, and the geographical studies which have been published help to confirm this knowledge.[33-35] Areas where asbestos was heavily used at appropriate times in the past effectively dominate the maps. Because the cases are known to occur many years after first exposure, these geographical patterns strongly support the earlier suggestion that internal migration does not greatly interfere with local mortality rates. Moreover, since mesothelioma of the pleura is rare outside these areas, there is unlikely to be another major cause in this country[36,37] although, because of the potential difficulty that the disease may be recognized and certified more readily if a history of asbestos exposure has been elicited, this interpretation should be viewed with some caution.

b *Lung Cancer*

Moving to one of the other respiratory cancers with large urban/rural ratios for both men and women—namely, lung cancer—it is pertinent to note that cigarette smoking habits have long, if not

always, been different in cities than in the country. Figure 2 shows graphically some data from surveys conducted by the Tobacco Research Council.[38] It can be seen that, since the early 1950s, both the proportion of cigarette smokers and also the quantity of manufactured cigarettes consumed per smoker have been higher among urban than rural dwellers in each sex. There is little change in the differences between the types of area over the years. For men there has been a gradual decline in the proportion of smokers, whereas the trend is slightly upwards for women. In both sexes the average number of manufactured cigarettes consumed per smoker has increased—rising by over 50% among women over a period of 20 years. If statistics on smoking habits for earlier periods of time were available, it would be possible, using the urban/rural lung cancer mortality ratios (see Table II), to estimate the relative risk of lung cancer in smokers compared to non-smokers, if the raised urban/rural ratios were taken to be entirely due to differential cigarette smoking habits. The result for men could be compared with, for example, the value found in the prospective study of British doctors.[39] Beral and her colleagues[40] have discussed the rationale behind converting population-based mortality rates into estimates of individual relative risk.

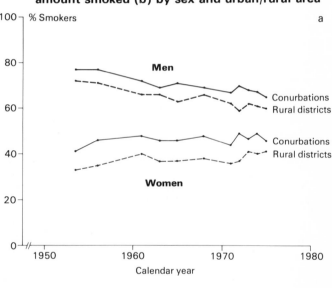

Fig. 2. Time-trends in % smokers (a) and average amount smoked (b) by sex and urban/rural area

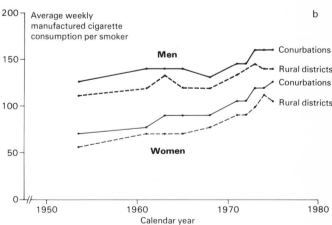

The pattern in Plate IV could be explained if, in particular, women in the south had taken up the cigarette habit at an earlier period of time, at an earlier age or had smoked more heavily than those in more northern parts of the country and Wales, but information is lacking on this point. Other authors have suggested that air pollution may also be relevant in explaining the elevated urban/rural ratios,[41–44] although according to a recent paper the air pollution factor may be less important now than in the past.[45] Smoking behaviour would seem to be pertinent also to the high urban/rural ratios for cancers of the larynx and pharynx[46] and for bladder cancer.[47] In the latter case, as well as for lung cancer, occupational factors are also likely to be important. However, occupation and smoking are correlated attributes (see Fig. 6.3 in Reference 48) and this is a complication for interpreting relationships between occupation and mortality for smoking-related cancers.

c Detection of Environmental Associations

A number of the relationships between potential causative factors and particular cancers have been discovered by astute observation or through serendipity—for example, nasal cancer in furniture makers and in boot and shoe manufacturers.[49,50] It seems plausible therefore that a systematic search between mortality and environmental data (general, occupational and personal) should yield clues to presently unsuspected causes.[51] The Occupational Mortality Decennial Supplement[48] is one such method—mainly in relation to occupation and industry. A recent collaborative report based on combining results from a number of European countries has pointed to the apparent high relative risk of lung cancer among butchers.[52] There are reasons to believe that this may have a viral origin[53] and further investigative studies are underway.

One method of searching the geographical differences in relation to environment has been alluded to earlier. Areas of high mortality can be compared in detail. A formal analysis of the industries, using data from the 1971 Census, in the five selected areas of highest nasal cancer mortality during 1968–78 revealed that, in addition to the expected concentrations of the furniture and leather industries, there were high levels of manufacture of women's and girls' tailored outerwear compared to England and Wales overall.[32] Tailoring was one of the occupations suggested as being at possible risk in a national survey of cases of nasal cancer,[54] but did not have a raised SMR in the Occupational Mortality Decennial Supplement.[48] Clothing workers, however, have been found to have a raised incidence of nasal cancer using Cancer Registry data in each sex, although the numbers of cases are small.[55]

An alternative to looking at the environment of high-mortality areas compared to the national average is to study their joint relationship over the whole range of each factor. Usual techniques for doing this would be correlation or regression analysis, but results given here are by a modification[87] of an associated method.[56] The result of this approach to the geographical distribution of nasal cancer in men and industry is shown in Table IV. Essentially the 1366 Local Authority areas are initially ranked in terms of the proportion of their male population who are employed in a particular industry, and then collated together into groups (20 in this case) which each contain the same number of expected nasal cancer deaths. An analysis is carried out to determine whether the number of observed deaths (or equivalently the observed/expected ratio) shows any significant trends through these groups. It can be seen from the Table that the furniture and upholstery industry comes at the head of the list, with leather goods

TABLE IV. Relationships between mortality (observed deaths/expected deaths) from nasal cancer in men during 1968–78 and the percentage of males employed in different industries in the 1366 local authority areas

Industrial unit*	Slope of relationship†	Chi-square test‡	
		Trend	Other sources of variation
Furniture and upholstery	11.64	20.02§	27.36
Glass	7.44	8.17§	24.78
Men's and boys' tailored outerwear	7.42	8.15§	19.83
Copper, brass and other copper alloys	7.30	7.87§	31.02**
Universities	7.16	7.58§	17.52
Leather goods	7.09	7.43§	22.41
Brushes and brooms	6.66	6.55∥	25.17
Brewing and malting	6.38	6.02∥	22.14
Dresses, lingerie, infant's wear	6.35	5.96∥	25.61
Women's and girls' tailored outerwear	6.31	5.88∥	34.98¶
Metal industries (n.e.s.)	6.25	5.77∥	15.84
Iron castings	6.15	5.59∥	25.33
Motor cycle, tricycle and pedal cycles	6.03	5.38∥	26.77
Miscellaneous manufacturing	6.02	5.35∥	27.08
Telegraph and telephone apparatus	5.77	4.91∥	19.17
Public houses	5.66	4.74∥	13.67
Mechanical handling equipment	5.33	4.20∥	22.19
Locomotive and railway track equipment	5.21	4.01∥	27.97
Domestic electrical appliances	5.19	3.99∥	31.04**

* Standard industrial classification.[57] Only the 19, out of a total of 207, industries with statistically significant positive trends are shown—in ranked order
† Standardized slope = increase in (100 × observed deaths/expected deaths) per standard deviation increase in the percentage working in the industry, and enables comparison across industrial units
‡ Trend, 1 degree of freedom
§ $P < 0.01$ ($X^2 > 6.63$): other sources of variation, 18 d.f.
∥ $P < 0.05$ ($X^2 > 3.84$)
¶ $P < 0.01$ ($X^2 > 34.81$)
** $P < 0.05$ ($X^2 > 28.87$)

and various sections of the tailoring industry being prominent. Industries where statistically significant trends are found, which may be of relevance in the light of raised nasal cancer among furnace and foundry workers,[54] are the manufacture of copper, brass and copper alloys, of iron castings and unspecified metal industries. Other industrial units which are related to nasal cancer include glass, brushes and brooms, brewing and malting (and public houses), and teachers in universities. When looking at 207 industries simultaneously, without in every case an *a priori* hypothesis, some statistically significant trends can be expected to emerge by chance alone and the last list of industries may contain such examples. On the other hand—since this should be regarded as a hypothesis-generating approach—a detailed look at industries raised in this way, particularly if the work is dusty or produces fumes, may be revealing.

d General Environmental Factors

More generally, a large number of potential aetiological factors have been associated with the variations in cancer mortality within England and Wales. These can be grouped broadly into those associated with the general and occupational environments, personal behaviour, and (rarely) genetics.

There are a number of examples of the first group of general environmental factors. One such, which caused some concern a few years ago, was the suggested relationship between fluoridation of water and cancer mortality of all sites. The possible connection was initially proposed in the United States,[58,59] but has subsequently been refuted.[60–62] In the UK, a suggestion was made that cancer rates in Birmingham, where the water had been fluoridated, had risen more rapidly than in unfluoridated Manchester over a period of time.[63,64] However, in a further examination of appropriate information, Birmingham subsequently was found to have suffered no increased mortality from cancer compared with cities where the water supply did not contain added fluoride.[65,66]

An area where the epidemiological evidence is not yet definitive is the possible role of environmental nitrates in human cancer.[67,68] A study of stomach cancer mortality in an English town with high nitrate concentration in the drinking water suggested high death rates from the disease.[69] However, a recent re-assessment[28] of this town and its surrounding areas indicated that the local population contained a high proportion of coal miners, whose stomach cancer rates are known to be high.[48] Another site of cancer thought to be possibly involved is the oesophagus, and this derives partly from the fact that the major source of nitrate intake into the human body is from food. The main items of dietary nitrate are vegetables, which themselves have been suggested to be protective against gastric cancer. A recent study of salivary nitrate secretion found higher levels in Oxford (low for stomach cancer) than in the north-east of England and north Wales (high for stomach cancer).[70] These salivary nitrate levels reflect green vegetable consumption, but are inversely related to stomach cancer rates. Thus, the evidence from epidemiological studies that nitrate is involved in the aetiology of stomach cancer is very weak (P Fraser, personal communication).

In the late 1970s, with the publication of a geochemical atlas containing the distribution on a 1 km grid scale of trace elements in soil over England and Wales,[71] there was a suggestion that cancer mortality (in particular, cancers of the lung and prostate)—as well as other morbidity and death rates—might be high in the village of Shipham in Somerset. This had been the site of an old zinc mine, and high levels of cadmium had built up in the soil where home-grown vegetables were produced. These high levels were distinctly noticeable in the geochemical atlas, but future epidemiological work did not find high cancer rates among Shipham residents.[72,73] Other uses of the geochemical atlas in relation to human health are discussed by Thornton and Webb.[74]

In the 1960s, there was a suggestion that an association might exist between the radium content of water supplies and local bone cancer mortality. This was investigated in England and Wales using mortality from primary bone tumours in 19 areas during 1951–53 and 1961–63, and figures for the long-term radioactivity measured in samples of drinking water. In neither set of mortality data was there any significant correlation.[75]

Other areas with particularly raised death rates which may be related to the local geology or soil composition include North Wales, which has high rates for cancer of the oesophagus, particularly in women, as well as stomach cancer. This was noted many years ago by Stocks,[4,76] and the excess levels still persist. Cattle feeding on bracken fern, which are also infected by a papilloma virus, have been shown to suffer a high incidence of alimentary tract cancer.[77,78] This may have relevance to man, and

a study of the relationship between the geographical distribution of bracken and cancer mortality is underway (C P Taylor *et al*, in preparation). It has been suggested that the recycling of water may be responsible for the high stomach cancer rates on the east side of London. However, a study taking into account the social class composition and the size of the boroughs with excess rates showed no relationship with water re-use.[79] As an example of the effect of climate, there is a known relationship between the mean hours of local sunshine and the incidence of malignant melanoma of the skin in the regions of England and Wales,[80] as well as in other countries (B Armstrong, this volume); but no similar association exists with mortality from other skin cancer[13] perhaps because the fatality is extremely low.

e *Personal Environmental Factors*

Turning to the relationships of cancer mortality to factors in the personal environment and behaviour, it is of interest to note how the geographical distributions for different cancers fit into the known epidemiology based on direct studies of individuals. For example, mortality rates from cancers of the ovary and breast are higher in many parts of the south than in the north—and in the former areas of the country there are proportionally more women of higher social class and lower family size. The latter two factors have been associated with these cancers in individual studies,[48,68,81] with higher rates in upper social class women and women having fewer children. On the contrary, cancer of the cervix shows the reverse distribution which again accords with expectation from epidemiological studies on individuals, although the number of sexual partners is more relevant than the number of children.[68]

On a regional basis there has been shown to be a relationship between both the consumption of vegetables (excluding potatoes) and levels of the pentose fraction of dietary fibre intake, but not total fibre, and large-bowel cancer mortality.[82] This supports other epidemiological evidence on a personal level in relation to the 'dietary fibre' hypothesis.[83] The feature of dietary intake with the largest regional variation in England and Wales is the consumption of fresh fruit and vegetables, and this may have important relevance to the distribution of cancer mortality (see, for example, Reference 84).

6 Conclusion

It is concluded that there is sufficient geographical variation of cancer by site between areas of England and Wales to make its study a worthwhile contribution to the detection of the causes of cancer, in conjunction with other standard epidemiological and laboratory methods.[46,85]

REFERENCES

1 Alderson MR. The geographical distribution of cancer. J R C Physicians Lond 1982; 16: 245–251
2 General Register Office. Supplement to the twenty-fifth Annual Report of the Registrar-General of Births, Deaths and Marriages in England (1851–1860). London: HMSO, 1864
3 Haviland A. The geographical distribution of heart disease and dropsy, cancer in females and phthisis in females in England and Wales. London: Smith, Elder, 1875
4 Stocks P. Distribution in England and Wales of cancer of various organs. Annual report of the British Empire Cancer Campaign 1936; 13: 239–280
5 Stocks P. Distribution in England and Wales of cancer of various organs. Annual report of the British Empire Cancer Campaign 1937; 14: 198–223

6 Stocks P. Distribution in England and Wales of cancer of various organs. Annual report of the British Empire Cancer Campaign 1939; 16: 308–343
7 Cruickshank DB. Regional influences in cancer. Br J Cancer 1947; 1: 109–128
8 Howe GM. National Atlas of Disease Mortality in the United Kingdom. London: Nelson, 1963
9 Howe GM. National Atlas of Disease Mortality in the United Kingdom. 2nd ed. London: Nelson, 1970
10 Howe GM. Mortality from selected malignant neoplasms in the British Isles: the spatial perspective. Soc Sci Med 1981; 15D: 199–211
11 Office of Population Censuses and Surveys. Area Mortality 1969–73. (Series DS, no 4) London: HMSO, 1981

12 Chilvers C, Adelstein A. Cancer mortality: the regional pattern. Popul trends 1978; 12: 4–9

13 Gardner MJ, Winter PD, Taylor CP, Acheson ED. Atlas of cancer mortality in England and Wales, 1968–78. Chichester: Wiley, 1983

14 Doll R. Atlas of Cancer Mortality in England and Wales, 1968–78. Chichester: Wiley, 1983; Preface

15 Cameron HM, McGoogan E. A prospective study of 1152 hospital autopsies: I. Inaccuracies in death certification. J Pathol 1981; 133: 272–283

16 Cochrane AL, Moore F. Death certification from the epidemiological point of view. Lancet 1981; 2: 742–743

17 Alderson MR, Bayliss RIS, Clarke CA, Whitfield AGW. Death certification. Br Med J 1983; 2: 444–445

18 Adelstein AM. Death certification and epidemiological research. Br Med J 1978; 2: 1229–1230

19 Diehl AK, Gau DW. Death certification by British doctors: a demographic analysis. J Epidemiol Community Health 1982; 36: 146–149

20 Royal College of Physicians and Royal College of Pathologists. Medical aspects of death certification. J R Coll Physicians Lond 1982; 16: 205–218

21 Freedman LS, Rubin SG. Limitations of mortality data as a guide to comparative lung cancer incidence within an urban area. Public Health 1979; 93: 111–116

22 Office of Population Censuses and Surveys. Cancer statistics, survival. Survival up to 1980 of cases of cancer registered in England and Wales during 1971–5. (Series MB1, no 9) London: HMSO, 1982

23 Fraser P, Beral V, Chilvers C. Monitoring disease in England and Wales: methods applicable to routine data-collecting systems. J Epidemiol Community Health 1978; 32: 294–302

24 Freedman LS. Variations in the level of reporting by hospitals to a Regional Cancer Registry. Br J Cancer 1978; 37: 861–865

25 Fox AJ, Goldblatt PO. Longitudinal study: socio-demographic mortality differentials, 1971–75. Office of Population Censuses and Surveys Series LS, no. 1. London: HMSO, 1982

26 Armstrong BK, Woodings TL, Stenhouse NS, McCall MG. Mortality from cancer in migrants to Australia—1962–71. NH and MRC Research Unit in Epidemiology and Preventive Medicine, Raine Medical Statistics Unit, Department of Medicine, University of Western Australia, 1983

27 Hewitt D. Vagaries of local mortality rates under the 1953–54 rules for transfer of deaths. Br J Prev Soc Med 1957; 11: 45–49

28 Davies JM. Stomach cancer mortality in Worksop and other Nottinghamshire mining towns. Br J Cancer 1980; 41: 438–445

29 Davies JM, Chilvers C. The study of mortality variations in small administrative areas of England and Wales, with special reference to cancer. J Epidemiol Community Health 1980; 34: 87–92

30 Muir CS. The evidence from epidemiology. In: Lenihan J, Fletcher WW, eds. Health and the Environment. London: Blackie, 1976

31 Barker DJP. Geographical variations in disease in Britain. Br Med J 1981; 283: 398–400

32 Gardner MJ, Winter PD, Acheson ED. Variations in cancer mortality among local authority areas in England and Wales: relations with environmental factors and search for causes. Br Med J 1982; 284: 784–787

33 Wagner JC, Gilson JC, Berry G, Timbrell V. Epidemiology of asbestos cancers. Br Med Bull 1971; 27: 71–76

34 Greenberg M, Lloyd Davies TA. Mesothelioma register, 1967–68. Br J Ind Med 1974; 31: 91–104

35 Gardner MJ, Acheson ED, Winter PD. Mortality from mesothelioma of the pleura during 1968–78 in England and Wales. Br J Cancer 1982; 46: 81–88

36 Gardner MJ. Tumour incidence after asbestos exposure in Great Britain—with special reference to the cancer risk of the non-occupational population. In: Fibrous dusts—measurement, effect, prevention. VDI: Berichte, 1983; 183–190

37 Acheson ED, Gardner MJ. The control limit for asbestos. London: HMSO, 1983

38 Tobacco Research Council. Statistics of smoking in the United Kingdom. (Research Paper I) 7th ed. London: Tobacco Research Council, 1976

39 Doll R, Peto R. Mortality in relation to smoking: 20 years' observations on male British doctors. Br Med J 1976; 2: 1525–1536

40 Beral V, Chilvers C, Fraser P. On the estimation of relative risk from vital statistical data. J Epidemiol Community Health 1979; 33: 159–162

41 Stocks P. On the relations between atmospheric pollution in urban and rural localities and mortality from cancer, bronchitis and pneumonia, with particular reference to 3:4 benzopyrene, beryllium, molybdenum, vanadium and arsenic. Br J Cancer 1960; 14: 397–418

42 Gardner MJ, Crawford MD, Morris JN. Patterns of mortality in middle and early old age in the County Boroughs of England and Wales. Br J Prev Soc Med 1969; 23: 133–140

43 Adelstein AM. Encouragement from recent statistics. In: Raven TW, ed. Outlook on cancer. New York: Plenum Press, 1977; 255–275

44 Lawther PJ, Waller RE. Trends in urban air pollution in the United Kingdom in relation to lung cancer mortality. Environ Health Perspect 1978; 22: 71–73

45 Chinn S, du V Florey C, Baldwin IG, Gorgol M. The relation of mortality in England and Wales 1969–73 to measurements of air pollution. J Epidemiol and Community Health 1981; 35: 174–179

46 Doll Sir R. Strategy for detection of cancer hazards to man. Nature 1977; 265, 589–596

47 Armstrong B, Doll R. Bladder cancer mortality in England and Wales in relation to cigarette smoking and saccharin consumption. Br J Prev Soc Med 1974; 28: 233–240

48 Office of Population Censuses and Surveys. Occupational Mortality 1970–72. (Series DS no 1) London: HMSO, 1978

49 Macbeth RG. Malignant disease in the paranasal sinuses. J Laryngol Otol 1965; 79: 592–612

50 Acheson ED, Cowdell RH, Jolles B. Nasal cancer in the Northamptonshire boot and shoe industry. Br Med J 1970; 1: 385–393

51 Alderson MR. Chemical carcinogenesis: whither epidemiology? Br Med Bull 1980; 36: 95–100

52 Fox AJ, Lynge E, Malker H. Lung cancer in butchers. Lancet 1982; 1: 165–166

53 Pegum JS. Lung cancer in butchers. Lancet 1982; 1: 561

54 Acheson ED, Cowdell RH, Rang EH. Nasal cancer in England and Wales: an occupational survey. Br J Ind Med 1981; 38: 218–224

55 Office of Population Censuses and Surveys. Cancer statistics registrations. Cases of diagnosed cancer registered in England and Wales, 1978. (Series MB1, no 10) London: HMSO, 1983

56 Selvin S, Merrill D, Sacks ST. An alternative to ecologic regression analysis of mortality rates. Am J Epidemiol 1982; 115: 617–623

57 Office of Population Censuses and Surveys. Standard Industrial Classification. London: HMSO, 1968

58 Burk D, Yiamouyannis J. Letter (21 July). Congressional Record 1975; 191: H7172–6. Washington DC: US Government Printing Office

59 Yiamouyannis J, Burk D. Letter (16 December). Congressional Record 1975; 191: H12731–4. Washington DC: US Government Printing Office

60 Oldham P, Newell DJ. Fluoridation of water supplies and cancer—a possible association? Appl Stat 1977; 26: 125–135

61 Kinlen L, Doll R. Fluoridation of water supplies and cancer mortality III: A re-examination of mortality in cities in the USA. J Epidemiol Community Health 1981; 35: 239–244

62 Chilvers C. Cancer mortality by site and fluoridation of water supplies. J Epidemiol Community Health 1982; 36: 237–242

63 Burk D. An open letter to Sir Emmanuel Kaye, CBE. 22 October, 1979

64 Burk D. Letter to an official at the Department of Health and Social Security, London, 5 November 1979

65 Cook-Mozaffari P, Bulusu L, Doll R. Fluoridation of water supplies and cancer mortality I: A search for an effect in the UK on risk of death from cancer. J Epidemiol Community Health 1981; 35: 227–232

66 Cook-Mozaffari P, Doll R. Fluoridation of water supplies and cancer mortality II: Mortality trends after fluoridation. J Epidemiol Community Health 1981; 35: 233–238

67 Fraser P, Chilvers C, Beral V, Hill MJ. Nitrate and human cancer: A review of the evidence. Int J Epidemiol 1980; 9: 3–11

68 Doll R, Peto R. The causes of cancer: quantitative estimates of the avoidable risks of cancer in the United States today. Oxford: University Press, 1981

69 Hill MJ, Hawksworth GM, Tattersall G. Bacteria, nitrosamines and cancer of the stomach. Br J Cancer 1973; 28: 562–567

70 Forman D, Al-Dabbagh S, Doll R. Regional variation in levels of secretion of salivary nitrates and nitrites. Preliminary report presented to Society for Social Medicine meeting, September, 1983

71 Imperial College of Science and Technology. Applied Geochemistry Research Group. The Wolfson geochemical atlas of England and Wales. Oxford: Clarendon Press, 1978

72 Philipp R, Hughes AO. Morbidity and soil levels of cadmium. Int J Epidemiol 1982; 11: 257–260

73 Inskip H, Beral V, McDowall M. Mortality of Shipham residents: 40-year follow-up. Lancet 1982; 1: 896–899

74 Thornton I, Webb JS. Geochemistry and health in the United Kingdom. Philos Trans R Soc Lond [Biol] 1979; 288: 151–168

75 **Boyd JT, Doll R, Hill GB, Sissons HA. Mortality from primary tumours of bone in England and Wales, 1961–63. Br J Prev Soc Med 1969; 23: 12–22**

76 Stocks P. Regional and local differences in cancer death rates. (General Register Office, Studies on Medical and Population Subjects, no 1) London: HMSO, 1947

77 Jarrett WFH, McNeil PE, Grimshaw WTR, Selman IE, McIntyre WIM. High incidence area of cattle cancer with a possible interaction between an environmental carcinogen and a papilloma virus. Nature 1978; 274: 215–217

78 Jarrett WFH. Bracken fern and papilloma virus in bovine alimentary cancer. Br Med Bull 1980; 36: 79–81

79 Beresford SAA. The relationship between water quality and health in the London area. Int J Epidemiol 1981; 10: 103–115

80 Swerdlow AJ. Incidence of malignant melanoma of the skin in England and Wales and its relationship to sunshine. Br Med J 1979; 2: 1324–1327

81 Newhouse ML, Pearson RM, Fullerton JM, Boesen EAM, Shannon HS. A case control study of carcinoma of the ovary. Br J Prev Soc Med 1977; 31: 148–153

82 Bingham S, Williams DRR, Cole TJ, James WPT. Dietary fibre and regional large-bowel cancer mortality in Britain. Br J Cancer 1979; 40: 456–463

83 Burkitt DP, Walker ARP, Painter NS. Effect of dietary fibre on stools and transit-times and its role in the causation of disease. Lancet 1972; 2: 1408–1411

84 Peto R, Doll R, Buckley JD, Sporn MB. Can dietary beta-carotene materially reduce human cancer rates? Nature 1982; 290: 201–208

85 Doll Sir R. The epidemiology of cancer. Cancer 1980; 45: 2475–2485

86 Gardner MJ, Winter PD. Mapping small area cancer mortality: a residential coding story. J Epidemiol Commun Health 1984; 38: 81–84

87 Gardner MJ, Winter PD. Extensions to a technique for relating mortality and environment—exemplified by nasal cancer and industry. Scand J Work Environ Health 1984; 10: In press

ritish Medical Bulletin (1984) Vol. 40, No. 4, pp. 329–334

THE GEOGRAPHIC PATHOLOGY OF CANCER OF THE OESOPHAGUS

NICHOLAS E DAY PhD

Unit of Biostatistics and Field Studies
Division of Epidemiology and Biostatistics
International Agency for Research
on Cancer

TABLE I. Incidence and mortality rates of oesophageal cancer per year per 10^5

Region	Male	Female	Reference
Africa			
Mozambique—Lourenc Marques	4.4	0.0	2
Nigeria—Ibadan	1.5	1.1	4
S. Africa—Natal African	40.9	12.3	3
Uganda—Kyandoro	1.8	1.1	2
Zimbabwe—Bulawayo African	63.8	2.2	4
North America			
Canada—Alberta	2.6	0.7	4
USA—Detroit: black	14.1	3.7	4
white	4.9	1.1	
Caribbean			
Puerto Rico	14.8	5.4	4
Latin America			
Brazil—Recife	5.2	1.6	4
Sao Paolo	13.1	2.2	4
Chile	–	–	4
Asia			
China	31.7	15.9	5
India (Bombay)	15.2	10.8	4
Japan	7.1	1.6	4
Singapore: Chinese	20.0	6.4	4
Indian	5.6	5.9	
Malay	2.0	3.7	
Europe			
England and Wales	5.5	2.9	6
Finland	5.2	3.9	4
France	14.1	1.1	6
Greece	2.0	0.7	6
Italy	8.6	0.8	6
Rumania	1.9	0.5	6
Spain	5.4	0.9	6
Switzerland	7.3	0.8	6

Cancer of the oesophagus, although relatively infrequent in most of western Europe and north America is, overall, one of the most common cancers in the world.

A recent estimate has placed it seventh in order of frequency of occurrence, both sexes combined.[1] Among the more common cancers, its distribution shows perhaps the most striking patterns of variation, making it the malignancy *par excellence* where geographical pathology should illuminate the aetiology.

In certain small localities the disease attains an incidence unequalled by any other fatal tumours anywhere in the world, yet within a matter of some hundred kilometres, the disease can have almost disappeared. These sharp gradients in incidence are a feature of the epidemiology of the disease, and are not only steeper, but also cover a wider range in incidence, than the local variations seen for other cancers (apart from such outstanding exceptions as the tumours associated with the Balkan nephropathy).

In this paper, I shall sketch the broad pattern of incidence of the disease, then examine in detail the incidence patterns in some of the regions where the disease is frequent. I conclude by discussing the extent to which these remarkable local variations in incidence have been exploited for aetiological studies, and with what success.

1   Worldwide Distribution

Cancer of the oesophagus is a rapidly fatal disease in the great majority of cases, so that mortality and incidence rates should be comparable. Table I gives a brief resume of available mortality and incidence rates, indicating the mean features of inter-country variation, with some indication of within-country differences. Salient features of the table are:

1 very low rates among females in many of the populations;
2 high or very high rates among male blacks in both South Africa and north America;
3 intermediate or high rates in the Caribbean and Latin America;

4 high rates in the Indian sub-continent;
5 very high rates for China, and in the migrant Chinese population.

These figures give an indication of the magnitude of the public health problem posed by the disease, and the countries where it is most keenly felt, but are of limited value for considering the aetiological implications. For the latter, finer detail is required.

2   China

Over 60% of the cases of oesophageal cancer occurring in the world each year are estimated to occur in China,[1] where it is the second most common cancer after stomach cancer. The national annual mortality rates for the two cancers are in fact very close (for stomach cancer, 32.3 per 100000 in males and 15.9 in females, as compared to 31.7 per 100000 and 15.9 respectively for the oesophagus (See Fig. 1)). The distribution of the two diseases over the country, however, are very markedly different. Stomach cancer is more common in the north and less common in the south, the changes in incidence are smooth, and in few counties is the disease rare. Oesophageal cancer, by contrast, is rare over large tracts of the country, the disease occurring mainly in a few sharply demarcated areas, in which the incidence rises to levels considerably higher than seen anywhere for stomach cancer.

The much greater variation seen in the distribution of oesophageal cancer than seen for other common tumours in China is shown in Table II. This variability arises not only from the occasional foci of very high incidence, but also from the large number of counties with particularly low incidence.

3   The Central Asian Oesophageal Cancer Belt

Westwards from the high-incidence area in northern Sinkiang, areas of extremely high incidence are seen in Kazakhstan,

FIG. 1. Mortality rates per 100000 for cancers of the stomach (left) and oesophagus (right) among females in the eastern half of the People's Republic of China

(from Atlas of Cancer Mortality in the People's Republic of China[5])

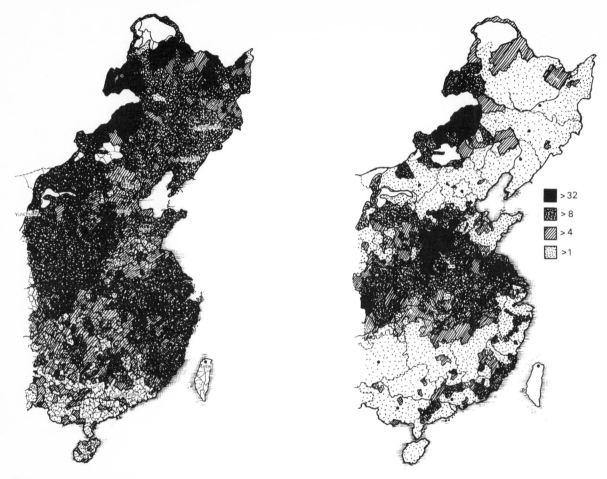

The corresponding rates for males show a similar pattern. Only the eastern half of the Republic is shown, the large regions of uninhabited desert in the western half reducing the interest in the rates. Of interest, however, are the high rates seen in the far north-west of the country, northern Xingiang, adjoining Kazakhstan in the USSR, where the population is mainly Kazakh.

TABLE II. Distribution by county of the incidences of the more common cancers in the People's Republic of China

(from Atlas of Cancer Mortality in the People's Republic of China[5])

Annual Crude Mortality per 100000	Number of counties					
	Males			Females		
	Oesophagus	Stomach	Liver	Oesophagus	Stomach	Cervix & uterus
<4	532	78	126	1071	305	362
4–	400	326	394	529	696	683
8–	532	666	1168	456	921	890
16–	549	821	615	206	394	376
32–	264	425	84	107	76	80
64–	103	76	5	23	–	1
128–	12	–	–	–	–	–
Total crude rate	19.7	20.9	14.5	9.9	10.2	10.0

Uzbekistan and Turkmenistan, in the Soviet Union; the north-east of Iran and northern Afghanistan.[7–11] These regions, together with western Sinkiang, form the centre of the old Turkic Kingdom of Uleg Beg and Timur, with Samarkand as capital. In all three countries, high rates of the disease are seen almost exclusively in the groups of Turkic origin, Turkoman, Uzbek and Kazakh, and not in the groups of Indo-European origin, Persian, Pathan and Russian.[8,10,11] The whole central Asian region is displayed in Fig. 2 with the rates for males. One can see, as in Fig. 1, not only the areas of very high incidence, but also the remarkably rapid fall-off to areas with low or moderate rates (the corresponding map displaying female rates is almost identical).

The area of this region which has been most extensively studied is northern Iran; Fig. 3 displays the incidence rates as recorded by the Caspian Cancer Registry. The series of analytic studies undertaken to exploit the range of incidences is described in a later section.

A noteworthy feature of the incidence pattern seen in China and central Asia is the parallelism between male and female rates.

FIG. 2. Age-standardized incidence rates per 100000 for cancer of the oesophagus among males in Central Asia

(From Day and Muñoz[12])

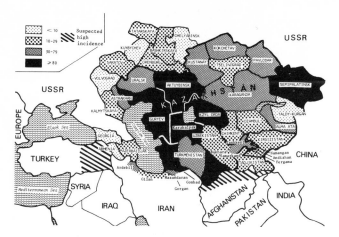

FIG. 3. Incidence rates for cancer of the oesophagus on the Caspian littoral of Iran

(From Mahboubi et al.[10])

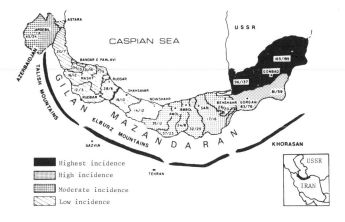

When the rates are high they are equally high in both sexes, with the highest rates sometimes seen in females. When the rates are low, there is typically a two- or three-fold male excess.

4 Chinese Migrant Population: Singapore

As can be seen from Fig. 1, incidence or mortality figures for Chinese living outside China can be used to assess the effect of migration only if their place of origin in China is known. For many Chinese populations outside China, such information is not fully available. An exception is Singapore, where the cancer registry has information both on place of origin of the family in China (that is, dialect group) and on whether the person was born in China or Singapore.[13] Most Chinese in Singapore come either from the south of Kwantung province (Cantonese speakers), from Fukkien province (Hokkien speakers) or from the neighbourhood of Swatow in north-east Kwantung province (Teochew speakers). The last two groups come from one of the areas shown in Fig. 1 as having exceptionally high incidence. The rates in Table III

TABLE III. Oesophageal cancer among Chinese in Singapore: age-standardized annual incidence rates, 1968–77

(from Shanmugaratnam et al.[13])

	Male	Female
By dialect group:		
Cantonese	4.5	2.2
Teochew	30.7	7.8
Hokkien	27.5	6.7
By place of birth:		
China	22.8	6.1
Singapore	7.0	2.2
Annual decrease in incidence over the period 1968–77	3.4%	11.0%
Age-adjusted incidence, 1968–72	20.1	6.4
Age-adjusted incidence, 1973–77	18.9	4.1

reflect these differences. Table III indicates also the first generation effect in oesophageal cancer incidence. Unlike cancer of the stomach, where the difference is minimal, Singapore-born Chinese have only 40% of the risk of China-born. The oesophagus, in fact, is the only site where the China-born have a substantially higher risk.

In addition to the differences by place of birth, the incidence is falling rapidly in all Chinese groups in Singapore, more rapidly in females (Table III). Among Singapore-born females, the disease has now become rare. The more rapid fall in females may explain why the sex ratio in Singapore Hokkien and Teochew is 4:1 (M:F) as compared to 1.5:1 in the Fukkien province on the mainland.

5 Africa

The epidemiology of oesophageal cancer in the African continent has been the subject of several recent reviews,[14–17] and will not be considered in detail here. Throughout north, west and central Africa, the disease is rare. In east and southern Africa, areas of high and low incidence are intermingled, with sharp gradients of incidences. Unlike China and Central Asia, however, in some of the areas of high interest only males are affected, as in Bulawayo (see Table I) or some regions round Lake Victoria.[16] In South Africa, particularly in the associated rural regions of the Transkei and the Ciskei, the incidence in females rises in parallel with that in males. There is also some evidence that the disease is of recent origin and has been increasing. Patterns of contrasting incidence in the Transkei have been extensively documented[18,19] but it seems that, in the areas formerly of low incidence in northern Transkei, the incidence has risen rapidly in the last fifteen years (Table IV).[20] The incidence patterns which generated extensive analytic work in the Transkei are in the process of disappearing. It is unclear whether differences in nutritional status and tobacco habits between the north and the south of the Transkei should be related to past, present or future differences in cancer incidence.

TABLE IV. Changing patterns of oesophageal cancer incidence in the Transkei

(from Van Rensburg et al.[20])

| | Annual rates per 100000 population | | | | | |
| | Males | | | Females | | |
	1955–59	1965–69	1981	1955–59	1965–69	1981
Northern Transkei	13	14	51	8	5	33
Southern Transkei	93	68	63	48	33	65

6 Europe

a *Males*

The major patterns of variation in Europe are seen for males, the incidence among females being low or very low in most of Europe (see Table I). Even in Europe, a striking feature of the epidemiology of the disease is the large variation, greater in relative terms than for most other cancers. Brittany and Normandy provide the most extreme examples.[21,22] The distribution by canton in Brittany and the Normandy departments of Calvados and Orne are shown in Fig. 4.[22] Data by canton have not yet been published for the other two departments with high rates, Manche and Mayenne, which would round out the picture. The rates in western Brittany and in the south east of Orne are similar to the average rates in France. In the foci of high incidence, the rates are five to ten times higher.

In Italy, the European country with the highest alcohol consumption after France, oesophageal cancer rates nowhere reach the levels seen in Brittany, but of the commoner cancers, the rates show the greatest variation.[23] Between the north-east and

FIG. 4. Age-standardized mortality rates per 100000 for cancer of the oesophagus among males in Normandy (above) and Brittany (below), 1958–66

(From Tuyns and Vernhes[10])

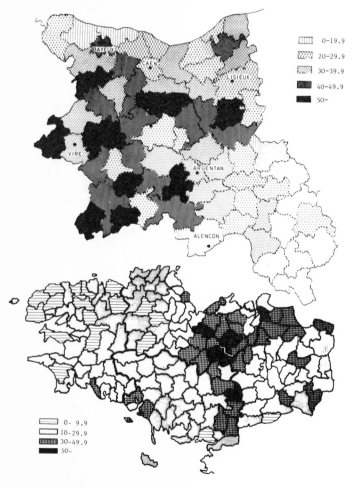

FIG. 5. Mortality rates per 100000 for cancer of the oesophagus in Italy

(From Cislaghi *et al.*[23])

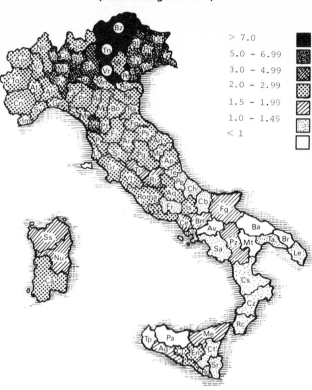

south, there is more than a sixfold difference (see Fig. 5),[23] compared to differences of only threefold for cancers of the stomach, colon, or lung.

Even in England and Wales, where oesophageal cancer in men is not unduly common and the geographical distribution is patchy, with no noteworthy trends, the relative difference between the 10th and 90th percentile of the rates by local authority region is greater than for the other common tumours illustrated in an atlas of cancer mortality.[24]

b *Females*

Among females in Europe, the picture is completely different. Throughout the Mediterranean region, including France and Italy, and central and eastern Europe, the disease is very rare (see Table I). Only in Scandinavia, particularly in the north, and in the British Isles is the disease seen with any frequency. In Scandinavia, the once relatively high rates have largely disappeared, as shown in Table V for Finland.[25–27] Higher rates are still seen in

TABLE V. Decreasing rates of oesophageal cancer among females in Finland: rates per 100000 people per year

(from Finnish Cancer Registry[25–27])

Year	Age standardized rate	Age group							
		45–49	50–54	55–59	60–64	65–69	70–74	75–79	80+
1954	6.4	2.9	7.6	12.1	25.9	41.6	62.1	91.2	95.2
1969	4.0	3.4	3.8	6.4	17.9	16.8	32.2	53.5	93.6
1979	2.6	0.0	0.7	8.5	8.9	13.5	24.8	37.1	56.2

northern Norway,[28] than in the rest of the country. In England and Wales, high rates are confined to parts of Wales and Cornwall, and to some extent Lancashire, with some indication of a belt of lower incidence running north-south through the centre of England.[24]

7 Discussion

The striking geographical variation in the incidence of oesophageal cancer poses two questions. To what extent can it be explained by known risk factors? And to what extent can it be exploited to give new insight into aetiology?

In Europe and north America, alcohol and tobacco use have been identified as agents in the aetiology of the disease. Case-control studies in Brittany and the United States indicate that perhaps 90% of the cases of the disease can be attributed to them.[12] Furthermore, the risk associated with heavy consumption of both is extremely high, people drinking more than 120 g of ethanol per day and smoking more than 30 g of tobacco being at some 150-fold greater risk of the disease than those drinking less than 40 g of ethanol and smoking less than 9 g of tobacco.[29] Among well nourished, non-drinking, non-smoking males in Europe and north America, oesophageal cancer virtually does not occur. Among drinkers and smokers, the risk rises considerably more sharply with rising alcohol consumption than with rising tobacco consumption, in fact approximately as the exponential of alcohol consumption but only the square root of tobacco consumption.[30] Much of the geographical distribution for males in Europe and north America can be explained in terms of alcohol consumption. North eastern Italy is known for its high rates of alcoholism[31] compared to southern Italy; Brittany and Normandy have higher mortality rates for alcoholism than most of France[32]; and studies in the Caribbean and among US blacks have related both factors, but particularly alcoholism, to the observed high rates.[33,34]

There are, however, further features not explicable in terms of alcohol and tobacco, which may have a bearing on the aetiology in the regions of the world where these two factors are of negligible importance. Within Brittany and Normandy, the variation in mortality by department is unrelated to mortality rates due to alcoholism,[32] supporting one's suspicion that the variation seen in Figure 3 cannot be due solely to differences in the quantity of alcohol consumption. This variation has, surprisingly, not been studied although there is an indication[35] of a geographic relationship with home distillery.[35] In Poland, alcohol and tobacco consumption have risen steadily since the war, reflected in sharply increasing mortality rates for cancers of the lung and larynx (W. Zatonsky, personal communication). Mortality from cancer of the oesophagus has been in slow but steady decline. In Puerto Rico and among US blacks, poor diet has been implicated[36,37] and a recent report suggests low vitamin C intake in Normandy may have a role to play.[38]

The low rates seen in females throughout most of Europe reflect the very low proportion of women who both drink and smoke heavily. The higher rates previously seen in the north of Scandinavia have been related to poor diet, as in the associated Patterson Kelly syndrome.[59] A similar nutritional background might be associated with the relatively high female rates in Wales.

In southern Africa, tobacco in various forms is clearly of importance,[40,41] but the relative risk seen in case-control studies seems far from sufficient to explain the major differences in incidence (even allowing for considerable misclassification in tobacco histories).

Throughout China, Soviet central Asia and northern Iran, alcohol and tobacco play a negligible role in determining the

TABLE VI. Geographic distribution of various factors in northern Iran, in regions of varying oesophageal cancer incidence

(from Iran/IARC study group[44])

Factor studied	Oesophageal cancer incidence		
	High	Medium	Low
Presence of morphine metabolite in the urine (% of adults over 35)	50	19	13
Cultivation of green vegetables (% of households)	14	61	67
% of households with low intake* of:			
Non-cereal protein	41	27	9
Vitamin A	37	6	10
Vitamin C	37	0	8
Riboflavin	27	2	4

* For definition of low intake, see original paper

geographical pattern of the disease.[42] In Singapore also, these two factors explain little of the differences between groups.[43]

In these latter regions, interest then focuses on the manner in which the observed large differences in risk can be exploited in studies of aetiology. A series of investigations expressly designed for this purpose was conducted in northern Iran from the end of 1973 until it was brought to an end in 1978 by civil unrest in the area. The initial studies demonstrated a strong geographical association between oesophageal cancer risk and low intakes of animal protein, vitamin A, vitamin C, and riboflavin, infrequent cultivation of green vegetables and high prevalence of opium use (see Table VI).[44] No association was seen with dietary consumption of volatile introsamines or polycyclic aromatic hydrocarbons, or intake of nitrate or nitrite. Examination of food, stored grain, and flour gave no indication of unusual fungal or mycotoxin contamination.[44–46]

The geographic studies thus pointed strongly to poor diet and opium as the factors which merited further investigation, and indicated equally strongly that further study of dietary contamination by known carcinogens was unlikely to be fruitful. Opium use was widespread throughout central Asia and much of China in the past, but present use is likely to be much reduced, and its role as a risk factor outside Iran is debatable. Some aspect of dietary improverishment however, is becoming an increasingly likely candidate as a major aetiological agent in the rest of Central Asia and in China.

Recent results from China parallel and extend the early findings from Iran, demonstrating deficiencies biochemically rather than by presumed intake (D E Thurnham et al, in preparation). Similar geographic patterns of micro-nutrient deficit have been reported from the Transkei.[20]

It is now a plausible hypothesis that micro-nutrient deficiencies or imbalance provide a unifying explanation of the epidemiology of oesophageal cancer.[15] The main evidence comes from geographic studies, exploiting the variation in incidence of the disease. Alcohol and tobacco, easy to study by conventional case-control means and useful to identify as visible targets for public health measures, may have clouded more basic aspects of the aetiology of the disease.

One would expect further geographical studies to provide a clearer picture of the precise nutritional profiles conducive to oesophageal cancer. A complementary approach is by means of short-term intervention studies using precursor lesions[47] as an endpoint. A study of this type is currently under way in China where the effect of diet supplements on lesions assumed to be early precursors of oesophageal cancer is being investigated.[48]

REFERENCES

1 Parkin DM, Stjernsward J, Muir CS: Estimates of the worldwide frequency of twelve major cancers. Bull WHO; 62

2 Doll R, Payne P, Waterhouse J. Cancer incidence in five continents, Vol. I. Berlin: Springer, 1966

3 Doll R, Muir CS, Waterhouse J. Cancer incidence in five continents, Vol. II. Berlin: Springer, 1971

4 Waterhouse J, Muir CS, Correa P, Powell J. Cancer incidence in five continents, Vol. III. Lyon: IARC Scientific Publications No 15, 1976

5 Atlas of cancer mortality in the People's Republic of China. Reijing: China Map Press, 1979

6 WHO. Age-adjusted rates for cancer for selected sites in 46 countries. Nagoya: Segi Institute of Cancer Epidemiology, 1975–76

7 Serenko AF, Tserkovnogo GF. Malignant tumours (statistical data from the USSR). Moscow: Medizina, 1974

8 Nugmanov SN, Kolycheva NI. Age, sex and ethnic characteristics of patients with oesophageal carcinoma in Kazakhstan, Epidemiology of malignant tumours. Alma Ata: Nauka, Kasakh SSR, 1970; 272–276

9 Nuryagdev SN. Epidemiology of malignant tumors in Kazakhstan. Epidemiology of malignant tumours. Alma Ata: Nauka, Kasahk SSR, 1970; 308–310

10 Mahboubi E, Kmet J, Cook PJ et al. Oesophageal cancer studies in the Caspian littoral of Iran: the Caspian cancer registry. Br J Cancer 1973; 28: 197–208

11 Sobin LH. Cancer in Afghanistan. Cancer 1969; 23: 678–688

12 Day NE, Muñoz N. Esophagus. In: Schottenfeld D, Fraumeni JF. Cancer epidemiology and prevention. Philadelphia: Saunders, 1982; 596–623

13 Shanmugaratnam K, Lee HP, Day NE. Cancer incidence in Singapore 1968–77. IARC Scientific Publications No 47. Lyon: IARC, 1983

14 Rose EF. Esophageal cancer in Transkei: the pattern and associated risk factors. In: Pfeiffer CJ, ed. Cancer of the esophagus. Vol. I. Cleveland: CRC Press Inc, 1982

15 van Rensburg SJ. Epidemiologic and dietary evidence for a specific nutritional predisposition to esophageal cancer. JNCI 1981; 67: 243–251

16 Cook PJ. Cancer of the oesophagus in Africa. Br J Cancer 1971; 25: 853–880

17 Oettle AG. Cancer in Africa, especially in regions south of the Sahara. JNCI 1964; 33: 383–439

18 Burrel RJW. Esophageal cancer among Bantu in the Transkei. JNCI 1962; 28: 495–514

19 Rose E. Esophageal cancer in the Transkei 1955–69. JNCI 1973; 51: 7–16

20 van Rensburg SJ, Benade AS, Rose EF, du Plessis JP. Nutritional status of African populations predisposed to esophageal cancer. Nutrition and Cancer 1983; 4: 206–216

21 Tuyns AJ, Masse LMF. Mortality from cancer of the oesophagus in Brittany. Internat J Epidemiol 1973; 2: 241–245

22 Tuyns AJ, Vernhes JC. La mortalité par cancer de l'oesophage dans les départements du Calvados et de l'Örne. Gastroenterol Clin Biol 1981; 5: 257–265

23 Cislaghi C, De Carli A, Morosini P, Puntoni R. Atlante della mortalita per tumori in Italia 1970–72. Rome: Lega Italiana per la Lotta Contro i Tumori, 1978

24 Gardner MJ, Winter, PD, Taylor CP, Acheson ED. Atlas of cancer mortality in England and Wales, 1968–78

25 Cancer Society of Finland, eds. Cancer incidence in Finland 1953–56. Helsinki: Finnish Cancer Registry publication no. 5, 1958

26 Cancer Society of Finland, eds. Cancer incidence in Finland 1969. Helsinki: Finnish Cancer Registry publication no. 20, 1971

27 Cancer Society of Finland, eds. Cancer incidence in Finland 1979. Helsinki: Finnish Cancer Registry publication no. 30, 1982

28 Norwegian Cancer Society, eds. Geographical variations in cancer incidence in Norway 1966–75. Oslo: Norwegian Cancer Registry, 1978

29 Tuyns AJ, Pequinot, G, Abbatucci JS. Le cancer de l'oesophage en Ille-et-Vilaine en fonction des niveaux de consommation d'alcool et de tabac. Des risques qui se multiplient. Bull Cancer 1977b; 64: 45–60

30 Breslow NE, Day NE. The analysis of case-control studies. Lyon: IARC Scientific Publications No. 32, 1980

31 Rossi M, Ancona E, Mastrangelo C et al. Rilievi epidemiologici sul cancro esofageo nella Regione Veneto. Minerva Medica 1982; 73: 1531–1540

32 Tuyns AJ. Cancer of the oesophagus: further evidence of the relation to drinking habits in France. Int J Cancer 1970b; 5: 152–156

33 Martinez I: Factors associated with cancer of the oesophagus, mouth and pharynx in Puerto Rico. JNCI 1969; 42: 1069–1094

34 Pottern LM, Morris LE, Blot WJ, Ziegler RG, Fraumeni JF. Esophageal cancer among black men in Washington DC: Alcohol, tobacco and other risk factors. JNCI 1981; 67: 777–783

35 Barrelier MT. Le cancer de l'oesophage en Basse-Normandie. These: Caen, 1974

36 Martinez I. Cancer of the esophagus in Puerto Rico, mortality and incidence analysis 1950–64. Cancer 1964; 17: 1279–1288

37 Ziegler RG, Morris LE, Blot WJ, Pottern LM, Hoover R, Fraumeni JF. Esophageal cancer among black men in Washington DC. II. Role of nutrition. JNCI 1981; 67: 1199–1206

38 Tuyns AJ. Protective effect of citrus fruit on esophageal cancer. Nutrition and Cancer 1983; 5: 195–200

39 Wynder EL. Etiological aspects of squamous cancers of the head and neck. JAMA 1971; 215: 452–453

40 Bradshaw E, Schonland M. Smoking, drinking and oesophageal cancer in African males of Johannesburg, South Africa. Br J Cancer 1974; 30: 157–163

41 Hewer J, Rose F, Ghadirian P et al. Ingested mutagens from opium and tobacco pyrolysis products and cancer of the oesophagus. Lancet 1978; ii: 494–496

42 Mahboubi E, Day NE, Ghadirian P et al. The negligible role of alcohol and tobacco in the etiology of esophageal cancer in Iran—a case-control study. In: Nieburgs H, ed. Prevention and detection of cancer. Part II. Detection. New York: Marcel Dekker, 1978, 1149–1159

43 de Jong UW, Breslow N, Goh Ewe Hong J et al. The relationship between the ingestion of hot coffee and intra-oesophageal temperature. Gut 1974; 13: 24–30

44 Iran/IARC Study Group. Esophageal cancer studies in the Caspian littoral of Iran: results of population studies—A prodrome. JNCI 1977; 49: 1127–1138

45 Cook-Mozafari P, Azordegan F, Day NE et al. Oesophageal cancer studies in the Caspian littoral of Iran: results of a case-control study. Br J Cancer 1979; 39: 293–309

46 Kmet J, McLaren DS, Siassi F. Epidemiology of oesophageal cancer with special reference to nutritional studies among the Turkoman of Iran. In: Tobin RB, Mehlman MA, eds. Advances in modern human nutrition. New York: Pathotex, 1981; 343

47 Muñoz N, Crespi M, Grassi A, Wang GO, Shen O, Ou ZC. Precursor lesions of oesophageal cancer in high-risk populations in Iran and China. Lancet 1982; 1: 876–879

48 International Agency for Research on Cancer: Annual Report 1983. Lyon: IARC, 1983; 51–52

British Medical Bulletin (1984) Vol. 40, No. 4, pp. 335–341

THE GEOGRAPHY OF CANCER OF THE STOMACH

D COGGON MA BM MRCP
E D ACHESON DM FRCP

MRC Environmental Epidemiology Unit
Southampton General Hospital
Southampton

Although in many parts of the world its incidence is now declining, cancer of the stomach remains important in North America and Australasia, in much of Europe, and in parts of Asia and South America. There are striking geographical differences in the incidence of stomach cancer both between and within countries, and over the past 40 years these differences have stimulated research into a wide range of possible aetiological and protective factors. However, despite extensive investigation, the geographical distribution of the disease is still only partially explained.

1 Classification

Almost all gastric cancers are carcinomas: lymphomas and sarcomas of the stomach are rare. Lauren has distinguished two main histological types of gastric carcinoma—'intestinal' characterized by large cells with a definite glandular pattern, and 'diffuse' in which the cells are poorly differentiated and rarely form glandular structures.[1] In recent years it has become apparent that these two types of carcinoma are epidemiologically distinct (see below). However, most epidemiological studies have not discriminated between the different histological varieties of stomach cancer.

2 Sources of Information

Information about the geographical distribution of stomach cancer is available from mortality statistics, from cancer registration data and from the findings of ad hoc surveys. Care is needed in the interpretation of apparent differences in incidence and mortality, particularly those which occur between countries with widely differing standards of medical care. A general discussion of the problems which arise in the comparison of international mortality and cancer registration statistics can be found in reviews by Alderson[2] and by Doll and colleagues.[3]

Inasmuch as the fatality rate of stomach cancer is high (even in countries with good medical facilities less than 10% of patients survive five years from the time of diagnosis) mortality is a good index of incidence. On the other hand, a diagnosis of gastric cancer can only be established with accuracy by expensive or invasive investigations, or by autopsy. Because of this errors in the certified cause of death are common. Clinical and autopsy diagnoses were compared in a survey carried out in 1959 at 75 British hospitals, and of 253 deaths attributed to stomach cancer by clinicians only 148 were confirmed as such by the pathologists.[4] At the same time, post-mortem examination revealed 86 cancers of the stomach which had not been diagnosed during life. Even when allowance is made for the incomplete sample of deaths studied (65% of all hospital deaths during the study period) the proportion of clinically undiagnosed gastric cancers was still at least 20%. The high frequency of errors, most of which resulted from confusion with tumours arising at other sites, is an indication of the need for caution when interpreting mortality data, although it should be noted that there was a tendency for mistakes to cancel each other, so that the total numbers of deaths ascribed to gastric cancer by the clinicians and pathologists were similar (253 and 234 respectively).

Diagnoses recorded by cancer registries are in general more accurate than those obtained from death certificates, but there are often doubts about the completeness with which registries ascertain their cases. This again may lead to errors when data from different sources are compared.

Despite these deficiencies, mortality and cancer registration statistics when viewed together reveal a consistent pattern and point to geographical differences in the frequency of stomach cancer that are too large to be explained by artifacts of the kind which have been discussed.

Unfortunately, mortality and registration data are still not available for many parts of the world, but useful information about disease patterns in these areas has sometimes been obtained from surveys of hospital admissions or examination of material referred to local pathology departments.

3 Descriptive Data

a Incidence and Mortality by Country

Table I shows age-standardized incidence rates for cancer of the stomach taken from the most recent edition of *Cancer Incidence in Five Continents*.[5] The figures are based upon information supplied

TABLE I. Cancer of stomach: age-standardized incidence rates per 100000 per year[5]

Cancer registry	Incidence		Cancer registry	Incidence	
	Male	Female		Male	Female
Japan—Miyagi	88.0	42.0	Czechoslovakia—	27.6	13.0
China—Shanghai	55.7	21.0	Western Slovakia		
India—Poona	8.8	7.7	Denmark	17.1	8.9
			Finland	29.3	15.3
Hawaii (Caucasian)	12.2	5.0	Germany FR—Hamburg	26.7	12.6
Hawaii (Japanese)	34.0	15.1	Norway	20.6	10.5
Hawaii (Hawaiian)	36.6	18.6	Sweden	18.3	9.5
Australia—	13.7	6.7	UK—Birmingham	22.1	10.1
New South Wales			Yugoslavia—Slovenia	42.0	18.0
Brazil—Sao Paulo	45.7	19.0			
Canada—Alberta	11.9	5.2	Senegal—Dakar	3.7	2.0
Colombia—Cali	46.3	27.3			
Jamaica—Kingston	17.7	9.3			
Puerto Rico	21.1	9.2			
USA—Connecticut	11.1	5.1			

TABLE II. Cancer of stomach: age-standardized death rates per 100000 per year—1976[6]

Country	Death rate Male	Death rate Female	Country	Death rate Male	Death rate Female
Hong Kong	17.0	7.2	Austria	29.2	15.0
Israel	13.7	7.1	Belgium	16.8	9.5
Japan	54.5	27.5	Bulgaria	28.6	15.1
Philippines	5.7	4.4	Denmark	12.8	7.0
Singapore	32.4	12.9	France	14.9	6.5
Thailand	1.4	0.6	Germany DR	25.9	12.3
Australia	11.8	5.9	Germany FR	25.5	13.2
New Zealand	14.6	6.2	Greece	13.1	7.8
			Hungary	35.8	16.8
Canada	11.9	5.5	Iceland	28.2	17.9
Chile	49.9	22.7	Malta	24.8	6.2
Costa Rica	45.7	22.2	Netherlands	20.5	9.2
Honduras	4.3	3.0	Norway	17.4	8.2
Nicaragua	1.9	0.5	Poland	35.0	13.6
Paraguay	19.5	9.3	Romania	28.8	12.8
USA	6.8	3.2	Spain	23.7	12.1
Uraguay	30.3	12.9	Sweden	15.3	8.0
Venezuela	27.8	17.4	Switzerland	18.4	7.9
			England and Wales	19.1	8.7
			Northern Ireland	18.3	10.3
			Scotland	19.1	10.2
			Yugoslavia	23.7	11.0
			Mauritius	17.1	8.8

TABLE III. Cancer of stomach: changes in age-standardized incidence rates at selected cancer registries

(after Doll *et al.*[3] and Waterhouse *et al.*[5])

Registry	Period A	Period B	% Change in incidence Period A to Period B Male	% Change in incidence Period A to Period B Female
Japan—Miyagi	1959–1960	1973–1977	−8	−12
Hawaii (Caucasian)	1960–1963	1973–1977	−5	−43
Hawaii (Japanese)	1960–1963	1973–1977	−23	−31
Hawaii (Hawaiian)	1960–1963	1973–1977	−28	+1
Canada—Alberta	1960–1962	1973–1977	−28	−26
Colombia—Cali	1962–1964	1972–1976	−16	+14
Jamaica—Kingston	1958–1963	1973–1977	−35	−15
Puerto Rico	1962–1963	1973–1977	−27	−34
USA—Connecticut	1960–1962	1973–1977	−38	−43
Denmark	1953–1957	1973–1976	−46	−56
Finland	1959–1961	1971–1976	−45	−48
Germany FR—Hamburg	1960–1962	1973–1977	−28	−35
Norway	1959–1961	1973–1977	−38	−44
Sweden	1959–1961	1971–1975	−31	−29
UK—Birmingham	1960–1962	1973–1976	−21	−33
Yugoslavia—Slovenia	1956–1960	1973–1976	−13	−29

by selected cancer registries, and are mostly for the period 1973–1977. The incidence is high in Japan, China, Colombia, Brazil, Yugoslavia, Hawaii (Japanese and Hawaiians) and Finland, and low in Senegal, India, Canada, the United States and Australia. In both men and women there is more than a 20-fold difference between the highest rate (Miyagi, Japan) and the lowest (Dakar, Senegal). Registration data from earlier years indicate that there is also a high incidence of gastric cancer in Iceland and in Chile.[3]

The mortality statistics presented in Table II were assembled by Segi[6] and reveal a pattern consistent with the incidence data. Death rates are high in Japan, Chile, Costa Rica and several central European countries, and low in the United States, Canada, Australia, Thailand and parts of central America. Mortality data also suggest a high incidence in several of the central Asian republics of the Soviet Union.[7]

Further information about the geographical distribution of stomach cancer has been gathered by Dunham and Bailar.[8] From analysis of hospital, biopsy and autopsy series it appears that the disease is rare in southern and south-east Asia and in most of Africa, although localized areas of high incidence have been reported in two mountainous regions of East Africa.[9]

Despite the large international differences in gastric cancer incidence and mortality, the sex ratio shows little geographical variation. Griffith has examined the sex ratio of gastric cancer mortality in detail[10] and found that in each of 24 countries the ratio increases from a value close to one at younger ages to reach a maximum of about two around the age of 60. At older ages the ratio declines. This remarkably constant pattern suggests that whatever is responsible for the international variation in stomach cancer incidence affects men and women in a similar manner throughout the world.

In most countries stomach cancer incidence and mortality are falling. Table III shows the changes in incidence that have been recorded since the 1950s and early 1960s by 14 of the registries which contribute to *Cancer Incidence in Five Continents*. The rates for Caucasian women in Hawaii are based on small numbers of cases and only in the women of Cali, Colombia has there been an increase of any consequence. In all other populations the incidence has declined. Furthermore, the extent of this decline is too great to

be attributed to improvements in diagnostic technique or changing fashions of diagnosis. Examination of age-specific rates reveals that in most places the fall in incidence has applied to all age groups. A notable exception, however, is Japan where the reduction has been on a smaller scale and confined to persons under the age of 70; among the elderly the incidence has gone up.

Mortality trends confirm the widespread fall in gastric cancer incidence and suggest that in most countries the decline is longstanding (Fig. 1). Exceptions are Japan where death rates did not start to fall until the late 1950s, and Portugal and Yugoslavia where mortality is, if anything, increasing. The apparent inconsistency between mortality and registration trends in Yugoslavia may have occurred because the cancer registry covers only the Slovenia region whereas the mortality data are for the country as a whole. It is known that there are important regional differences in the incidence of stomach cancer within Yugoslavia (see below).

b Geographical Differences Within Countries

In addition to the large international differences in the incidence and mortality of stomach cancer, important geographical variations in its frequency have been demonstrated within countries. Plate I shows the pattern of gastric cancer mortality in men during the years 1968–78 for the 1366 local authority areas of England and Wales (the distribution for women is very similar). The high incidence of stomach cancer in North Wales has been recognized for at least 50 years.[11] In addition, the map shows clusters of high mortality in the industrial areas of Tyneside, Lancashire, South Wales and the West Midlands, and in East London.

In the United States cancer mortality has been mapped by county for the period 1950–69.[12] Death rates from cancer of the stomach are elevated in many of the major cities and also in areas characterized by low socio-economic class (e.g. certain counties in Pennsylvania and Kentucky). There is in addition a cluster of rural counties with increased mortality in the northern states of Wisconsin, Michigan, Minnesota and the Dakotas, and a further focus of high mortality in New Mexico and Colorado.

An atlas of mortality from cancer and other major diseases has recently been published for Japan[13] and confirms earlier observations of high death rates in the north-western part of Honshu.[14,15]

FIG. 1. Cancer of the stomach: mortality trends for males by country 1931–75

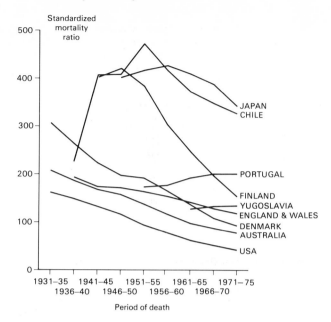

The same standard rates have been used to calculate all the standardized mortality ratios[2]

In the United States, death rates from stomach cancer are elevated in migrants from Scandinavia, the Soviet Union and central Europe—places where the disease is known to be more common.[25] This may explain the cluster of rural counties with high mortality in Minnesota and neighbouring states, since many of the inhabitants of these counties are of Russian, Austrian, German or Scandinavian descent.[12]

Among Chinese residents of the USA, mortality from stomach cancer is lower than that in the Chinese populations of Taiwan, Hong Kong and Singapore.[26] The rates for Chinese born in the United States are close to those of white Americans. The mortality of first generation immigrants is somewhat higher, but probably nearer to that of white Americans than to rates in their places of birth.

The pattern for Japanese migrants to the United States is similar in that they experience death rates from gastric cancer intermediate between those in Japan and those in American whites.[27] Unlike the Chinese, however, their mortality, particularly in the older age groups, is closer to that of their birthplace than to that of their adopted country. Mortality rates of Japanese born in the USA are higher than those of US whites but, in men at least, are lower than those of first-generation immigrants. Particular attention has been paid to the Japanese living in Hawaii, where a case-control study has shown that migrants from areas of Japan with the highest incidence of stomach cancer continue to display an elevated risk (as compared with migrants from other parts of Japan) in their new homeland.[28] This difference does not occur in their offspring however.

The results of studies in other countries are consistent with those from the USA. In Manitoba, Canada, high death rates from stomach cancer have been observed in immigrants from Scandinavia, Iceland and the Ukraine, with lower mortality in their children.[29] In Israel the incidence is higher in Jews of European extraction than in those coming from Africa and Asia, and is higher in new immigrants than in those who have lived in the country for ten or more years.[30] European migrants to Australia have higher mortality rates from stomach cancer than native Australians, but again their excess risk is reduced with increasing duration of residence.[31]

Migration within countries has also been studied. In Santiago, Chile, stomach cancer is more common in persons who spent their early life in regions of the country where the incidence is high,[32] and in Cali, Colombia, the risks of gastric carcinoma in immigrant groups reflect the incidence of the disease in the areas from which they originate.[17] The last finding is of special interest because it applies to persons who have moved to Cali from places with a lower incidence as well as to migrants from high-risk areas.

In contrast stomach cancer mortality is relatively low in the southern island of Kyushu.

An analysis of mortality for the period 1957–71 showed that in Chile death rates from stomach cancer were highest in three agricultural provinces lying about 200 miles south of Santiago.[16] Mortality in the extreme north and south of the country was less than half as high.

In Colombia, another country with a high incidence of stomach cancer, the highest rates occur in the mountainous regions of the interior, while the disease is less frequent in coastal areas.[17]

Regional differences in stomach cancer incidence and mortality have also been described in Iceland, where the disease is most common in the north-western part of the island,[18] in Yugoslavia where the frequency is higher in the alpine and Panonic regions of Slovenia than in the Adriatic coastal area,[19] and in Czechoslovakia,[20] the Netherlands,[21] Belgium[22] and China.[23]

In contrast to the marked regional variations in stomach cancer incidence, urban–rural differences are generally small and show no consistent pattern from one country to another. For example, in England and Wales (see pp. 320–328) and in the United States[24] mortality is higher in cities and large towns, but in Iceland[18] and the Netherlands[21] there is, if anything, an excess in rural areas.

c *Migrant Studies*

Understanding of geographical variation in the incidence of disease is often aided by the study of migrant populations. There have been many such investigations of stomach cancer, most of them concerning persons who have moved from high- to low-risk areas. These studies suggest that migrants carry a risk intermediate between that of their country of origin and that of their adopted country, and that the incidence in their offspring is often further displaced towards that of the host nation.

d *Histology*

There is now good evidence that the two main histological varieties of gastric carcinoma differ in their epidemiology. In particular, it appears that geographical differences in the frequency of stomach cancer are more marked for intestinal-type tumours. Thus, for example, review of surgical material from Mexico City and from three cities in Colombia has indicated an excess of diffuse carcinoma in areas with a low incidence of gastric cancer, while the intestinal type was predominant in high-risk areas.[33] These findings accord with those from a study of Japanese populations in Hawaii and in Miyagi, Japan, in which the estimated incidence of diffuse carcinomas was the same in both places, but the rates for intestinal-type tumours were substantially lower in Hawaii.[34]

Further support comes from observations of migrant groups. In

Connecticut, USA intestinal-type carcinomas were found to be relatively more common in migrants from Europe, the Soviet Union, China and South America than in persons born in countries with a lower incidence of gastric cancer such as the United States.[35] Similarly, in a study based on the Israel cancer registry, a higher frequency of intestinal-type tumours was seen in migrants from Eastern Europe than in migrants from Asia and in subjects born in Israel;[36] and in Santiago, Chile, the association found between stomach cancer and residence in high-risk areas during early life applied only to intestinal-type carcinomas.[32] A study of migrants groups in Cali, Colombia, was less conclusive, but this may have been because the number of cases observed was too small.[17]

The theory that intestinal-type tumours predominate in populations at high risk of stomach cancer has been challenged by Kubo,[37] but his failure to confirm the findings of other workers probably stems from differences in methodology.

4 Factors Underlying the Geographical Distribution of Stomach Cancer

a *Genetic*

Genetic predisposition to cancer of the stomach has long been recognized in that persons with blood group A have an increased risk of developing the disease. A recent study has suggested that the association applies principally to diffuse carcinomas[34] but, against this, the relative risk appears remarkably constant from one place to another and is, if anything, higher in countries where stomach cancer is more common (N E Day, personal communication). If the association were limited to diffuse carcinomas, one would expect the overall effect to be strongest in low-incidence areas where a greater proportion of tumours are of the diffuse type. The possibility that genetic factors contribute to the higher incidence of stomach cancer in Wales than in England has been explored in two investigations. The first showed a correlation of mortality rates in Welsh counties and county boroughs with levels of 'Welshness' as measured by the proportion of Welsh-speaking people in each area and by the proportion of people with Welsh surnames.[38] The second was a case-control study of gastric cancer in Swansea in which an excess of Welsh surnames was found among the case group.[39] These findings are compatible with the hypothesis that Welsh people are genetically predisposed to stomach cancer, but they could also be explained by cultural differences between the Welsh and the English.

Although genetic susceptibility may have some effect on the geographical distribution of stomach cancer, the fact that its incidence is often much lower in migrant populations than in their countries of origin would imply that environmental factors exert a more important influence. Furthermore, the reduction in incidence among first-generation immigrants is usually less marked than that in their offspring, suggesting either that these environmental factors operate early in life, or alternatively that they are cultural phenomena which lose their impact as successive generations adopt the ways of their new homeland.

b *Climate*

Wynder has pointed out that the incidence of stomach cancer tends to be high in countries with climatic conditions typical of higher latitudes and is lower in countries with tropical climates.[19] However, this association with climate is only loose and does not, for example, explain the much higher incidence of the disease in central Europe than in Canada. If climate does exert an influence on the occurrence of stomach cancer it is probably mediated through its effect on diet.

c *Geology*

During the 1950s and early 1960s, investigators sought hard to explain the high death rates from stomach cancer in North Wales, and much of this early research was directed at possible geological risk factors. Analysis of soil samples taken from gardens in North Wales and the adjacent English county of Cheshire showed a correlation between the organic content of soil in 66 administrative areas and mortality from gastric cancer in those districts.[40] More detailed examination of individual cases suggested that the risk of stomach cancer was highest in persons who had resided for long periods on a particular type of soil with intermediate organic content.[40] Surveys carried out in the Netherlands[41] and in Japan[14] have also demonstrated high rates of stomach cancer in areas with peaty soils containing high concentrations of organic matter. In addition, the Japanese investigation indicated a possible association with volcanic soils, and the high levels of volcanic activity in countries where gastric cancer is most common have been noted by other authors.

Attention has also focused on trace elements in the soil. In particular, a case-control study carried out in North Wales, Cheshire and Devonshire revealed high zinc/copper ratios in samples taken from the gardens of stomach cancer patients.[42] Against this it has been pointed out that in the English village of Shipham where the soil contains high concentrations of zinc and low concentrations of copper, the incidence of gastric cancer is low.[43]

A requirement of theories relating the incidence of stomach cancer to geological features is that there should be a plausible biological mechanism whereby such factors might produce tumours. Possible explanations include the absorption of harmful substances as a result of direct contact with the soil (in most cases this would be occupational) or the ingestion of carcinogens in locally grown vegetables. These two possibilities were explored by Stocks.[44] He found that in North-West Wales, mortality from stomach cancer was elevated in men who had worked on farms or in quarries (as compared with other workers), but that there was no corresponding excess in the wives of agricultural workers or in farmers living in Cheshire where the risk factor was assumed to be absent from the soil. However, he was unable to demonstrate a clear association between stomach cancer and possession of a vegetable garden or eating vegetables from it.

Another way in which local geology might influence the occurrence of stomach cancer is through its effect on drinking water. Millar measured concentrations of uranium oxide in the water supplies of houses in North Wales where there had been a death from stomach cancer, but found them no higher than expected.[45] A relationship with drinking water was found, however, in a case-control study carried out in Japan.[46] This showed an association between stomach cancer and the prolonged use of well-water, although the chemical composition of water supplies was not examined in detail. The effects of nitrate in drinking water are considered under the heading of diet (see below).

Despite much research no geological factor has yet been shown to have a definite role in the aetiology of stomach cancer, and the contribution of such factors to its geographical distribution remains unclear.

d Occupation

The high incidence of stomach cancer in farmers and quarrymen of North Wales has already been mentioned, and it has been suggested that an area of high gastric cancer mortality in Utah may be attributable to the local coalmining industry.[47] However, the uniformity of the ratio of male-to-female incidence from one country and region to another argues against a major role for occupational factors in determining the geographical distribution of the disease.

e Diet

In recent years interest in the epidemiology of gastric cancer has centred largely on the influence of dietary factors. One proposed aetiological agent is salt. Joossens has shown a correlation between mortality from stomach cancer and cerebrovascular accidents at both a national and regional level, and has suggested that salt may be the causal factor linking the two diseases.[48] More direct evidence for this theory comes from Japan where geographical correlations have been demonstrated between stomach cancer mortality and the concentration of salt used in soy-bean paste,[15] and also with intake of salted food.[49] In a nutritional survey of four Colombian villages known to have different rates of stomach cancer, there was again a suggestion of excessive salt consumption in the higher-risk communities.[50] In addition, several case-control studies have shown associations between stomach cancer and salty foods.[15,28,51]

Other methods of food preservation have also come under suspicion. In Iceland, which has a high incidence of stomach cancer, large quantities of smoked meat and fish are eaten, and singed sheep heads are a special local dish. These foods contain polycyclic aromatic hydrocarbons, some of which are known to be carcinogenic. Comparison of dietary habits in two rural areas of Iceland, one with a high mortality from stomach cancer and one with a low mortality, did not show any difference in the consumption of smoked food, but singed meat was eaten more often in the high-risk area.[52] If techniques of food preservation are involved in the aetiology of stomach cancer, the increasing use of refrigeration over the course of this century may have contributed to the widespread decline in the incidence of the disease.

Much attention has been given to the possible role of N-nitroso compounds in the pathogenesis of stomach cancer. Like polycyclic aromatic hydrocarbons, many of these compounds are potent animal carcinogens. Small quantities occur preformed in certain foodstuffs, but interest has centred more on their endogenous formation from dietary nitrate.[53] Most ingested nitrate is excreted unchanged in the urine, but a proportion is converted by bacteria in the saliva and gastric juice to nitrite. The latter may then react with dietary amines (which are present in many food items) to produce N-nitroso compounds. If this mechanism were important in the generation of tumours, one would expect to find an association between gastric cancer and dietary intake of nitrate, most of which comes from vegetables and drinking water.

In 1973 Hill and colleagues reported that mortality from stomach cancer was excessive in Worksop, an English town with high levels of nitrate in its water supply.[54] The magnitude and significance of this excess have since been questioned,[55] and an attempt to correlate stomach cancer mortality in 32 rural districts of Eastern England with levels of nitrate in public water supplies has yielded inconsistent results.[56] However, a geographical correlation between the risk of stomach cancer and nitrate in drinking water has been demonstrated in Colombia.[57] Also, in a comparison of two Danish towns, there was a higher incidence of stomach cancer in the city with the greater concentration of nitrate in its water.[58] In Chile, which has rich natural deposits of saltpetre, nitrate fertilizers have been used on an enormous scale. Analysis of death rates from stomach cancer in provinces of Chile has shown a high correlation with the use of nitrate fertilizers[59] and with per-capita cumulative exposure to these products.[16]

When more direct measures of nitrate intake have been used, the relationship to gastric cancer incidence has been less clear. A survey of four population groups in Colombia has indicated a correlation between gastric cancer risk and urinary excretion of nitrate.[57] On the other hand, measurement of nitrate concentrations in urine samples from school children in four areas of Chile showed the highest levels in a region of low stomach cancer mortality.[60] Concentrations of salivary nitrite were similar in all four areas and the investigators concluded that exposure to nitrates does not on its own explain the geographical distribution of gastric cancer in Chile. Preliminary results from a British survey are also against a simple relationship between nitrates and stomach cancer in that they show higher levels of salivary nitrate and nitrite in subjects from the Oxford region (a low-gastric-cancer-incidence area) than in the north-east of England or North Wales (high-incidence areas) (D Forman personal communication).

As early as 1947 Stocks postulated that the high mortality from stomach cancer in North Wales might be related to the low consumption of fresh milk and vegetables in that area,[11] and a negative association between gastric cancer and milk consumption has since been demonstrated in a large Japanese case-control study.[15]

A protective effect of fresh fruit and vegetables has been suggested by studies from several countries. In an Icelandic survey, intake of vitamin C was lower in a region with high mortality from stomach cancer than in a low-incidence area.[52] Case-control studies in the USA,[51] Norway[51] and Japan,[46] and in Japanese residents of Hawaii[28] have all shown negative associations with the consumption of certain uncooked vegetables, and comparison of high and low risk populations in Colombia has also pointed to a protective action of vegetables and fruit.[50]

Analyses of stomach cancer mortality and incidence by country have revealed a positive correlation with cereal consumption[61] and negative correlations with consumption of meat and fat,[62] but these findings have received only limited support from studies of individual patients.

Of all the dietary relationships which have been investigated, a harmful effect of salt and a protective action of fresh fruit and vegetables are perhaps most likely to influence the geographical distribution of stomach cancer.

5 Conclusions

The precise causes of stomach cancer are still largely unknown, but it seems certain that the disease results from the interplay of many factors. On the basis of current epidemiological knowledge, Correa and colleagues have proposed a unifying theory of its pathogenesis.[63] They postulate a chain of events which starts with injury to the gastric mucosa, caused for example by dietary factors, pernicious anaemia or gastroenterostomy. This leads to a reduction in gastric acidity with a consequent increase in the bacterial reduction of nitrate which in turn results in the increased formation of carcinogenic N-nitroso compounds. This model appears plausible, but it has yet to be proved valid.

Of the many postulated risk factors, those related to diet are perhaps most likely to explain the geographical distribution of stomach cancer. Conclusive identification of these factors is difficult, however, because the aspects of diet which determine the large geographical differences in disease frequency probably vary little within most communities, and their effects are therefore not apparent in case-control studies. At the same time, studies which examine the relationship of gastric cancer to diet by comparing countries or regions are unable to disentangle the effects of individual foods because their consumption is correlated one with another. For this reason, particular effort has gone into the search for populations with abnormally heterogeneous diets (e.g. certain migrant groups) in which case-control studies might be more productive.

A further obstacle to our understanding of stomach cancer is the long latent period between first exposure to a carcinogen and the eventual development of a tumour. In an attempt to overcome this problem, a search has been made for precursor lesions which might act as early markers for the disease process. One suggestion is that benign gastric ulcer predisposes to stomach cancer, but efforts to correlate mortality from the two diseases have been generally unrewarding. More promising however, is the recent discovery of an association between gastric cancer and intestinal metaplasia of the stomach.[17,57,64,65]

It is to be hoped that this finding, together with a search for communities with unusually heterogeneous dietary practices will in time lead to a better understanding of stomach cancer, and in particular its remarkable geographical distribution.

REFERENCES

1 Laurén P. The two histological main types of gastric cancer: diffuse and so-called intestinal-type carcinoma: an attempt at a histo-clinical classification. Acta Pathol Microbiol Scand 1965; 64: 31–49

2 Alderson M. International mortality statistics. London: Macmillan, 1981

3 Doll R, Payne P, Waterhouse J, eds. Cancer incidence in five continents (UICC technical report I). Berlin: Springer Verlag, 1966

4 Heasman MA, Lipworth L. Accuracy of certification of cause of death. (GRO studies on medical and population subjects No 20). London: HMSO, 1966

5 Waterhouse J, Muir C, Shanmugaratnam K, Powell J, eds. Cancer incidence in five continents. Vol IV (IARC Scientific publications no 42) Lyon: International Agency for Research on Cancer, 1982

6 Segi M. (In collaboration with Hattori H, Noye H, Segi R.) Age-adjusted death rates for cancer for selected sites (A—classification) in 40 countries in 1976. Nagoya: Segi Institute of Cancer Epidemiology, 1981

7 Doll R. The geographical distribution of cancer. Br J Cancer 1969; 23: 1–8

8 Dunham LJ, Bailar JC III. World maps of cancer mortality rates and frequency ratios. JNCI 1968; 41: 155–203

9 Burkitt DP. A study of cancer patterns in Africa. In: British Postgraduate Medical Federation. Scientific Basis of Medicine. Annual Reviews. London: University of London Press, 1969; 82–94

10 Griffith GW. The sex ratio in gastric cancer and hypothetical considerations relative to aetiology. Br J Cancer 1968; 22: 163–172

11 Stocks P. Regional and local differences in cancer death rates. (GRO studies on medical and population subjects no 1). London: HMSO, 1947

12 Hoover R, Mason TJ, McKay FW, Fraumeni JF. jr. Cancer by county: new resource for etiologic clues. Science 1975; 189: 1005–1007

13 The Research Committee on Geographical Distribution of Diseases (Chairman Dr. I Shigematsu). National atlas of major disease mortalities for cities, towns and villages in Japan: All causes of death, cancer, cardiovascular disease, diabetes mellitus, liver cirrhosis and tuberculosis 1969–1978. Tokyo: Japan Health Promotion Foundation, 1981

14 Segi, M, Kurihara M. Cancer in Japan from the viewpoint of geographical pathology. Tohoku J Exper Med 1960; 72: 169–193

15 Hirayama T. The epidemiology of cancer of the stomach in Japan with special reference to the role of diet. UICC Monogr Ser 1967; 10: 37–49

16 Armijo R, Coulson AH. Epidemiology of stomach cancer in Chile—The role of nitrogen fertilizers. Int J Epidemiol 1975; 4: 301–309

17 Correa P, Cuello C, Duque E. Carcinoma and intestinal metaplasia of the stomach in Colombian migrants. JNCI 1970; 44: 297–306

18 Sigurjonsson J. Geographical variations in mortality from cancer in Iceland, with particular reference to stomach cancer. JNCI 1966; 37: 337–346

19 Wynder EL, Kmet J, Dungal N, Segi M. An epidemiological investigation of gastric cancer. Cancer 1963; 16: 1461–1496

20 Gregor O, Toman R, Prusová F, Drnková V, Pastorová J. Geographical distribution of stomach cancer in Czechoslovakia. Gut 1969; 10: 150–154

21 Tromp SW. The geographical distribution of cancer of the stomach in the Netherlands (Period 1946–52). Br J Cancer 1956; 10: 265–281

22 Verhasselt Y. Geography of stomach cancer in Belgium. An approach. Geogr Med 1981; 11: 104–115

23 Xu G-W. Gastric cancer in China: a review. J R Soc Med 1981; 74: 210–211

24 Haenszel W. Variation in incidence of and mortality from stomach cancer, with particular reference to the United States. JNCI 1958; 21: 213–262

25 Haenszel W. Cancer mortality among the foreign-born in the United States. JNCI 1961; 26: 37–132

26 King H, Haenszel W. Cancer mortality among foreign- and native-born Chinese in the United States. J Chron Dis 1973; 26: 623–646

27 Haenszel W, Kurihara M. Studies of Japanese migrants. 1. Mortality from cancer and other diseases among Japanese in the United States. JNCI 1968; 40: 43–68

28 Haenszel W, Kurihara M, Segi M, Lee RKC. Stomach cancer among Japanese in Hawaii. JNCI 1972; 49: 969–988

29 Choi NW, Entwistle DW, Michaluk W, Nelson N. Gastric cancer in Icelanders in Manitoba. Israel J Med Sci 1971; 7: 1500–1508

30 Tulchinsky D, Modan B. Epidemiological aspects of cancer of the stomach in Israel. Cancer 1967; 20: 1311–1317

31 McMichael AJ, McCall MG, Hartshorne JM, Woodings TL. Patterns of gastro-intestinal cancer in European migrants to Australia: the role of dietary change. Int J Cancer 1980; 25: 431–437

32 Armijo R, Orellana M, Medina E, Coulson AH, Sayre JW, Detels R. Epidemiology of gastric cancer in Chile: 1—case-control study. Int J Epid 1981; 10: 53–56

33 Muñoz N, Correa P, Cuello C, Duque E. Histologic types of gastric carcinoma in high- and low-risk areas. Int J Cancer 1968; 3: 809–818

34 Correa P, Sasano N, Stemmermann GN, Haenszel W. Pathology of gastric carcinoma in Japanese populations: Comparisons between Miyagi prefecture, Japan, and Hawaii. JNCI 1973; 51: 1449–1459

35 Muñoz N, Connelly R. Time trends of intestinal and diffuse types of gastric cancer in the United States. Int J Cancer 1971; 8: 158–164

36 Muñoz, N, Steinitz R. Comparative histology of gastric cancer in migrant groups in Israel. Israel J Med Sci 1971; 7: 1479–1487

37 Kubo T, Tsunoda H, Tanaka S, Soga J. Geographical pathology of gastric carcinoma: a comparative study on histological types between high and low mortality areas in Japan. Gann 1981; 72: 235–244

38 Ashley DJB. Gastric cancer in Wales. J Med Genet 1969; 6: 76–79

39 Ashley DJB, Davies HD. Gastric cancer in Wales. Gut 1966; 7: 542–548

40 Stocks P, Davies RI. Epidemiological evidence from chemical and spectrographic analyses that soil is concerned in the causation of cancer. Br J Cancer 1960; 14: 8–22

41 Tromp SW, Diehl JC. A statistical study of the possible relationship between cancer of the stomach and soil. Br J Cancer 1955; 9: 349–357

42 Stocks P, Davies RI. Zinc and copper content of soils associated with the incidence of cancer of the stomach and other organs. Br J Cancer 1964; 18: 14–24

43 Philipp R, Hughes AO, Robertson MC. Stomach cancer and soil metal content. Br J Cancer 1982; 45: 482

44 Stocks P. A study of cancer mortality in farming, quarrying, mining and other occupations in North Wales and Cheshire. Br J Cancer 1961; 15: 701–711

45 Millar IB. Gastro-intestinal cancer and geochemistry in North Montgomeryshire. Br J Cancer 1961; 15: 175–199

46 Haenszel W, Kurihara M, Locke FB, Shimuzu K, Segi M. Stomach cancer in Japan. JNCI 1976; 56: 265–274

47 Matolo NM, Klauber MR, Gorishek WM, Dixon JA. High incidence of gastric carcinoma in a coal mining region. Cancer 1972; 29: 733–737

48 Joossens JV, Kesteloot H, Amery A. Salt intake and mortality from stroke. New Eng J Med 1979; 300: 1396

49 Sato T, Fukuyama T, Suzuki T *et al.* Studies of the causation of gastric cancer. 2. The relation between gastric cancer mortality rate and salted food intake in several places in Japan. Bull Inst Publ Health 1959; 8: 187–198

50 Correa P, Cuello C, Fajardo LF, Haenszel W, Bolaños O, de Ramirez B. Diet and gastric cancer: Nutrition survey in a high-risk area. JNCI 1983; 70: 673–678

51 Bjelke E. Epidemiologic studies of cancer of the stomach, colon and rectum, with special emphasis on the role of diet. Scand J Gastroenterol 1974; 9 supp 31: 1–253

52 Dungal N, Sigurjonsson J. Gastric cancer and diet. Br J Cancer 1967; 21: 270–276

53 Fraser P, Chilvers C, Beral V, Hill MJ. Nitrate and human cancer: a review of the evidence. Int J Epidemiol 1980; 9: 3–11

54 Hill MJ, Hawksworth G, Tattersall G. Bacteria, nitrosamines and cancer of the stomach. Br J Cancer 1973; 28: 562–567

55 Davies JM. Stomach cancer mortality in Worksop and other Nottinghamshire mining towns. Br J Cancer 1980; 41: 438–445

56 Fraser P, Chilvers C. Health aspects of nitrate in drinking water. The Science of the Total Environment 1981; 18: 103–116

57 Cuello C, Correa P, Haenszel W *et al.* Gastric cancer in Colombia. I. Cancer risk and suspect environmental agents. JNCI 1976; 57: 1015–1020

58 Jensen OM. Nitrate in drinking water and cancer in northern Jutland, Denmark, with special reference to stomach cancer. Ecotoxicol Environ Safety 1982; 6: 258–267

59 Zaldívar R, Robinson H. Epidemiological investigation on stomach cancer mortality in Chileans: association with nitrate fertilizer. Z Krebsforsch 1973; 80: 289–295

60 Armijo R, Gonzalez A, Orellana M, Coulson AH, Sayre JW, Detels R. Epidemiology of gastric cancer in Chile: II—Nitrate exposures and stomach cancer frequency. Int J Epid 1981; 10: 57–62

61 Hakama M, Saxén EA. Cereal consumption and gastric cancer. Int J Cancer 1967; 2: 265–268

62 Armstrong B, Doll R. Environmental factors and cancer incidence and mortality in different countries with special reference to dietary practices. Int J Cancer 1975; 15: 617–631

63 Correa P, Haenszel W, Tannenbaum S. Epidemiology of gastric carcinoma: review and future prospects. Nat Cancer Inst Mongr 1982; 62: 129–134

64 Correa P, Cuello C, Duque E *et al.* Gastric cancer in Colombia. III. Natural history of precursor lesions. JNCI 1976; 57: 1027–1035

65 Haenszel W, Correa P, Cuello C *et al.* Gastric cancer in Columbia. II. Case-control epidemiolgic study of precursor lesions. JNCI 1976; 57: 1021—1026

British Medical Bulletin (1984) Vol. 40, No. 4, pp. 342–345

CANCER OF THE LIVER

PAULA COOK-MOZAFFARI MA BLitt

MRC External Staff
University of Oxford

SCHALK VAN RENSBURG BVSc DVSc

National Research Institute for Nutritional Diseases
Tygerberg, South Africa

1 Incidence in men
2 Incidence in women
3 Incidence in migrant populations
4 Time trends
5 Risk factors
    a Aflatoxin
    b Hepatitis B virus
    c Alcohol
    d Other risk factors
References

Primary liver cancer (PLC) is common in much of Asia and Africa and rare in northern Europe and north America. For a disease that is common in areas of the world where medical services are limited, the all-age incidence rates are likely to be biased by underdiagnosis among the elderly. In discussing levels of incidence, therefore, truncated rates (for the age group 35–64)[1-4] are used. In 1969, Doll[5] recommended that geographical comparisons for PLC should be restricted even further, to persons under 45 years of age, because it is difficult, at older ages, to distinguish genuine primary tumours from misdiagnosed secondary growths, given the propensity of tumours of the lung, intestine, and stomach to metastasize to the liver. However, the advent of needle biopsies and alpha-fetoprotein estimation have facilitated the diagnosis of PLC and it has seemed legitimate now to extend comparisons at least up to 65 years. This has the advantage of distinguishing different levels of incidence within regions of moderate frequency where the numbers at younger ages are too low to give stable rates. In many poorer parts of the world where there may still be a high proportion of clinical diagnoses, malignancies at the sites that metastasize to the liver are themselves rare and most liver tumours are likely to be genuine primary carcinomas.[6]

1   Incidence in Men

Incidence levels for men in different parts of the world at ages 35–64 years are summarized in Table I. Most of the information is taken from the four volumes of *Cancer Incidence in 5 Continents*.[1-4] Further indications of incidence are available from a survey of cancer frequency in Africa south of the Sahara (P Cook-Mozaffari and D P Burkitt, in preparation); from a survey of cancer incidence among workers in the gold mines of South Africa,[7,8] and from surveys of the occurrence of PLC undertaken in conjunction with aetiological investigations.[6,9-12] Supplementary information on incidence patterns is also available from mortality statistics.[6,13-15] The prognosis for PLC is so poor that the figures will not be biased by differential levels of treatment and cure. Estimations of incidence levels from all these sources are set out in Table I.

The one region of the world for which use of truncated incidence rates for the age group 35–64 does not correctly represent the very high levels of incidence that occur is Mozambique. This happens because between the ages of 20 and 50 the age-specific rates are at a similar level, and then decrease at older ages,[11] instead of showing the sharp increase with age that is usual for epithelial tumours. The same shape of age curve has been observed both in the city of Maputo (formerly Lourenco Marques) and in the Province of Inhambane. There is no indication from incidence data that this shape of age curve occurs anywhere else in the world. The incidence of PLC for Maputo in men aged 15–24 is 55 times the rate for men of the same age in Senegal and 100–230 times the rates in the Chinese populations of Hong Kong, Singapore, and Shanghai compared with the two to three-fold excess indicated by the truncated rates for the age group 35–64. The incidence among adolescents and young adults in Maputo is exceptional for any type of cancer anywhere in the world, being higher than the rate for lung cancer observed in London among men thirty years older.[1] Great care was taken to exclude non-residents from the incidence figures for Maputo[16] and the rate for other types of cancer at young ages are as low as would be expected from incidence rates elsewhere in the world.

TABLE I. Approximate level of incidence for PLC in different parts of the world

		Age-standardized incidence per 100 000 for men aged 35–64			
<4	4–	12–	25–	50–	100–
Canada	USA (blacks)	Southern Uganda*	Southern Nigeria	Dakar, Senegal†	Maputo, Mozambique
USA (whites)	USA (Latin)	North-west Tanzania*	Southern Ivory Coast*	Northern Ivory Coast*	Bulawayo, Zimbabwe
Northern Europe	Caribbean*	Botswana	Most of East Africa*	North-west Uganda*	Taiwan
UK	South America	Lesotho	Most of Malawi and Zambia*	Southern Malawi*	
South Africa (whites)	Western Europe	Swaziland (High veld)	Most of South Africa	Natal, South Africa	
New Zealand (non-Maori)	Central Europe	Singapore (Indian)	Swaziland (Middle veld)	Swaziland (Low veld)	
Australia	South Africa (coloured)	Southern Europe	Singapore (Malayan)	Inhambane, Mozambique	
	South Africa (Indian)	Northern Japan (Hokkaido)*	Southern Japan (Kyushu)*	Singapore (Chinese)	
	Bombay, India	New Zealand (Maori)	Hawaii (Hawaiians)	Hong Kong†	
		West-central China‡	North-eastern China‡	Shanghai, China†	
			East-central China‡	Coastal China south of Shanghai‡	

* Estimates of incidence include liver tumours of unspecified origin (WHO International Classification of Diseases 7th Edition, Code 156 and 8th Edition, Code 197.8)
† Liver tumours of unspecified origin not included; true incidence of PLC may be higher
‡ Not clear whether liver tumours of unspecified origin are included; true incidence of PLC may be higher

2 Incidence in Women

The incidence of PLC is almost always lower in women than in men. There is considerable variation in the ratio of male-to-female rates. The ratios for white populations fall mostly in the range 1.0 to 2.4, those for blacks in the range 2.5 to 7.9 and those for Chinese and Japanese populations in the range 1.5 to over 10.[1-4] It is not clear whether these differences represent genuine variation or different patterns of attendance at hospital in the different ethnic groups.

3 Incidence in Migrant Populations

Elevated rates occur in Chinese people who have migrated to the USA, but are less than those recorded in China, Hong Kong or Singapore. The US rates for Chinese men vary from 11.4 per 100 000 in Hawaii to 41.0 in the San Francisco Bay area. Mortality data show that the risk is highest in foreign-born Chinese living in America with male rates that are 11 times those of white Americans and female rates that show a five-fold excess.[17] Among American-born Chinese the increased risk is only of the order of 2.7 fold for men and 2.1 fold for women. In Israel the incidence of PLC among Jews born in Africa or Asia (6 per 100 000 for men[2-4]) is similar to the rate for non-Jews living in Israel and three times the rate among Jews who were born in Europe or America.

4 Time Trends

Analysis of year-by-year death rates for young adults in the UK has shown a slight elevation of rates for women in the age groups 20–29, 30–39 and 40–49 in the years 1977 to 1981 that was not apparent for men[18] and that occurred after a long period of stability. The figures for 1982 strengthen the impression of an increase (D Forman, personal communiction). No such increase has been observed in the USA, Australia or the Federal Republic of Germany.

In southern Africa the successive stages of the mine-workers' survey give evidence of a decreasing incidence for PLC.[7,8] Between 1964–71 and 1972–79 the incidence among mine-workers from Mozambique declined by 40% while among mine-workers from other parts of southern Africa a decrease of 18% occurred.

5 Risk Factors

a Aflatoxin

During the early 1960s, outbreaks of liver disease, including cancer, in poultry and in hatchery-reared rainbow trout in the USA and Europe were found to have been due to feed and fishmeal made from peanuts contaminated by aflatoxin-producing moulds. Subsequent animal experiments established the carcinogenicity of the aflatoxins and demonstrated that aflatoxin B_1 is one of the most potent known hepatocarcinogens.[19] In 1965, Oettlé[20] suggested that mycotoxins were the most likely cause of the high rates of PLC that occurred in Africa and, toward the end of the 1960s, field studies were set up to investigate the extent to which aflatoxins were consumed. Surveys in Swaziland, Uganda, Kenya, Mozambique and Thailand[21] indicated a geographical association within each country between contamination levels of samples of foodstuffs purchased from markets, samples of home-stored goods, and plate-samples of food ready for consumption. In Mozambique contamination was so severe that, if laboratory rats were fed the food consumed by humans there, most would be expected to develop PLC within a year or two. The number of areas studied within each country was small but international comparison of all the data available from plate-sample surveys indicated a strong geographical correlation between contamination levels and the incidence of PLC.[11,21] The type of foodstuff consumed is an important determinant of the quantity of aflatoxin ingested. Peanuts are particularly liable to contamination and are a dietary staple in Mozambique while in the relatively low-incidence area of southern Uganda and north-west Tanzania, bananas are the staple carbohydrate, leaving less room in the diet for the grains and beans that were found to be contaminated in the Ugandan survey. A further instance of a geographical association between the incidence of PLC and aflatoxin contamination levels has recently been reported from China[22] and stronger confirmation of an aetiological role has come from a case-control study in the Phillipines where the mean contamination level of dietary items was established and individual levels of consumption determined retrospectively.[23] No increased risk was apparent, however, in a case-control study in Hong Kong.[24]

One area exists that would seem to be anomalous for the geographical association between PLC incidence and aflatoxin ingestion. The south-eastern states of the United States have a climate that is very similar to that of Mozambique and the plains of south-eastern China. Some of the most economically disastrous outbreaks of aflatoxin contamination of major agricultural crops ever reported have concerned US corn[25,26] and aflatoxin has been found, sometimes at high levels, in the liver of both PLC patients and control populations from the southern states of the USA.[27] A preference for corn bread and grits (coarse-ground cornmeal) in the southern states of America could have led to an intake of aflatoxin as high as in the areas of high contamination in Asia or Africa[28] and yet both incidence and mortality data show an incidence for PLC that is only low to moderate.

b Hepatitis B Virus (HBV)

Areas of highest incidence for PLC are also endemic or hypo-endemic for hepatitis infections and a causal association has long been suspected.[29] Concurrently with the work on aflatoxin, in the early 1970s, it became apparent that signs of past HBV infection were more common in HCC patients than in control populations although methodology at that time did not reveal the true prevalence of infection particularly in patients with PLC (a review of early studies is given by Prince et al. 1975[30]). Advance in technology for the detection of HBV and carefully planned case-control studies have subsequently indicated that persons with signs of chronic active HBV infection are at very high risk for the development of PLC.[31,32] A much higher proportion of patients has always been found to be positive for the various markers of HBV in Africa and Asia than in Europe or America.[6] Since PLC patients are on average older in Europe and America, a part of this difference, but probably not all, may be due to the decline in the prevalence of carrier status that occurs with age in the general population,[30,31,33] and which seems to reflect loss of markers rather than a cohort effect. A prospective study in Taiwan has indicated that the relative risk is as high as 200-fold with all but one case of PLC occurring among persons who were chronic carriers at the start of the investigation.[15] The latter result, together with the discovery of viral DNA incorporated into the host-genome[34] even in PLC patients (from a European population) who have no detectable serological markers for HBV,[35] suggests that a history of HBV infection may be an initiating factor in the development of most cases of PLC. It has also been suggested that HBV infection may be a sufficient factor and that aflatoxin may have little carcinogenic effect in man.[36] This argument was based on calculations that showed a similar risk of HCC in carriers of HBV in the USA and Mozambique. However, comparable calculations have been made for as many populations as possible where both the incidence of PLC and the prevalence of HBV carrier status in the general population can be established (Cook-Mozaffari and Van Rensburg, in preparation) and these indicate a wide variation in risk among carriers especially in the different African and Asian territories for which data are available. Very high values for Mozambique contrast with a low risk in Botswana, Lesotho, southern Japan, among New Zealand Maoris and in Greenland.

The strong geographical association that exists between PLC incidence and the contamination of food samples by aflatoxin despite the crude nature of the measures of incidence[11,21] and a complete lack of association with HBV infection at higher levels of prevalence for hepatitis B surface antigen (HBsAg) suggest that in areas where PLC is common the level of aflatoxin contamination of foodstuffs may be the more important determinant of the geographical pattern of variation for PLC. The areas of particularly low risk for PLC among carriers of HBV, in Botswana, Lesotho, New Zealand and Greenland, are either too hot and dry or too cold for the growth of aflatoxin-producing mould.

The precise relationship between HBV infection and aflatoxin contamination as risk factors in the development of PLC requires further elucidation. In-vitro experiments suggest that human livers may be relatively resistant to aflatoxin carcinogenesis,[19] reinforcing the postulate that damage by HBV infection may be a necessary initiating factor. On the other hand, the work in Greenland indicates that carrier status for HBV gives little increased risk of developing PLC in the absence of some potentiating factor. This, however, is not supported by the geographical correlation that has been demonstrated between the prevalence of HBsAg and PLC mortality in the different districts of Greece[15] in a part of the world where the dry summers of the Mediterranean climate are very unlikely to favour the development of aflatoxin. The incidence of PLC among different ethnic groups in Singapore and New Zealand, among immigrants from different countries to Israel, among Chinese immigrants to the USA and in different geographical regions of Japan likewise suggest a heightened risk due to difference in HBsAg prevalence.[37–39] The higher rates of maternal transmission of HBV that have been observed for the Chinese compared with other racial groups in the UK[40] are of interest in this context and further exploration of different levels of infectivity among carriers might help explain some of the geographical anomalies in the occurrence of PLC in association with HBV.

The exceptionally high incidence of PLC among adolescents and young adults in Mozambique would seem to suggest that, whatever their role in isolation, together, HBV carriage and aflatoxin consumption have a very potent effect. The flattening of the age curve that has been observed in Mozambique probably indicates that there are insufficient susceptible individuals in the population for the very high levels of aflatoxin ingested there to have their full carcinogenic potential.[11]

A study from South Africa has shown that the incidence of PLC among mine-workers from Mozambique drops after a year at the mines.[41] This and the universal decline of PLC incidence that has been observed in recent decades in Mozambique could reflect changes in food habits that lessen the intake of aflatoxin and suggest that the latter may be having a late-stage effect in the development of PLC.[11] If this were so then swifter intervention might be implemented, in areas of the world where aflatoxin is a risk factor, by dietary reform for susceptible individuals than by the vaccination programmes that are being intensively de-

veloped.[42] The 11-fold risk differential that remains between Chinese who have emigrated to the USA and white Americans suggests a limit to the efficiency of intervention through the elimination of aflatoxin from the diet. However, comparison of the incidence rates for Taiwan* and for US whites (160 and 2 per 100000) indicates that the risk differential before emigration may have been as high as 80-fold.

c Alcohol

It has long been apparent that in western societies persons with micro-nodular cirrhosis caused by a long history of excessive alcohol intake are at increased risk for the development of PLC, while in Africa cirrhosis is mostly macro-nodular and is rarely related to alcohol.[19] It has been assumed that in the West there are two pathways for the development of PLC, one associated with alcohol and the other with HBV carrier status, and that this is the explanation of the much lower prevalence of HBV markers (c. 20–30%) that has repeatedly been found among PLC patients in Europe and the USA than in patients from Africa and Asia.[6] This assumption is called in question by the discovery of viral DNA incorporated into the tumour cells of every one of a group of PLC patients from France, all of whom had a history of heavy alcohol intake and many of whom had no serum markers for HBV.[34] A secondary finding of the study was that a series of patients with liver damage due to alcohol but no evidence of PLC had a higher prevalence of serum HBsAg than the general population (i.e. blood donors). It seems possible, therefore, that the statistical associations of HCC with alcoholic cirrhosis that have been noted are an artefact due to the greater likelihood of HBV infection among those with an excessive intake of alcohol. Alternatively, the results of a Scottish study, that showed a high prevalence of HBsAg among patients with alcoholic cirrhosis but not in patients suffering from alcoholism who had normal livers, suggested to the authors that the outcome of HBV infection is modified in the chronic alcoholic, with the development of chronic hepatitis and cirrhosis instead of the recovery of normal liver structure.[43] The role which alcohol plays in contributing to the raised incidence of PLC in central and southern Europe is, therefore, not as yet clear. These are also regions which have a higher prevalence of HBV than is found in northern Europe.[38]

d Other Risk Factors

Case-control studies in Greece[44] and in Hong Kong[24] have demonstrated an increased risk of PLC among cigarette smokers that was independent of alcohol intake. The effect was apparent only for patients who had no serum markers to indicate active HBV infection and, amongst the latter in Greece, the effect was most marked for those without cirrhosis. On the assumption that all patients had at some stage been HBV carriers and that the cirrhosis reflected an interaction between HBV infection and alcohol consumption, it could be either that cigarette smoking is an unnecessary additional factor in those with gross liver damage (due either to chronic hepatitis alone or to chronic hepatitis plus alcohol) or that a low cigarette consumption, possibly even passive smoking, exerts a maximal effect on livers dmaged in these ways.

Many other associations of a weaker nature have been observed. One study has shown an elevated risk for farm workers and for workers in the dry-cleaning and petrol-station service industries[45] while there is a heightened risk of hepatobiliary cancer mortality in US counties where the chemical industry is most highly concentrated.[46]

---

* The Taiwan figure may indicate more accurately the true incidence of PLC in the high risk areas of China than the figures quoted in Table I (see footnote to Table I).

The higher risk of PLC among men than women throughout the world may reflect a hormonal effect. There is growing evidence that changing the hormonal balance by the use of oral contraceptives may result in a small increase in risk.[18] The higher ratio of male-to-female incidence that has been observed in African and Asian populations could in part reflect an interaction with aflatoxin consumption since it is well established experimentally that testosterone promotes and oestradiol inhibits aflatoxin hepatocarcinogenesis.[47,48]

REFERENCES

1 Doll R, Payne P, Waterhouse J, eds. Cancer incidence in five continents. Vol. I. Berlin: Springer Verlag, 1966; (UICC Technical Report) 219

2 Doll R, Muir C, Waterhouse J, eds. Cancer incidence in five continents. Vol. II. Berlin: Springer Verlag, 1970; (UICC Technical Report) 388

3 Waterhouse J, Muir C, Correa P, Powell J, eds. Cancer incidence in five continents. Vol. III. Lyon: IARC Scientific Publications No. 15, 1976; 584

4 Waterhouse J, Muir C, Shanmugaratnam K, Powell J, eds. Cancer incidence in five continents. Vol. IV. Lyon: IARC Scientific Publications No. 42, 1982; 812

5 Doll R. The geographical distribution of cancer. Br J Cancer 1969; 33: 1–8

6 Munoz N, Linsell A. Epidemiology of primary liver cancer. In: Correa P, Haenzel W, eds. Epidemiology of cancer of the digestive tract. The Hague: Martinus Nijhoff, 1982; 161–195

7 Harington JS, McGlashan ND, Bradshaw E, Geddes EW, Purves LR. A spatial and temporal analysis of four cancers in African gold miners from southern Africa. Br J Cancer 1975; 31: 665–678

8 Bradshaw E, McGlashan ND, Fitzgerald D, Harington JS. Analyses of cancer incidence in black gold miners from southern Africa (1964–79). Br J Cancer 1982; 46: 737–748

9 Keen P, Martin P. Is aflatoxin carcinogenic in man? The evidence in Swaziland. Trop Geog Med 1971; 23: 44–53

10 Tuyns AJ, Loubière R, Duvernet-Battesti Fr. Regional variations in primary liver cancer in Ivory Coast. J Natl Cancer Inst 1971; 47: 131–135

11 Van Rensburg SJ, Cook-Mozaffari P, Van Schalkwyk DJ, Van der Watt JJ, Vincent T, Purchase IF. Hepatocellular carcinoma and dietary aflatoxin in Mozambique and Transkei. Int J Cancer; In press

12 Beasley RP, Hwang LY, Lin CC, Chien CS. Hepatocellular carcinoma and hepatitis B virus. Lancet 1981; 2: 1129–1132

13 The Research Committee on Geographical Distribution of Diseases, eds. National atlas of major disease mortalities for cities, towns and villages in Japan. Tokyo: Jiji Press, 1981; 51

14 The Editorial Committee, eds. Atlas of cancer mortality in the People's Republic of China. Shanghai: China Map Press, 1979; 99

15 Trichopoulos D, Papaevangelou G, Violaki M, Vissoulis Ch, Sparrow L, Manousos ON. Geographic correlation between mortality from primary hepatic carcinoma and prevalence of hepatitis B surface antigen in Greece. Br J Cancer 1976; 34: 83–87

16 Prates MD, Torres FO. A cancer survey in Lourenco Marques, Portuguese East Africa. J Nat Cancer Inst 1965; 35: 729–757

17 King H, Locke FB. Cancer mortality among Chinese in the United States. J Natl Cancer Inst 1980; 65: 1141–1148

18 Forman D, Doll R, Peto R. Trends in mortality from carcinoma of the liver and the use of oral contraceptives. Br J Cancer 1983; 48: 349–354

19 Falk H. Liver. In: Schottenfeld D, Fraumeni JF, eds. Cancer epidemiology and prevention. Philadelphia: WB Saunders, 1982; 668–682

20 Oettlé AG. The aetiology of primary carcinoma of the liver in Africa: a critical appraisal of previous ideas with an outline of the mycotoxin hypothesis. S Afr Med J 1965; 39: 817–825

21 Linsell CA, Peers FG. Aflatoxin and liver cell cancer. Trans Roy Soc Trop Med Hyg 1977; 71: 471–473

22 Yeh FS, Yan RC, Mor CC, Liu YK, Yang KC. Research on etiological factors of hepatocellular carcinoma in Guangxi, China. Proceedings of the Thirteenth International Cancer Congress, Seattle, 1982; 340

23 Bulatao-Jayme J, Almero EM, Castro MaCA, Jardeleza MaTR, Salamat LA. A case-control dietary study of primary liver cancer risk from aflatoxin exposure. Int J Epidemiol 1982; 11: 112–119

24 Lam KC, Yu MC, Leung JWC, Henderson BE. Hepatitis B virus and cigarette smoking: risk factors for hepatocellular carcinoma in Hongkong. Cancer Res 1982; 42: 5246–5248

25 Lillehoj EB, Fennell DI, Kwolek WF. *Aspergillus flavus* and aflatoxin in Iowa corn before harvest. Science 1976; 193: 495–496

26 McMillan WM, Wilson DM, Widstrom NW, Gueldner RC. Incidence and level of aflatoxin in pre-harvest corn in south Georgia in 1978. Cereal Chem 1980; 57: 83–84

27 Siraj MY, Hayes AW, Unger PD, Hogan, GR, Ryan NJ, Wray BB. Analysis of aflatoxin B_1 in human tissues with high-pressure liquid chromatography. Toxicol Appl Pharmacol 1981; 58: 422–430

28 Stoloff L. Aflatoxin as a cause of primary liver-cell cancer in the United States: a probability study. Nutr—Cancer 1983; 5: 165–186

29 Steiner PE. Cancer of the liver and cirrhosis in trans-Saharan Africa and the United States of America. Cancer 1960; 13: 1085–1166

30 Prince AM, Szmuness W, Michon J et al. A case control study of the association between primary liver cancer and hepatitis B infection in Senegal. Int J Cancer 1975; 16: 376–383

31 Kew MC, Desmyter J, Bradburne AF, Mcnab GM. Hepatitis B virus infection in southern African blacks with hepatocellular cancer. J Nat Cancer Inst 1979; 62: 517–520

32 Trichopoulos D, Tabor E, Gerety RJ et al. Hepatitis B and primary hepatocellular carcinoma in a European population. Lancet 1978; 2: 1217–1219

33 Szmuness W, Hirsh RL, Prince AM, Levine RW, Harley EJ, Ikram H. Hepatitis B surface antigen in blood donors: further observations. J Infect Dis 1975; 131: 111–118

34 Shafritz DA, Shouval D, Sherman HI, Hadziyannis SJ, Kew MC. Integration of hepatitis B virus DNA into the genome of liver cells in chronic liver disease and hepatocellular carcinoma. N Engl J Med 1981; 305: 1067–1073

35 Bréchot C, Nalpas B, Courouce AM et al. Evidence that hepatitis B virus has a role in liver-cell carcinoma in alcoholic liver disease. N Engl J Med 1982; 306: 1384–1387

36 Prince AM, quoted by Lutwick LI. Relation between aflatoxin, hepatitis B virus and hepatocellular carcinoma. Lancet 1979; i: 755–757

37 Eliakim M. The epidemiology of viral hepatitis in Israel. Isr J Med Science 1978; 15: 248–256

38 Szmuness W. Hepatocellular carcinoma and the hepatitis B virus: evidence for a causal association. Prog Med Virol 1978; 24: 40–69

39 Asano M, Kato H, Yoshimoto K et al. Primary liver carcinoma and liver cirrhosis in atomic bomb survivors, Hiroshima and Nagasaki 1961–75 with special reference to hepatitis B surface antigen. J Natl Cancer Inst 1982; 69: 1221–1227

40 Derso A, Boxall EH, Tarlow MJ, Flewett TH. Transmission of HBsAg from mother to infant in four ethnic groups. Br Med J 1978; 1: 949–952

41 Purves LR. Primary liver cancer in man as a possible short duration seasonal cancer. S Afr J Science 1973; 69: 173–178

42 Blumberg BS, London WT. Hepatitis B virus: pathogenesis and prevention of primary cancer of the liver. Cancer 1983; 50: 2657–2665

43 Pettigrew NM, Goudie RB, Russell RI, Chaudhuri AKR. Evidence for a role of hepatitis virus B in chronic alcoholic liver disease. Lancet 1972; 2: 724–725

44 Trichopoulos D, MacMahon B, Sparros L, Merikas G. Smoking and hepatitis B negative primary hepatocellular carcinoma. J Natl Cancer Inst 1980; 65: 111–114

45 Stemhagen A, Slade J, Altman R, Bill J. Occupational risk factors and liver cancer. Am J Epidemiol 1983; 117: 443–454

46 Hoover R, Fraumeni JF. Cancer mortality in US counties with chemical industries. Environ Res 1975; 9: 196–207

47 Akao M, Kuroda K. Enhancing and inhibitory effects of some stilbene and steroid compounds on induction of hepatoma in rats fed 3′-methyl-4-(dimethylamino)azobenzene. Gann 1978; 69: 375–382

48 Mainigi KD, Campbell TC. Effect of sex differences on sub-cellular distribution of aflatoxin in F—344 rats treated with various risk-modifying factors. Toxicol Appl Pharmacol 1981; 58: 236–243

British Medical Bulletin (1984) Vol. 40, No. 4, pp. 346–350

MELANOMA OF THE SKIN

BRUCE K ARMSTRONG D Phil FRACP

NH & MRC Research Unit in
Epidemiology and Preventive Medicine
Department of Medicine
University of Western Australia

1   Worldwide variation in incidence of melanoma
2   Variation in incidence of melanoma within regions of the world
3   Inconsistency in patterns of melanoma incidence by latitude
4   Effects of other geographic or climatic factors
5   Effects of ethnic differences in sun sensitivity
6   Effects of migration from low-incidence to high-incidence areas
7   Nature of individual exposure to the sun and the u.v.-dose-response relationship
8   Other causal variables
9   Conclusion
    References

In the first comprehensive analysis of the geography of cutaneous melanoma in Caucasians, Lancaster[1] noted that mortality from the disease was particularly high in Australia and South Africa as compared with the parts of Europe from which their populations originated; that mortality in Australia, New Zealand and the United States of America increased with proximity to the equator; and that within Europe melanoma was more common in Norway and Sweden than elsewhere, the converse being true of France and Italy. He interpreted these data as suggesting the hypothesis that sunlight is a cause of malignant melanoma; an idea which, apparently, was current in Australia at the time but had been given no formal exposition. He made no attempt to explain the apparently anomalous relationship between latitude and melanoma in Europe.

While geographic variation in melanoma frequency generally does suggest the sunlight hypothesis, there are inconsistencies in the relationship between the two both between and within countries. In this paper we will examine some of these inconsistencies and see whether or not they can be reconciled with the sunlight theory

1   Worldwide Variation in Incidence of Melanoma

The recorded incidence of malignant melanoma varies from a low of about 0.2 cases per 100000 annually in parts of Japan to a high of nearly 40 per 100000 in Queensland, Australia.[2,3] While there are problems of comparability between quoted rates, particularly in the inclusion or exclusion of in-situ disease (nearly 30% of cases in Queensland), there seems little doubt that the true range of variation is not less than about one hundred-fold.

Figure 1 shows the relationship between latitude of residence and incidence of melanoma as determined for about the same calendar period by cancer registries reporting in Cancer Incidence in Five Continents, Volume IV.[2] The incidence data plotted are those based on populations of predominantly Caucasian origin.

The latitude plotted is that estimated to pass through the 'centre of gravity' of the registry population. There is no clear inverse relationship between melanoma incidence and latitude. In fact, for both males and females the data are best fitted by a quadratic relationship between melanoma and latitude with a minimum at about 52° of latitude. In fitting these curves, several outlying points were omitted: Hawaii whites, Israel Jews, and the Spanish populations of New Mexico, Navarra and Zaragoza. Their exclusion will be justified below and, in any case, serves only to improve the fit of the statistical models without altering their form greatly.

2   Variation in Incidence of Melanoma Within Regions of the World

The position for Europe is clear from Fig. 1. The inverted parabola for the world as a whole is determined mainly by the parabolic relationship within Europe. To the south, there are comparatively high rates in Switzerland, Hungary, Romania, France and the north of Italy (latitudes 45 to 48° north), then low rates between latitudes 48 and 55° north and then rising rates into the more northerly parts of the continent (Scotland, Finland, Denmark, Sweden and Norway).

Variations in melanoma incidence within countries of Europe do not conform to the pattern which might be expected from Fig. 1. Melanoma incidence increases along a north to south gradient in all countries from which relevant data have been reported: England and Wales,[4] Norway,[5] Sweden[6] and Finland.[7] Gradients from south to north might have been expected in Norway, Sweden and Finland (all between latitudes 55 and 70° north) given the pattern of Fig. 1. Within Britain, however, Scotland (latitude 55 to 59°) is anomalous, and consistent with Fig. 1, in having a higher incidence of melanoma than any part of England and Wales. Urban–rural gradients (to lower rates of melanoma in the rural areas) may explain the north–south gradients in Finland and Norway but do not appear to do so in Sweden.

The geographical distribution of melanoma in North America has been studied extensively. Since the vast majority of North Americans live below latitude 52° north, a north–south gradient would be expected from Fig. 1 and has been observed.[8,9] Neither longitude nor altitude appeared to correlate with melanoma mortality.[8] In several studies, an attempt was made to express the effects of latitude in terms of received ultraviolet (u.v.) radiation. Elwood *et al.*[8] calculated an epidemiological index of annual u.v. dose, which incorporated latitude and estimates of atmospheric ozone concentration and cloud cover, for each Canadian province and U.S. state. This index was highly negatively correlated with latitude (r = −0.89) and positively correlated with melanoma mortality (r = 0.67 in males and 0.56 in females) but not as strongly as was latitude itself (r = −0.78 and −0.72 respectively). Similar results were obtained for melanoma incidence and mortality in the centres covered by the Third National Cancer Survey.[9] In correlating actual measured annual u.v. dose with melanoma incidence in four centres of the Third National Cancer Survey, Fears *et al.*[10] again found a significant positive association similar in strength to that previously observed with estimated monthly totals in erythema-producing u.v. light.[9] Baker-Blocker,[11] however, found no association between measured u.v. irradiation and melanoma mortality in 18 United States counties although there were sizeable correlations between melanoma mortality and latitude (negative), and latitude and u.v. (also negative), in these counties. The u.v. measurements were obtained through several different agencies using two different types of meter, although with highly correlated readings. In

FIG. 1. Association of incidence of malignant melanoma in Caucasian populations with latitude of residence

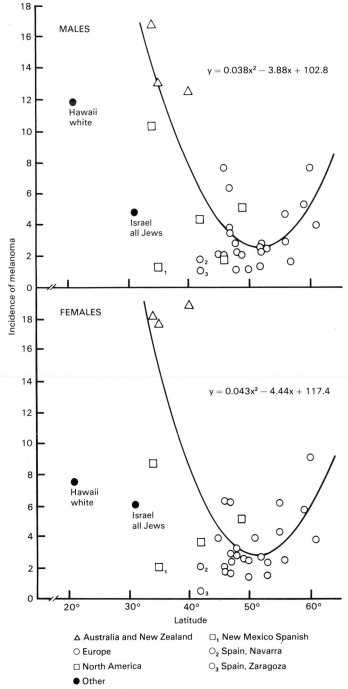

Australia and New Zealand
Europe
North America
Other

$\square_1$ New Mexico Spanish
$\bigcirc_2$ Spain, Navarra
$\bigcirc_3$ Spain, Zaragoza

Incidence data are age-standardized to the world population and taken from Waterhouse *et al.*[2] Only rates based on ten cases or more have been included. For countries with more than one registry, the two with the highest and lowest rate for each sex have been selected.

addition, some southern counties with appreciable proportions of Spanish origin residents were included in the analysis.

Geographical gradients of melanoma in Australia too are somewhat contradictory. For the country as a whole, as reported

by Lancaster originally in 1956,[1] mortality rises with proximity to the equator; this appears to be the pattern also in incidence data, insofar as they are available. The relative positions of the states, with respect to mortality, were more or less maintained between 1950 and 1977 in spite of two- to three-fold increases in absolute rates of death from melanoma. Within Queensland and Western Australia, however, states of Australia which span, respectively, 19 and 21 degrees of latitude, opposite gradients have been observed. In an early report from the Queensland Melanoma Project,[13] the highest crude incidence rate was in the coastal south of Queensland with somewhat lower rates in the coastal north and a clear north-to-south gradient in inland areas. The largest difference was between coastal (high incidence) and inland (low incidence) areas. In a more recent and more rigorous analysis based on incidence data from 1979/80, there was little difference in age-standardized melanoma incidence between north and south coastal regions and a small south to north gradient in inland areas.[14] The largest difference, as before, was between coastal and inland areas (high to low). In Western Australia, in two recent time periods (Table I), melanoma incidence has been appreciably lower in the north (i.e. nearer the equator) than the south. Within the south itself there was little evidence of an urban (Perth) or coastal (Perth and the south-west) excess.

3 Inconsistency in Patterns of Melanoma Incidence by Latitude

Assuming the truth of the sunlight theory of melanoma, an assumption which has not gone unchallenged,[16] there are clear inconsistencies in the patterns of melanoma incidence by latitude in Caucasian races. The most outstanding is the unexpectedly high incidence of melanoma in some populations in the far north of Europe (Fig. 1). A south to north gradient beyond latitude 52° north is not evident, however, within the countries showing these high rates (Norway, Sweden and Finland); indeed the opposite may be true. In Australia as a whole, the expected south to north gradient is seen but it is not present in the two states spanning the greatest range of latitude (Queensland and Western Australia). Only in North America is the expected latitude gradient consistently observed although even here doubts have been raised as to whether there is a parallel correlation between melanoma incidence and received u.v. irradiation.

If the sunlight theory is to be retained these inconsistencies require explanation. Possible explanations lie in: effects of other geographical or climatic factors (e.g. humidity, cloud cover, air pollution, altitude, longitude, air temperature, air-ground-air reflectance, etc); ethnic differences in sun sensitivity; the effects of migration from low-incidence to high-incidence areas; the nature

TABLE I. Age-standardized incidence of preinvasive and invasive cutaneous malignant melanoma by region of Western Australia, 1975–76 and 1980–81

(data from Holman *et al.*[18] and unpublished observations)

Region	Latitude	Average annual bright sunlight hours	Incidence per 100000 Males 1975–76	Males 1980–81	Females 1975–76	Females 1980–81
South-west	32°–35°S	6.5	30.9 (23)*	32.3 (30)	41.2 (30)	43.6 (39)
South central	32°–35°S	7.4	12.4 (6)	45.2 (25)	27.8 (14)	41.7 (23)
Perth city	32°S	7.5	30.1 (201)	35.2 (282)	28.6 (206)	33.8 (289)
Midlands and south-east	26°–34°S	8.8	24.5 (18)	20.6 (15)	29.6 (20)	43.9 (29)
North	14°–30°S	9.6	16.9 (10)	16.5 (16)	19.0 (10)	24.2 (19)

* Numbers of cases in brackets

of individual exposure to the sun and the u.v. dose–response relationship; and other non-u.v.-related variables with an overriding causal effect.

4 Effects of Other Geographic or Climatic Factors

Other geographical or climatic factors may modify the relationship between latitude and u.v. dose.[17] Their potential importance is illustrated in Fig. 2 which shows the distribution of average daily total erythemal dose of u.v. over Australia in mid-summer. For most of the country, erythemal dose is no greater in the tropics than it is below latitude 32° south. In Queensland, the dose is more or less the same along the whole of the populated coast. This lack of correlation between u.v. irradiation and latitude in summer (there is almost perfect correlation in winter) is explained by cloud cover in summer in the tropics. It has been advanced as a possible explanation for the latitude inconsistency and coastal excess of melanoma in Queensland[14] and it could also explain the latitude inconsistency in Western Australia.

Both altitude and longitude may modify the u.v. dose received;[18] u.v.-B irradiation increases by 2% per 304.8 metres rise in altitude and, in the United States at least, there is a west-to-east gradient in thickness of the atmospheric ozone layer resulting in potentially higher u.v. doses in more westerly parts of the country. It should be recalled, however, that in taking these variables into account, Elwood *et al.*[8] were unable to improve or eliminate the latitude correlation with melanoma mortality. Altitude and longitude appeared uncorrelated with melanoma mortality in their study and, in a separate study, melanoma mortality was found to be higher at low than high altitudes in mountainous areas of the United States.[19]

While air pollution may reduce the absorbed u.v. dose at ground level,[17] its effects on geographical variation would be difficult to

estimate. Any substantial effect of air pollution is rendered unlikely by the commonly observed urban excess of melanoma.

Other geographical or climatic factors which may be relevant are probably only important in interaction with behavioural variables: warm air temperature encourages unclad exposure; the reflection of u.v. from white sand and snow is important to those who participate in beach and snow sports; and long summer days (24 hours of summer daylight in Arctic Greenland give the same u.v. dose as a tropical day)[20] will only be important if the amount of time spent outdoors is proportionally increased. These issues will be considered in more detail below.

5 Effects of Ethnic Differences in Sun Sensitivity

Melanoma in pigmented races, including the lightly pigmented Asian races is infrequent, does not vary appreciably with latitude, and shows a relative predilection for the feet—a comparatively rare site in white races.[21] It is commonly held that natural pigmentation of the skin protects against melanoma. This view is supported by studies of individuals.[22] Ethnic factors therefore may be important in explaining inconsistencies in the geography of melanoma in Caucasians assuming that, in some areas, appreciable interbreeding with pigmented races has occurred, or that increased cutaneous pigmentation has evolved in response to long residence in a sunny climate.[21]

Four outliers were excluded from the mathematical modelling of the points in Fig. 1, partly on the grounds of racial pigmentation: Spain, Navarra and Zaragoza; New Mexico, Spanish; and Israel, all Jews. Compared with most Europeans, Spaniards are fairly heavily pigmented and, historically, have had periods of interbreeding with North African races; the Spanish of New Mexico have, in addition, the pigmentary results of interbreeding with American Indians who are at low risk of melanoma,[23] and the Jews of Israel have their origins in Asia and Africa as well as Europe and America. Melanoma rates in Jews from Asia and Africa are substantially lower than in those from Europe and America.[24]

Racial pigmentation, or lack of it, is commonly advanced as the explanation for high rates of melanoma in Scotland and Scandinavia.[25] Recent results in people born in Western Australia[26] failed to show any appreciable difference in risk of melanoma between those of Celtic origin and those of other British origin. Those of Southern European origin, however, mainly Italian and Greek, had approximately a third the risk of melanoma as in those of mainly British origin. The difference was reduced appreciably but not eliminated by adjustment for measured degree of skin pigmentation. A north-to-south gradient in skin pigmentation in Europe, therefore, may contribute to explanation of the south-to-north gradient in melanoma risk.

6 Effects of Migration from Low-Incidence to High-Incidence Areas

The effects of migration of Caucasian races on melanoma risk have been studied in detail in Israel and Australia. Movshovitz and Modan[27] reported the highest rates in Israel as being among those born in Israel of European or American origin; rates among those who migrated to Israel from Europe or America were appreciably lower. Anaise *et al.*[24] further showed that among the immigrants from Europe and America incidence was highest in those who had lived in Israel the longest. Immigrant groups in Australia also have lower incidence and mortality rates of melanoma than native-born Australian;[12,15] mortality in immigrants rises with increasing time since migration but remains appreciably below that of native-born Australians even after long-term residence. A contradictory pattern was reported from

FIG 2. Distribution of average daily total erythemal dose of ultraviolet light over Australia in January

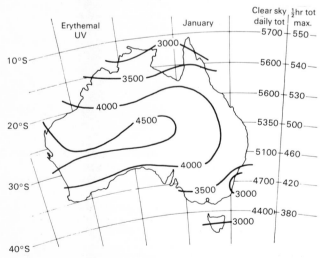

Columns to the right of the map represent daily total erythemal dose, assuming a clear sky, and the 1/2 hour total dose received at noon. One thousand erythemal units correspond to 1/2 hour exposure to $1\,Wm^{-2}$ per nm bandwidth at 300 nm.

Map reprinted with permission of the authors and the editor of the Australian Journal of Dermatology[17]

Hawaii—substantially higher incidence rates in Caucasian immigrants than in Caucasians born in Hawaii.[28] This apparent contradiction has been attributed to Southern European or mixed-race ancestry in the Hawaiian-born.[29]

The most direct explanation of the results reported from Israel and Australia is that risk of melanoma in migrants increases progressively with accumulated exposure to the new environment. An alternative model has been put forward as a result of study of place of birth and time since migration in a case-control study in Western Australia.[26] As expected, melanoma risk was higher in native-born Australians than immigrants of a similar ethnic mix. Age at arrival in Australia, however, rather than duration of residence in Australia, appeared to be the important time variable. Those who did not come to Australia before the age of 15 years showed no increase in risk of melanoma with increasing length of residence. It appears, therefore, that the environment in the first 15 years of life may be the most important in determining lifetime risk of melanoma.

Migration may explain some of the inconsistencies in the geographical distribution of melanoma which have been described above. It may, for example, partly explain the anomalously low rates among Israeli Jews (Fig. 1) because of the substantial proportion of migrants in the population of Israel (52% of the population on which the incidence rates in Fig. 1 are based[2]). Internal migration may contribute to the anomalous distribution of melanoma in Western Australia and perhaps Queensland. The north of Western Australia is populated predominantly by people born elsewhere in Australia, or elsewhere in the world, who have come to the north only in adult life. It is doubtful whether migration, except perhaps in the past and through genetic change, has had much effect on melanoma rates in Europe.

7 Nature of Individual Exposure to the Sun and the U.V.-Dose–Response Relationship

As mentioned above, a number of geographical or climatic factors may influence the amount and nature of individual exposure to the sun; they include particularly air temperature and proximity to the sea or another large expanse of water. In addition cultural and other social factors, which vary geographically, may be important: clothing habits, traditional sporting and leisure pursuits, amount of leisure time, the affluence to enjoy leisure in ways involving substantial sun exposure, etc.

The importance of these factors geographically has not been measured but is suggested by several observations. There is a direct relationship between socio-economic status and risk of melanoma, in that risk increases (cross-sectionally at least) with increasing affluence.[15] In addition, melanoma is paradoxically related to outdoor work with highest risk in those who work indoors and lowest risk in those who work outdoors.[15,30] A recent study from New Zealand suggests that the effect of socio-economic status may explain the apparent effect of indoor work.[31] These data have been taken to suggest that melanoma risk is increased more by intermittent (and therefore usually recreational) exposure to the sun than it is by more continuous exposure. Indeed, regular daily exposure to the sun may lead either to protective behaviour or

sun-induced skin pigmentation which may then actually lower risk. Measures of intermittent individual exposure to the sun do show a positive relationship with melanoma[32] and, as would be expected from this hypothesis, those who tan well are at lower risk of melanoma than those who tan poorly.[36] This interaction between exposure and protection has led to the theory that as frequency of sun exposure increases, risk of melanoma varies in the form of parabola—i.e. beyond a certain frequency, variable from one individual to another depending on skin type, risk may actually fall as sun exposure increases.[32] If this model is correct then, in particular situations, cultural and social factors could override the effects of latitude of residence.

The possible importance of these factors to the high rates of melanoma in Scandinavia has been raised by Eklund and Malec.[6] They suggested that sun-seeking holidays abroad may be an important risk factor in Sweden and, indeed, found a correlation between the frequency of issue of passports and incidence of melanoma in 16 regions of the country. It is possible that the infrequent but intense sun exposure received in this manner by the fair-skinned Scandinavians may be more important, in terms of melanoma risk, than the more continuous exposure received by their generally less affluent southern neighbours.

8 Other Causal Variables

Non-solar factors postulated as possibly relevant to melanoma have been reviewed recently by Hinds.[33] They include trauma, diet, hormones, occupation (other than the indoor/outdoor dichotomy), viruses and drugs. On present evidence, none of them can be put forward seriously as a possible alternative to the sunlight theory in explaining geographical variation in incidence of melanoma in Caucasians. Therefore, if some other factor is responsible, it is unknown at present.

9 Conclusions

While the incidence of melanoma in Caucasians generally increases with proximity to the equator, the reverse gradient north of latitude 52° north in Europe and inconsistencies in the relationship in other geographical areas suggest that latitude and the predicted parallel variation in received u.v. dose do not provide the whole explanation for geographic variation in melanoma incidence. There are a number of other factors, however, which by modifying received u.v. dose at any particular latitude, or affecting population susceptibility to u.v. or population pattern of exposure to u.v., may account for these inconsistencies. As regards Europe, where the main inconsistency lies, it would seem reasonable to attribute the south-to-north gradient observed in melanoma risk to a gradient in the opposite direction in skin pigmentation and a more intermittent pattern of sun exposure in those from the north. This latter applies particularly to Scandinavians; whether it applies also to Scots is not clear. While factors unrelated to the sun may influence risk of melanoma, there appears to be no need to postulate a role for them in geographical variability of the disease in Caucasians. Indeed, no other known factor is probably strong enough to explain more than a small part of the variation.

REFERENCES

1 Lancaster HO. Some geographical aspects of the mortality from melanoma in Europeans. Med J Aust 1956; 1: 1082–1087
2 Waterhouse J, Muir C, Shanmugaratnam K, Powell J, eds. Cancer Incidence in Five Continents. Vol IV. Lyon: International Agency for Research on Cancer, 1982. (IARC Scientific Publication no 42)
3 Green A. Incidence and reporting of cutaneous melanoma in Queensland. Aust J Dermatol 1982; 23: 105–109
4 Swerdlow AJ. Incidence of malignant melanoma of the skin in England and Wales and its relationship to sunshine. Br Med J 1979; 2: 1324–1327

5 Magnus K. Incidence of malignant melanoma of the skin in Norway, 1955–70. Variations in time and space and solar radiation. Cancer 1973; 32: 1275–1286

6 Eklund G, Malec E. Sunlight and incidence of cutaneous malignant melanoma. Effect of latitude and domicile in Sweden. Scand J Plast Reconstr Surg 1978; 12: 231–241

7 Teppo L, Pakkanen M, Hakulinen T. Sunlight as a risk factor of malignant melanoma of the skin. Cancer 1978; 41: 2018–2027

8 Elwood JM, Lee JAH, Walter SD, Mo T, Green AES. Relationship of melanoma and other skin cancer mortality to latitude and ultraviolet radiation in the United States and Canada. Int J Epidemiol 1974; 3: 325–332

9 Fears TR, Scotto J, Schneiderman MA. Skin cancer, melanoma, and sunlight. Am J Public Health 1976; 66: 461–464

10 Fears TR, Scotto J, Schneiderman MA. Mathematical models of age and ultraviolet effects on the incidence of skin cancer among whites in the United States. Am J Epidemiol 1977; 105: 420–427

11 Baker-Blocker A. Ultraviolet radiation and melanoma mortality in the United States. Environ Res 1980; 23: 24–28

12 Armstrong BK, Holman CDJ, Ford JM, Woodings TL. Trends in melanoma incidence and mortality in Australia. In: Magnus K, ed. Trends in cancer incidence: causes and practical implications. (Proceedings of a symposium held in Oslo, Norway, 1980.) Washington DC: Hemisphere Publishing Corporation, 1982; 399–417

13 Herron J. The geographical distribution of malignant melanoma in Queensland. Med J Aust 1969; 2: 892–894

14 Green A, Siskind V. Geographical distribution of cutaneous melanoma in Queensland. Med J Aust 1983; 1: 407–410

15 Holman CDJ, Mulroney CD, Armstrong BK. Epidemiology of pre-invasive and invasive malignant melanoma in Western Australia. Int J Cancer 1980; 25: 317–323

16 Cutchis P. On the linkage of solar ultraviolet radiation to skin cancer. Washington, DC: US Department of Transportation, 1978 (Institute for Defence Analyses Paper P-1342)

17 Barton IJ, Paltridge GW. The Australian climatology of biologically effective ultraviolet radiation. Aust J Dermatol 1979; 20: 68–74

18 Schreibner MM, Bozzo PD, Moon TE. Malignant melanoma in southern Arizona. Increasing incidence and sunlight as an etiologic factor. Arch Dermatol 1981; 117: 6–11

19 Amsel J, Waterbor JW, Oler J, Rosenwaike I, Marshall K. Relationship of site-specific cancer mortality rates to altitude. Carcinogenesis 1982; 3: 461–465

20 Kromann NP, Nielsen NH, Hansen JPH. Skin cancer in Greenland 1955–1974. J Cancer Res Clin Oncol 1983; 105: 76–78

21 Crombie IK. Racial differences in melanoma incidence. Br J Cancer 1979; 40: 185–193

22 Elwood JM, Gallagher RP, Hill GB, Spinelli JJ, Pearson JCG, Threlfall W. Pigmentation and skin reaction to sun as risk factors for cutaneous melanoma: Western Canada melanoma study. Br Med J 1984; 288: 99–102

23 Menck HR, Henderson BE, Pike MC, Mack T, Martin SP, SooHoo J. Cancer incidence in the Mexican-American. J Natl Cancer Inst 1975; 55: 531–536

24 Anaise D, Steinitz R, Hur NB. Solar radiation: a possible etiological factor in malignant melanoma in Israel. A retrospective study (1960–1972). Cancer 1978; 42: 299–304

25 MacKie RM, Hunter JAA. Cutaneous malignant melanoma in Scotland. Br J Cancer 1982; 46: 75–80

26 Holman CDJ, Armstrong BK. Pigmentary traits, ethnic origin, benign naevi and family history as risk factors for cutaneous malignant melanoma. J Natl Cancer Inst 1984; 72: 257–266

27 Movshovitz M, Modan B. Role of sun exposure in the etiology of malignant melanoma: epidemiologic inference. J Natl Cancer Inst 1973; 51: 777–779

28 Hinds MW, Kolonel LN. Malignant melanoma of the skin in Hawaii, 1960–1977. Cancer 1980; 45: 811–817

29 Lee JAH. Melanoma and exposure to sunlight. Epidemiol Rev 1982; 4: 110–136

30 Beral V, Robinson N. The relationship of malignant melanoma, basal and squamous skin cancers to indoor and outdoor work. Br J Cancer 1981; 44: 886–891

31 Cooke KR, Skegg DCG, Fraser J. Socio-economic status, indoor and outdoor work and malignant melanoma. Int J Cancer: In press

32 Holman CDJ. Risk factors in the causation of human malignant melanoma of the skin. Perth, Western Asutralia: University of Western Australia, 1983. 595 pp. Thesis

33 Hinds MW. Nonsolar factors in the etiology of malignant melanoma. Natl Cancer Inst Monogr 1982; 62: 173–178

British Medical Bulletin (1984) Vol. 40, No. 4, pp. 351–354

BREAST CANCER

M C PIKE PhD

R K ROSS MD*

Imperial Cancer Research Fund
Cancer Epidemiology and Clinical Trials Unit
Radcliffe Infirmary, Oxford

1 Menarche, first full-term pregnancy, menopause
  and post-menopausal weight
2 Diet
3 Endogenous hormones
  a Oestrogens
  b Prolactin
  c Progesterone
4 Summary
  References

There is more than a six-fold difference between those countries with the highest and lowest reported breast cancer rates (Table I).[1,2] Japan, China and black Africa have the lowest rates of breast cancer, while the highest rates are observed in the USA, Canada and certain parts of Western Europe.

Studies of Japanese migrants to Hawaii have shown that Japanese Americans have breast cancer rates intermediate between those of Japan and the USA, and at young ages their rates more closely resemble those of the USA than those of Japan.[3] The cumulative breast cancer rate of Japanese in Hawaii is now almost as high as the cumulative rate for the UK (Table I). Other areas in the USA with large groups of Japanese migrants have shown similar shifts in breast cancer rates. For example, under age 55 the incidence of breast cancer in Japanese women in Osaka is about one-fifth that of white women in Los Angeles, whereas Japanese women in Los Angeles have rates that are within 20% of the rates of whites. Over age 55 the rates in Osaka are one-eighth the rates in Los Angeles, while the rates of Japanese Americans are some four-fold higher than the rates in Osaka, but still only half the rates in Los Angeles whites. Similar shifts in rates are evident in Chinese migrants to the USA (Table I).

Breast cancer rates of African blacks are also greatly affected by migration. Blacks in Africa have breast cancer rates that are only approximately 15% of the rates of US whites (Table I), whereas blacks in the USA have overall breast cancer rates that are three-quarters of the rates of US whites (Table I) and, in fact, up to age 40 breast cancer rates of US blacks are actually higher than those of US whites.[4]

These dramatic effects of migration on breast cancer rates clearly show that environmental (probably dietary) and/or behavioural factors are the major determinants of the marked international variation in breast cancer occurrence. Epidemiological studies have identified four major risk factors for breast cancer—early menarche, late first full-term pregnancy (FFTP), late menopause and post-menopausal weight. Before one can undertake serious discussion of the possible effect of any other factor as an explanation, or partial explanation, of a particular aspect of the pattern of breast cancer occurrence in different groups, one needs to consider whether these four risk factors by themselves offer an adequate explanation.

1 Menarche, First Full-Term Pregnancy, Menopause and Post-Menopausal Weight

Early menarche, late FFTP and late menopause are generally accepted as the three major risk factors for breast cancer.[5] The higher breast cancer risk among women with an earlier menarche is, for a variety of reasons, most pronounced at young ages:[6] Table II shows the two-fold increased risk for menarche at age 11 or younger as compared with menarche at age 13 or older that was found in a study of women under age 33.[7] With regard to late FFTP, MacMahon *et al.*[8] in their international case-control study found that women with a FFTP under age 20 had about one-half the risk of nulliparous women, but that nulliparous women did not have as high a risk as women whose FFTP was after age 35 (see Table II). Single women and nulliparous married women had the same risk. Finally, Trichopoulos *et al.*[9] estimated that women whose natural menopause (last menstrual period) occurred before age 45 had only one-half the risk of women whose menopause occurred after age 55 (see Table II). They also demonstrated the same effect with bilateral oöphorectomy.

TABLE I. Cumulative incidence rates[1,2] of breast cancer in different countries

Population	0–64	0–74	Population	0–64	0–74
	Cumulative incidence rates %			Cumulative incidence rates %	
Hawaii, USA (White)	6.1	10.0	Sao Paulo, Brazil	4.0	6.0
Hawaii, USA (Hawaiian)	5.6	9.8	Norway	3.6	5.5
San Francisco Bay Area, USA (White)	6.1	9.3	Hawaii, USA (Japanese)	3.9	5.3
Geneva, Switzerland	5.3	8.3	Finland	2.9	4.4
British Columbia, Canada	5.4	8.1	Warsaw, Poland	2.8	4.1
San Francisco Bay Area, USA (Black)	4.7	7.2	Cali, Columbia	2.4	3.5
			Puerto Rica	2.2	3.2
New Zealand (White)	4.5	6.9	Singapore (Chinese)	1.7	2.4
Israel	4.4	6.7	Shanghai, PRC	1.5	2.2
Oxford, UK	4.3	6.5	Miyagi, Japan	1.3	1.9
New Zealand (Maori)	4.4	6.4	Ibadan, Nigeria	1.0	1.5
Hawaii, USA (Chinese)	4.3	6.3	Osaka, Japan	1.0	1.4
			Dakar, Senegal	0.9	1.3

TABLE II. Effects of age at menarche, age at first full-term pregnancy (FFTP), age at menopause, and post-menopausal weight on breast cancer risk

Risk Factor			Relative risk
Menarche	Age:	–11	1.00
		12	0.90
		13+	0.50
FFTP	Age:	–19	0.83
		20–24	1.00
		25–29	1.30
		30–34	1.57
		35+	2.03
		Nullips	1.67
Menopause	Age:	40–44	1.00
		45–49	1.27
		50–54	1.47
		55–59	2.03
Post-menopausal weight	Kg:	–59	1.00
		60–69	1.61
		70+	1.81

* Visiting from the Department of Preventive Medicine, University of Southern California School of Medicine, Los Angeles, USA.

Post-menopausal weight has recently been established as a risk factor. The results of de Waard *et al.*[10] for Dutch women aged 60–69 are shown in Table II. They found an approximately 40% increase in risk for a 10 kg increase in post-menopausal weight, and their findings are supported by the results of the large American Cancer Society cohort study.[11]

The distribution of age at menopause (last menstrual period) appears to vary very little between populations,[12] but there are large differences in the distributions of the other risk factors. We and our colleagues made a detailed study of the extent to which such differences between Japanese women and US white women could explain the large differences between their breast cancer rates.[6] Age at FFTP did not differ greatly between the two populations, but Japanese females born around 1900 had an average age at menarche 2.4 years later (16.4 as compared to 14.0 years) and they weighed on average 21.5 kg less (46.9 as compared to 68.4 kg) at age 70 than the 1900 cohort of US white women. These differences have steadily decreased over the years, but Japanese females born in 1940 still had menarche 1.3 years later (14.4 compared to 13.1 years) and at age 30 they weighed 8.2 kg less (49.5 compared to 57.7 kg) than comparable US white women. These major differences between Japan and the USA accounted for as much as two-thirds of the difference in the observed breast cancer rates in the two countries, but the ratio of the adjusted rates was still around 2.5, and it was clear that the established risk factors (menarche, FFTP, menopause and post-menopausal weight) could not provide the complete explanation.

This study comparing breast cancer rates of Japanese and US white women is the only detailed study, which takes into account cohort-specific distributions of the four risk factors, that has been done. A less detailed study has, however, been carried out of the relationship between age at menarche and (pre-menopausal) weight with the mortality and incidence rates of 26 countries.[13] This study found that, although breast cancer mortality and incidence rates were strongly correlated with age at menarche ($r = -0.59$ and -0.69) and weight ($r = 0.78$ and 0.62), certain dietary factors were more strongly associated with breast cancer risk. This study also concluded, although more tentatively, that the established risk factors could not provide the complete explanation of the international differences in breast cancer rates.

2 Diet

Much attention has been focused on dietary differences, particularly fat consumption, to explain both the international pattern of breast cancer occurrence and the changes in rates with migration.[13–15] International breast cancer mortality rates are particularly highly correlated with per capita consumption of fat ($r = 0.93$) and animal protein ($r = 0.85$).[13] There is a wealth of evidence that nutrition has profound effects on the breast cancer risk factors of age at menarche and weight, but these correlations of fat and animal protein with international breast cancer mortality rates remained highly significant after statistical adjustment for their effects on age at menarche and (pre-menopausal) weight. The multiple correlation coefficient of international breast cancer mortality rates with age at menarche and weight was 0.82, and this increased to 0.96 when fat, and 0.90 when animal protein, was taken into account.[13] Hirayama[16] also found that breast cancer mortality rates in various regions of Japan were highly correlated with fat consumption. When international breast cancer incidence, rather than mortality, rates are considered, the relative importance of fat and animal protein are reversed, but the magnitude of the correlation coefficients are again very high ($r =$

0.84 and 0.88).[13] The international correlations between per capita consumption of fat and animal protein (and certain other dietary constituents such as meat) are so high that it is not possible to confidently disentangle their separate effects.

Although the results of case-control studies have supported a role for fat consumption in the aetiology of breast cancer, the studies have found only small differences between cases and controls generally no larger than the differences in total calorie consumption.[17,18] We believe that further progress in evaluating these dietary factors is most likely to come from a deeper understanding of how they might influence breast cancer risk at a cellular level.

3 Endogenous Hormones

a *Oestrogens*

The association of breast cancer with age at menarche and age at menopause almost certainly implies that ovarian activity is an important determinant of breast cancer risk, and suggests a possibly critical role for oestrogens. Case-control studies show that exogenous oestrogens, given as hormone replacement therapy to menopausal and post-menopausal women, increase the risk of breast cancer;[19,20] and both pre-menopausal and post-menopausal breast cancer cases have elevated oestrogen levels.[21] This role for oestrogens is also strongly supported by the extensive studies of the role of oestrogens in the occurrence of mammary tumours in rodents.[22]

In the early 1970s MacMahon and his colleagues conducted a series of studies on teenagers and young women to investigate whether some aspect of oestrogen metabolism underlay the large differences in breast cancer rates between Asia and North America. They were aware that the Asian girls chosen for study would have to be a group who would themselves experience low breast cancer rates, so they chose their study populations to be 'as similar as possible to women now in the breast cancer age range',[23] an important part of study design too often ignored. Although they initially reported their results in terms of the relative amounts of various urinary oestrogen metabolites,[23] their results can also be interpreted in terms of absolute total urinary oestrogen levels which probably reflect total serum oestrogen levels quite well.[21] In the comparison of teenage girls, they found that in overnight urines collected on the morning of day 21 of the cycle total urinary oestrogen levels were 36% higher in the North Americans. The levels were also elevated in such samples collected on the morning of day 10 of the cycle, but only by 9%. These differences might have been related to the later menarche in the Japanese girls, but larger differences were found in older women, where the effects of late menarche should have disappeared: in nulliparous women aged 20–24, total urinary oestrogen levels in the North American women were 49% higher on day 21 and 38% higher on day 10; similar differences were found in parous women in their thirties.

Oestradiol (E2), the most important of the circulating oestrogens, exists in plasma either in a 'free' state, or bound to sex-hormone binding globulin (SHBG) or more loosely to albumin.[24] Based on a variety of data, it is generally believed that the portion bound to SHBG is unavailable to tissues; the status of the portion bound to albumin is, however, the subject of some dispute. If oestrogens are an important factor in the aetiology of breast cancer, then free or non-SHBG bound E2 should show a clearer relation to breast cancer risk than total E2. A number of recent case-control studies have found this to be true.[24,25] There is evidence that the decreased risk of breast cancer associated with early FFTP and the increased risk associated with increased post-menopausal weight are both mediated, at least in part, by long-term alterations in

SHBG levels: SHBG levels are raised after FFTP[26] and are negatively correlated with weight.[24]

Moore and his colleagues[27] recently reported their preliminary investigations into whether differences in E2 binding have a role in producing the widely different breast cancer rates in Britain and Japan. They found that British women had a higher percentage of free E2 and of non-SHBG bound E2 than Japanese women: the percentage of free E2 was 10% higher (1.8% cf 1.6%) and the percentage of non-SHBG bound E2 was 52% higher (70% cf 46%) in British women. Although the Japanese women were approximately 10 kg lighter than the British women, this explained only a small fraction of the differences between the two groups of women. There appeared rather to be a diminished affinity of albumin for E2 in Japanese women.

b *Prolactin*

One of the hormone changes that accompanies puberty is an increase in prolactin levels. Prolactin is a critically important hormone in mammary carcinogenesis in the rat,[15] and in man, prolactin, in association with oestrogen, directly affects the growth of breast epithelium. Case-control studies and studies of daughters of breast cancer patients support a role for prolactin in the aetiology of breast cancer,[28,29] and a decrease in prolactin levels could be part of the mechanism by which FFTP reduces breast cancer risk.[30]

Studies comparing prolactin levels in countries with different breast cancer rates have, however, not found higher daytime prolactin levels in the countries with high breast cancer rates.[31] Prolactin levels have, however, marked diurnal variation and much further work is needed before one can be certain that there are not major differences in peak prolactin levels, which occur a few hours before waking, that could be an important factor in determining the variation in international breast cancer rates.

For a time it appeared that prolactin might provide the link between dietary fat and breast cancer. Rats fed on a high-fat diet have elevated prolactin levels, and drugs which block prolactin secretion abolish the difference in tumour yield which normally occurs between rats on low and high-fat diets, when they are given a carcinogen.[15] Hill and Wynder[32] found that peak nocturnal prolactin levels fell by half in seven female nurses who reduced their fat intake from 40% to 33% of calories for two weeks, but another small study failed to confirm this finding,[33] and an international study found no difference in circulating prolactin levels between Japanese and American girls with a two-fold difference in fat consumption.[31]

c *Progesterone*

We noted above that there is substantial evidence suggesting that elevated oestrogen levels increase breast cancer risk. That elevated levels of the other major ovarian hormone, progesterone, may also be an important factor in increasing breast cancer risk has only recently been deduced.

Table II showed that nulliparous women do not have quite as high a breast cancer risk as women whose FFTP is delayed to their late thirties. This very important observation was long thought to be anomalous, but it is now realized that the result is due to FFTP having two effects—an initial harmful effect, which is then, given sufficient time before menopause, more than compensated for by a long-term beneficial effect.[6] A possible cause of the initial harmful effect of FFTP may be the tremendous growth of breast epithelium during the first pregnancy; in fact, the breast cancer risk factors of age at menarche, age at FFTP, and age at menopause, as well as the

initial harmful effect of FFTP, may all be understood in terms of their effects on breast tissue cell kinetics.[6]

The mitotic activity of breast epithelium varies markedly during the normal menstrual cycle, with peak activity occurring late in the luteal phase.[34] This suggests that progesterone, at least in the presence of oestrogen, induces mitotic activity in breast epithelium. This effect of progesterone would be in sharp distinction to its effect on endometrial tissue, where the peak mitotic activity is in the follicular phase of the cycle. It strongly agrees, however, with the experimental findings that progesterone induces ductal growth in rodent breast tissue,[35] and with Dao's[22] conclusions from his experimental studies that 'the minimal hormonal combination necessary for initiation of carcinogenesis is ... estrogen, and progesterone. It appears that ... the target cell must be in an active proliferative state'.

If progesterone does increase breast cancer risk, then regular ovulatory cycles should be more common in breast cancer patients than in controls. Short cycles should also be more common in breast cancer patients than in controls, because differences in cycle length are almost completely due to differences in the length of the follicular phase,[36] so that the shorter the cycle length the greater the proportion of time a women spends in the luteal phase with its associated high progesterone levels. Although few studies have addressed these issues, they all provide support for this role for progesterone.[37–39]

Henderson *et al.*[37] in their study of young breast cancer cases found that the rapid onset of regular cycles after menarche was associated with a doubling of breast cancer risk; and these investigators also found that a rapid onset of regular cycles was more common in daughters of breast cancer patients than in daughters of control women.[38]

Only Olsson *et al.*[39] appear to have addressed the issue of cycle length directly—they found that breast cancer patients recalled having significantly shorter cycles than controls (median: 26.4 days cf 28.6 days).

Finally, MacMahon *et al.*[40] have recently reported that the rapid onset of regular cycles is more common in countries with high breast cancer rates. It may also be noted that the median cycle length of 30 year-old women in the USA appears to be approximately 1.6 days shorter than that of similarly aged Japanese women.[41]

4 Summary

There has been slow but steady progress over the last two decades in our understanding of the aetiology of breast cancer. The large variation in international rates, particularly that between the low rates in Japan and the high rates in the UK and USA, and the sharp changes in rates with migration, have provided the stimulus to much valuable work. Hormones appear to hold the key to the understanding of the human disease, just as they do in certain animal species.

At present it appears that the factors most likely involved in the explanation of the major differences in rates between different population groups are: (1) age at menarche and frequency of ovulation; (2) post-menopausal weight; and (3) oestrogen levels and the percentage of E2 bound to SHBG.

During this century the age at menarche has progressively decreased both in the UK and USA and in many other areas of the world. In a series of extensive cross-sectional studies, Tanner[42] and others demonstrated that age at menarche is directly related to childhood growth patterns: attainment of a critical body weight to height ratio appears necessary for menarche to occur. The increase in breast cancer that accompanies a decline in average age at menarche may be inevitable: but the average age at menarche can be increased through a reduction in childhood obesity and an increase in strenuous physical activity;[43] and the frequency of ovulation (after menarche) decreased by an increase in strenuous physical activity.[43]

The increase in breast cancer that accompanies increased post-menopausal weight adds another good reason for avoiding obesity. The basis of the increased risk associated with increased weight is in all likelihood mediated by the increased oestrogen levels and the decreased SHBG levels caused by increased weight.

The recent findings of Moore *et al.*[27] that a very high percentage of E2 is bound to SHBG in Japanese women is potentially the key to explaining much of the difference between Japanese and US

breast cancer rates that cannot be explained by the major risk factors of menarche and post-menopausal weight. The basis of this difference in binding of E2 is not understood: 'weight alone probably does not explain [the] findings . . . Whether the difference . . . relates to genetic differences in the structure of albumin . . . or to factors such as dietary intake of lipids or other substances remains to be determined'.[27]

Much further work is needed to discover a fuller range of factors that influence both age at menarche and frequency of ovulation—international studies, not only comparing the UK or USA to Japan but to other parts of Asia and Africa, should be fruitful. Further international studies of the nature of E2 binding in different populations are particularly needed. The relation of binding to diet is likely to be a most interesting and rewarding field of study.

REFERENCES

1 Doll R, Muir C, Waterhouse J, eds. Cancer incidence in five continents: Volume II—1970. International Union Against Cancer. New York: Springer-Verlag, 1970

2 Waterhouse J, Muir C, Shanmugaratnam K, Powell J, eds. Cancer incidence in five continents: Volume IV. Lyon: IARC Sci Publ No. 42, 1982

3 Haenszel W, Kurihara M. Studies of Japanese migrants. I. Mortality from cancer and other diseases among Japanese in the United States. J Natl Cancer Inst 1968; 40: 43–68

4 Gray GE, Henderson BE, Pike MC. Changing ratio of breast cancer incidence rates with age of Black females compared with White females in the United States. J Natl Cancer Inst 1980; 64: 461–463

5 MacMahon B, Cole P, Brown J. Etiology of human breast cancer: a review. J Natl Cancer Inst 1973; 50: 21–41

6 Pike MC, Krailo MD, Henderson BE, Casagrande JT, Hoel DG. 'Hormonal' risk factors, 'breast tissue age' and the age-incidence of breast cancer. Nature 1983; 303: 767–770

7 Pike MC, Henderson BE, Casagrande JT, Rosario I, Gray GE. Oral contraceptive use and early abortion as risk factors for breast cancer in young women. Br J Cancer 1981; 43: 72–76

8 MacMahon B, Cole P, Lin TM *et al.* Age at first birth and breast cancer risk. Bull WHO 1970; 43: 209–217

9 Trichopoulos D, MacMahon, B, Cole P. Menopause and breast cancer risk. J Natl Cancer Inst 1972; 48: 605–613

10 de Waard F, Cornelis HP, Aoki K, Yoshida M. Breast cancer incidence according to weight and height in two cities of the Netherlands and in Aichi Prefecture, Japan. Cancer 1977; 40: 1269–1275

11 Lew EA, Garfinkel L. Variations in mortality by weight among 750 000 men and women. J Chron Dis 1979; 32: 563–576

12 Hoel DG, Wakayashi T, Pike MC. Secular trends in the distribution of the breast cancer risk factors: menarche, first birth, menopause and weight in Hiroshima and Nagasaki, Japan. Am J Epidem 1983; 118: 78–89

13 Gray GE, Pike MC, Henderson BE. Breast cancer incidence and mortality rates in different countries in relation to known risk factors and dietary practices. Br J Cancer 1979; 39: 1–7

14 Armstrong B, Doll R. Environmental factors and cancer incidence and mortality in different countries, with special reference to dietary practices. Int J Cancer 1975; 15: 617–631

15 Carroll KK. Experimental evidence of dietary factors and hormone-dependent cancers. Cancer Res 1975; 35: 3374–3383

16 Hirayama R. Epidemiology of breast cancer with special reference to the role of diet. Prev Med 1978; 7: 173–195

17 Miller AB, Kelly A, Choi NW, Matthews V, Morgan RW, Munan L, Burch JD, Feather J, Howe GR, Jain M. A study of diet and breast cancer. Am J Epidem 1978; 107: 499–509

18 Nomura A, Henderson B, Lee J. Breast cancer and diet among the Japanese in Hawaii. Am J Clin Nutr 1978; 31: 2020–2025

19 Hoover R, Gray LA, Cole P, MacMahon B. Menopausal estrogens and breast cancer. N Engl J Med 1976; 295: 401–405

20 Ross RK, Paganini-Hill A, Gerkins VR. A case-control study of menopausal estrogen therapy and breast cancer. J Am Med Assoc 1980; 243: 1635–1639

21 MacMahon B, Cole P, Brown JB, Paffenbarger R, Trichopoulos D, Yen S. Urine estrogens, frequency of ovulation and breast cancer risk: case-control study in premenopausal women. J Natl Cancer Inst 1983; 70: 247–250

22 Dao TL. The role of ovarian steroid hormones in mammary carcinogenesis. In: Pike MC, Siiteri PK, Welsch CW, eds. Banbury Report 8: Hormones and breast cancer. New York: Cold Spring Harbor Laboratory, Cold Spring Harbor, 1981

23 MacMahon B, Cole P, Brown JB, Aoki K, Lin K M, Morgan R W, Woo N-C. Urine estrogen profiles of Asian and North American women. Int J Cancer 1974; 14: 161–167

24 Siiteri PK, Hammond GL, Nisker JA. Increased availability of serum estrogens in breast cancer: a new hypothesis. In: Pike MC, Siiteri PK, Welsch CW, eds. Banbury Report 8: Hormones and breast cancer. New York: Cold Spring Harbor Laboratory, 1981

25 Moore JW, Clark GM, Bulbrook RD *et al.* Serum concentrations of total and non-protein bound oestradiol in patients with breast cancer and in normal controls. Int J Cancer 1982; 29: 17–21

26 Bernstein L, Pike MC, Ross RK, Judd HL, Brown JB, Henderson BE. Estrogen and sex-hormone binding globulin levels in nulliparous and parous women. J Natl. Cancer Inst; In press

27 Moore JW, Clark GMG, Takatani O, Wakabayashi Y, Hayward JL, Bulbrook RD. Distribution of 17(beta)-estradiol in the sera of normal British and Japanese women. J Natl Cancer Inst 1983; 71: 749–754

28 Henderson BE, Pike MC. Prolactin—an important hormone in breast neoplasia? In: Pike MC, Siiteri PK, Welsch CW, eds. Banbury Report 8: Hormones and breast cancer. New York: Cold Spring Harbor Laboratory, 1981

29 Levin PA, Malarkey WB. Daughters of women with breast cancer have elevated mean 24-hour prolactin (PRL) levels and a partial resistance of PRL to dopamine suppression. J Clin Endocrinol Metab 1981; 53: 179–184

30 Yu MC, Gerkins VR, Henderson BE, Brown JB, Pike MC. Elevated levels of prolactin in nulliparous women. Br J Cancer 1981; 43: 826–831

31 Gray GE, Pike MC, Hirayama T *et al.* Diet and hormone profiles in teenage girls in four countries at different risk to breast cancer. Prev Med 1982; 11: 108–113

32 Hill P, Wynder E. Diet and prolactin release. Lancet 1976; ii: 806–807

33 Gray GE, Pike MC, Henderson BE. Dietary fat and plasma prolactin. Am J Clin Nutr 1981; 34: 1160–1162

34 Anderson TJ, Ferguson DJP, Raab GM. Cell turnover in the 'resting' human breast: influence of parity, contraceptive pill, age and laterality. Br J Cancer 1982; 46: 376–382

35 Dulbecco R, Henahan M, Armstrong B. Cell types and morphogenesis in the mammary gland. Proc Natl Acad Sci USA 1982; 79: 7346–7350

36 Aksel S. Hormonal characteristics of long cycles in fertile women. Fertil Steril 1981; 36: 521–523

37 Henderson BE, Pike MC, Casagrande JT. Breast cancer and the oestrogen window hypothesis. Lancet 1981; ii: 363

38 Henderson BE, Gerkins V, Rosario I, Casagrande JT, Pike MC. Elevated serum levels of estrogen and prolactin in daughters of patients with breast cancer. N Engl J Med 1975; 293: 790–795

39 Olsson H, Landin-Olsson M, Gullberg B. Retrospective assessment of menstrual cycle length in patients with breast cancer, in patients with benign breast disease, and in women without breast disease. J Natl Cancer Inst 1983: 70: 17–20

40 MacMahon B, Trichopoulos D, Brown J *et al.* Age at menarche, probability of ovulation and breast cancer risk. Int J Cancer 1982; 29: 13–16

41 Treloar AE, Boynton RE, Behn BT, Brown BW. Variation of the human menstrual cycle through reproductive life. Int J Fertil 1967; 12: 77–126

42 Tanner JM. Growth at adolescence. Oxford: Blackwell Scientific, 1962

43 Frisch RE, von Gotz-Welbergen AV, McArthur JW. Delayed menarche and amenorrhea of college athletes in relation to age of onset of training. J Am Med Ass 1981; 246: 1559–1563

British Medical Bulletin (1984) Vol. 40, No. 4, pp. 355–358

KAPOSI'S SARCOMA

M S R HUTT MD FRCP FRCPath

*Geographical Pathology Unit
Department of Histopathology
St Thomas's Hospital Medical School
London*

1 Sporadic Kaposi's sarcoma
   a Europe
   b North America
   c Asia and the Far East
   d Other parts of the world
2 Endemic Kaposi's sarcoma of Africa
3 Coexistence of Kaposi's sarcoma and other tumours
4 Kaposi's sarcoma in patients on immunosuppressive therapy
5 Epidemic Kaposi's sarcoma in patients with acquired immunodeficiency syndrome (AIDS)
6 Conclusions
  References

In 1872 Moricz Kaposi described an independent entity of 'Idiopathic multiple pigmentsarcoma of the skin' in five patients seen in the Dermatology Department in Vienna, a city then preeminent in the medical world.[1] He later amended the name to 'Idiopathic multiple haemorrhagic sarcoma'[2] to indicate the vascular origin of the tumour which consisted of fusiform spindle cells and a new rich growth of capillaries. The tumour was characterized by the development of skin nodules or plaques, usually starting on the hands or feet, but occasionally also involving the viscera.

During the next 80 years numerous case reports and reviews were published in Europe and North America. These did little to add to Kaposi's original description of the lesions, but emphasized that it was a very rare tumour occurring predominantly in elderly men and usually running a prolonged clinical course, though occasionally showing more aggressive features with visceral metastases.[3]

There is now a vast literature on the histogenesis of this tumour. Although the histological diagnosis is usually easy, argument has raged about the cell of origin. As a result of modern histochemical, electron microscopic, and immunocytochemical techniques it is generally agreed that Kaposi's sarcoma is a tumour arising from a pluripotential angioformative cell, or angioblast. The cells of the tumour show features of venous endothelial, fibroblastic, smooth muscle, and perithelial cell differentiation.[4–6]

1 Sporadic Kaposi's Sarcoma

a *Europe*

In 1897 de Amicis[7] described 12 patients seen in Northern Italy. This relatively high frequency in people of Italian extraction was confirmed by later reports. Dorfell reported 16 cases seen personally and reviewed the European literature.[8] There were 356 cases of whom 111 were Italians, 50 Russians, 20 Poles, 45 Jews, 12 Austrians, 8 Armenians, 7 Hungarians and 5 Germans. The relatively high incidence in Ashkenazic Jews and in the populations of Southern Europe, particularly Italy was noted by other authors.[9] By contrast very few cases were described in the United Kingdom, Scandinavia and other parts of north and west Europe.[10] In all regions the disease occurred predominantly in elderly males, though occasionally cases were seen in childhood.

b *North America*

Sporadic reports of Kaposi's sarcoma in the USA appeared in the first 75 years of this century, though the tumour only accounted for 0.02% of all malignancies.[11] McCarthy and Pack (1950)[12] described 36 cases of whom 83% were of Jewish origin. By contrast, there were no Jews in a series of 50 cases reviewed by Cox and Helwig (1959);[12] this may, however, reflect differences in the ethnic proportions in the regions from which the material was derived. It was at first thought that Kaposi's sarcoma was rare in the black populations of the USA but 11 of the 50 patients described by Cox and Helwig were black.[12] These authors also confirmed that the general clinical features of the tumour were similar in all racial groups. Sporadic Kaposi's sarcoma occurs predominantly in elderly men, the skin lesions are often multifocal and usually present on the extremities, most commonly on the feet or hands. Other skin sites and mucous membranes may be involved. The tumour usually runs a relatively benign course, though occasional patients have a progressive disease with widespread metastases. Cox and Helwig[12] noted that 8 out of 50 patients were alive and tumour-free 8 years after the initial diagnosis. The recent epidemic of cases is discussed in Section 5.

c *Asia and the Far East*

Throughout this whole area Kaposi's sarcoma occurs only sporadically and in most regions is extremely rare even in countries which are ecologically similar to subsaharan Africa. A few cases have been described in Papua New Guinea, a country where Burkitt's lymphoma is endemic, but the proportional frequencies are much lower than in Africa.

d *Other Parts of the World*

Sporadic cases have been described in South America and Australia. The tumour does not appear to be common in the tropical region of Amazonia.

2 Endemic Kaposi's Sarcoma of Africa

Although many Western doctors working in Africa in the early part of this century thought that cancer was rare, others, such as Sir Albert Cook in Uganda, recognized that cancer was not infrequent in the indigenous black population, but that the pattern (site and type) was very different from that seen in Europe.[13] In 1934 Smith and Elmes[14] reported the results of a histopathological survey of 500 malignant tumours submitted to their laboratory in Nigeria. Among these they drew specific attention to 10 cases of Kaposi's sarcoma in black males over the age of 30 years. During the next 37 years large numbers of cases were described in the countries of Africa lying south of the Sahara. These observations led to the organization of the first international symposium on Kaposi's sarcoma which was held in Kampala, Uganda in 1961.[15] At about the same time Lothe[10] published a thesis on Kaposi's sarcoma in Ugandan Africans in which he described 211 cases, by far the largest series ever reported. At this symposium it became apparent that Kaposi's sarcoma was endemic in large areas of subsaharan Africa, though the distribution of cases was uneven. There is an

FIG. 1. Map of Africa showing proportional frequencies of Kaposi's sarcoma (male and female combined)

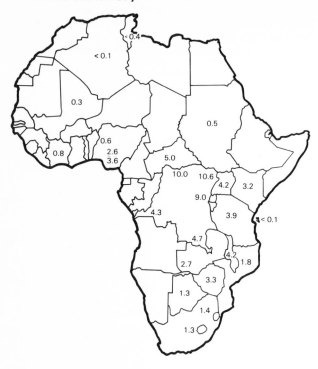

epicentre of high frequency in Eastern Zaire where the tumour accounts for over 10% of all malignancies (Fig. 1). Proportional frequencies are also high in neighbouring countries, particularly in western Uganda. The tumour is endemic in southern Sudan but not in Khartoum or other parts of north Africa.

In most of the countries in the equatorial belt of Africa the tumour accounts for over 3% of all malignancies and in some it is the fourth or fifth commonest tumour in men. Kaposi's sarcoma is also seen in the countries of west and southern Africa though the relative frequencies are slightly lower. While the clinical features are similar to many cases seen in Europe, with a predominance of nodular skin lesions and a relatively benign course, more aggressive skin lesions behaving like other sarcomas are also seen and visceral involvement is commoner. In contrast to Europe and North America many cases present in the third or fourth decades. In African children the tumour sometimes presents with multiple gross lymphadenopathy. Such cases run a rapidly progressive course with widespread metastases. In 1980 a second international symposium on Kaposi's sarcoma was held in Uganda to review the clinical and epidemiological features in Africa in the light of another 20 years of African experience with this tumour.[16] The overall distribution of the tumour in the countries of subsaharan Africa was confirmed by the addition of over 1000 cases. Local differences in proportional frequency within countries such as Uganda,[17] Tanzania,[18] and Kenya[19] were apparent. In all endemic areas the tumour occurs mainly in males, but the male:female ratios increase with age from 1.7:1 in the first decade (lymphadenopathic type) to 15:1 or more in those over 60 years.[16,18] The management of the various clinical types of the disease seen in Africa was discussed.[16]

4 Kaposi's Sarcoma in Patients on Immunosuppressive Therapy

In 1969 Siegal *et al.*[22] reported a case of visceral disseminated Kaposi's sarcoma in a renal transplant patient who died 10 months after the operation. Since that time a series of reports have been published in similar patients.[23,24] Several cases have also been described following the use of immunosuppressive drugs for the treatment of malignant lymphomas or autoimmune diseases.[25,26] Kleppe *et al.*[24] observed that 6 (14.6%) of the 41 patients on whom information was available on treatment antedating the development of the tumour were receiving corticosteroids and two of these also were given azathioprine.

5 Epidemic Kaposi's Sarcoma in Patients with Acquired Immunodeficiency Syndrome (AIDS)

In 1981 Gottlieb *et al.*[27] published a paper entitled 'a preliminary communication on extensively disseminated Kaposi's sarcoma in young homosexual men'. This paper was soon followed by others describing a syndrome of acquired immunodeficiency resulting in the development of multiple bacterial, viral, fungal, and protozoal infections, and/or in the occurrence of Kaposi's sarcoma. The majority of these patients came from the homosexual populations of California or New York. By June 1983, 1641 cases of AIDS had been recorded at the US Centres for Disease Control, 1532 of these were in males. Twenty-six per cent presented with Kaposi's sarcoma alone, 51% with the opportunistic infection *Pneumocystis carinii* pneumonia (PCP), 8% with both and 15% with other infections.[28] It is now apparent that four major populations are at risk for the development of AIDS.[29,30] About 75% of patients are homosexual males, 13% intravenous drug abusers, 6% immigrants from Haiti, 0.7% haemophiliacs who have received multiple infusions of anti-haemophilic globulin[31] and about 5% have no specific risk factors. The great majority affected are men, but AIDS has also been reported in women.

Clinically, Kaposi's sarcoma in many patients with AIDS occurs in young men and runs a rapidly progressive course quite unlike the sporadic cases previously seen in the USA. The initial lesions may occur in many different sites and systemic spread is common. The earliest skin lesions are often difficult to diagnose both clinically and histopathologically.[32] Since AIDS and its complications were recognized as a syndrome, reports of its occurrence have come from many European countries including Denmark, France, Holland, Switzerland and the United Kingdom, though in none of these countries has it assumed epidemic proportions.[33-37]

Epidemiological studies on patients with AIDS and Kaposi's sarcoma have shown that its occurrence is particularly related to certain groups of highly promiscuous homosexuals and that case-to-case sexual contact is frequent. In some cases occurring in Denmark there was a history of the patient visiting homosexual communities in the USA or being visited by such individuals in Denmark.[34] The occurrence in haemophiliacs and drug addicts also suggested that AIDS and possibly Kaposi's sarcoma are due to infective agents transmitted through blood.

6 Conclusions

The clinical, histopathological, and epidemiological evidence outlined in the previous sections indicates that Kaposi's sarcoma is an entity which can be differentiated from other tumours of vascular or soft tissue origin. It occurs in four forms. Sporadic cases, which are seen in many different parts of the world, usually affect elderly men and run a relatively benign course. Endemic Kaposi's sarcoma is confined to the black populations of subsaharan Africa, and has an epicentre of high incidence in eastern Zaire and adjacent countries; it often affects young men and may run an aggressive course. Kaposi's sarcoma also occurs with an unusual frequency in patients receiving immunosuppressive therapy. Epidemic Kaposi's sarcoma associated with AIDS occurs mainly in certain homosexual populations in the United States, but also affects other groups and is now seen in Europe and other parts of the world; this type also shows male dominance and often runs an aggressive course.

The geographical and ethnic distribution of sporadic Kaposi's sarcoma suggests that both genetic and environmental factors are involved in the aetiology.[20] The relatively high incidence in Italians and Jews, both in Europe and in the USA, points to a specific ethnic susceptibility but this cannot entirely explain the higher frequency in other groups living in southern Europe or the very low frequency in northern Europe. There is no explanation of the male dominance in these sporadic cases.

The endemic situation in Africa has puzzled epidemiologists and cancer researchers since its distribution became apparent in the 1960s. The tumour affects black populations of quite different ethnic origin; in Uganda Kaposi's sarcoma occurs in tribes of Bantu, Nilotic, and Hamitic origin. The African evidence points to the predominance of environmental factors in its aetiology.[11,16] Attempts have been made to link the distribution map of the tumour to the prevalence of a variety of parasitic diseases such as onchocerciasis and malaria, to regions of rainforest and high rainfall, to specific vectors and to other environmental factors such as natural radiation and trauma. While it is true that the highest frequency does occur in rainforest regions, the tumour also occurs in regions of savannah and bush scrub. Contrary to some suggestions, the distribution maps of Kaposi's sarcoma and Burkitt's lymphoma in Africa have significant differences as, for example, in south west Uganda where the former is very common and the latter is very rare.

An intriguing feature of the tumour in Africa is the widening sex-ratio with each decade, so that in patients over 45 years the ratios are as high or higher than in the sporadic cases. This suggests that there is an endogenous, probably hormonal, influence in the aetiology.[4]

The role of immunosuppression in the aetiology of Kaposi's sarcoma was suggested by the observation that these patients had a significant incidence of second tumours, particularly malignant lymphoma. This was strengthened by the occurrence of cases in renal transplant patients and those receiving immunosuppressants for other reasons. A debate followed as to whether the induction of the tumour was related directly to immunological mechanisms acting on the putative cell of origin, or whether the immuno-suppression predisposed to an oncogenic viral infection. Studies on immunosuppressed cases in Europe and North America showed that there was an association between Kaposi's sarcoma and cytomegalic virus (CMV) as judged by significant differences in antibody titres to the virus in cases and controls.[38,39] CMV-related antigens have been demonstrated in 22% of tumour biopsies, CMV-DNA sequences in 30%[21] and virus-specific RNA in 50% of tumours.[40,41]

Studies of CMV in African patients showed high titres of antibodies to CMV, comparable to those found in American cases, but there was no significant difference between these titres and age-sex matched African controls.[21]

The epidemic of AIDS, with its high frequency of a particularly malignant form of Kaposi's sarcoma[32] or the development of multiple opportunistic infections associated with immunodepression, stimulated new interest in this neglected malignancy. AIDS is characterized by specific defects in the T-lymphocyte population. These include T-lymphopenia, reduced T helper cell (leu-3, OKT4) to T suppressor cell (leu-2 OKT8) ratios, and cutaneous anergy. This is usually due to an absolute deficiency in T helper (OKT4) cells, though in some studies T suppressor cells have been raised.[42,43] The epidemiological evidence suggests that this defect in AIDS is due to an as-yet unidentified virus which is transmitted through the blood, and that the epidemic in the USA resulted from the introduction of this agent into a community whose life-styles were conducive to its transmission. An alternative hypothesis is that the immunosuppression of AIDS is due to the effects of multiple infections similarly transmitted.[44] The high frequency of CMV infections in AIDS, African patients, and immunosuppressed patients with this tumour, taken in conjunction with the demonstration of CMV-DNA and RNA in the tumour cells provides strong evidence that this virus may be implicated in the aetiology of Kaposi's sarcoma. Other infective agents, such as the human T-cell leukaemia-lymphoma virus have also been isolated from AIDS patients, but the role of this virus in the aetiology of either AIDS or Kaposi's sarcoma is uncertain.[44]

The role of genetic factors in the aetiology of Kaposi's sarcoma has been substantiated by recent observations.[45] Friedman-Kein *et al.* showed that the major histocompatibility antigen HLA-DR5 occurs with high frequency (over 60%) in patients with epidemic (AIDS) and sporadic (classical) forms of the tumour; this contrasts with control frequencies of only 23%. It is also significant that HLA-DR5 has a higher frequency in blacks, Italians and Jews living in New York than in other ethnic groups.[45] An increased frequency of HLA-DR5 has also been demonstrated in the lymphoadenopathic stage of AIDS suggesting that this genotype may predispose to the development of immunodeficiency.[46] The occurrence of AIDS in previously healthy Africans from Zaire, now living in Europe,[47] and in one European doctor who developed AIDS on returning to Denmark from working in Central Africa,[48] provides a possible link between endemic African Kaposi's sarcoma and the epidemic form associated with AIDS. The unravelling of these complex genetic and environmental factors associated with the development of this unusual tumour are providing new insights into the development of malignancies.

ADDENDUM

Since this paper was written, a human retrovirus, lymphadenopathy virus (LAV), has been described in France in patients with AIDS.[49,50] LAV is similar, if not identical, to the human retrovirus HTLV-III isolated from cases of AIDS in the United States.[51] The evidence suggests that this retrovirus is an aetiological agent of AIDS.

REFERENCES

1 Kaposi M. Idiopathisches multiples Pigmentsarkom der Haut. Arch Dermatol Syph 1872; 4: 265–273
2 Kaposi M. Zur Nomenclatur des idiopathischen Pigmentsarcoms Kaposi. Arch Dermatol Syph 1894; 29: 164

3 Rothman S. Some clinical aspects of Kaposi's sarcoma in the European and North American population. In: Ackerman LV, Murray JF, eds. Symposium on Kaposi's sarcoma. Unio Internationalis Contra Cancrum. Basel: Karger, 1962; 18: 51–58

4 Templeton AC. Kaposi's sarcoma. In: Sommers, Rosman. Pathology annual. New York: Appleton-Century-Crofts, 1981; 16: part 2, 315–336

5 Harrison AC, Kahn LB. Myogenic cells in Kaposi's sarcoma; An ultrastructural study. J Pathol 1978; 124: 157–160

6 Sterry W, Steigleder G-K, Bodeux E. Kaposi's sarcoma: venous capillary haemangioblastoma. A histochemical and ultrastructural study. Arch Dermatol Res 1979; 266: 253–267

7 De Amicis T. Die Sarkomatose der Haut. Monatsh Prakt Dermatol 1897; 25: 309–331

8 Dörfell J. Histogenesis of multiple idiopathic haemorrhagic sarcoma of Kaposi. Arch Dermatol Syph 1932; 26: 608–634

9 Mierzecki H. Sarcoma idiopathicum multiplex Kaposi. Arch Dermatol Syph 1932; 165: 577–584

10 Lothe F. Kaposi's sarcoma in Uganda Africans. Acta Pathol Microbiol Scand 1963; suppl 161

11 McCarthy WD, Pack GT. Malignant blood vessel tumors. A report of 56 cases of angiosarcoma and Kaposi's sarcoma. Surg Gynecol Obstet 1950; 91: 465–482

12 Cox FH, Helwig AB. Kaposi's sarcoma. Cancer, 1959; 12: 289–298

13 Davies JNP, Elmes S, Hutt MSR, Mtimavalye LAR, Owor R, Shaper L. Cancer in an African Community 1897–1956. An analysis of the records of Mengo Hospital, Kampala, Uganda. Br Med J 1964; 1: 259–264 & 336–341

14 Smith EC, Elmes BGT. Malignant disease in natives of Nigeria: an analysis of five hundred tumours. Ann Trop Med Parasitol 1934; 28: 461–512

15 Ackerman LV, Murray JF, eds. Symposium on Kaposi's sarcoma. Unio Internationalis Contra Cancrum. Basel: Karger, 1962

16 Olweny CLM, Hutt MSR, Owor R. Kaposi's sarcoma. 2nd Kaposi's sarcoma symposium, Kampala, 1980. Antibiotics and Chemotherapy Basel: Karger, 1981; 29

17 Taylor JF, Smith PG, Bull D, Pike MC. Kaposi's sarcoma in Uganda: Geographic and Ethnic distribution. Br J Cancer 1972; 26: 483–497

18 Bland JM, Mutoka C, Hutt MSR. Kaposi's sarcoma in Tanzania. East Afr J Med Res 1977; 4: 47–53

19 Kungu A, Gatei DG. Kaposi's sarcoma in Kenya. In: Olweny CLM, Hutt MSR, Owor R. Kaposi's sarcoma. 2nd Kaposi's Sarcoma Symposium, Kampala, 1980. Antibiotics and Chemotherapy. Basel: Karger, 1981; 29: 38–55

20 Oéttle, AG. Geographical and racial differences in the frequency of Kaposi's sarcoma as evidence of environmental or genetic causes. In: Ackerman, LV, Murray JF eds. Symposium on Kaposi's sarcoma. Unio Internationalis Contra Cancrum. Basel: Karger, 1962; 18: 17–54

21 Giraldo G, Beth E, Kyalwazi SK. Etiological implications on Kaposi's sarcoma. In: Olweny CLM, Hutt MRS, Owor R. Kaposi's sarcoma. 2nd Kaposi's sarcoma symposium, Kampala, 1980. Antibiotics and Chemotherapy. Basel: Karger, 1981; 29: 12–29

22 Siegel JH, Janis R, Alper JC, Schutte H, Robbins L, Blaufox MD. Disseminated visceral Kaposi sarcoma. JAMA 1969; 207: 1493–1496

23 Myers BD, Kessler E, Levi J, Pick A, Rosenfeld JB, Tikvah P. Kaposi sarcoma in kidney transplant recipients. Arch Intern Med 1974; 133: 307–311

24 Hardy MA, Goldfarb P, Levine S et al. De novo Kaposi's sarcoma in renal transplantation. Case report and brief review. Cancer, 1976; 38: 144–148

25 Klepp O, Dahl O, Stenwig JT. Association of Kaposi's sarcoma and prior immunosuppressive therapy. Cancer, 1978; 42: 2626–2630

26 Mazzaferri EL, Penn GM. Kaposi's sarcoma associated with multiple myeloma. Arch Intern Med 1968; 122: 521–525

27 Gottlieb GJ, Ragaz A, Vogel JV et al. A preliminary communication on extensively disseminated Kaposi's sarcoma in young homosexual men. Am J Dermatopathol 1981; 3: 111–114

28 Centers for Disease Control. Update on acquired immunodeficiency syndrome (AIDS). United States M.M.W.R. 1983; 32: 309–311

29 Centers for Disease Control. Update on acquired immune deficiency syndrome (AIDS). United States M.M.W.R. 1982; 31: 507–514

30 Centers for Disease Control. Opportunistic infections and Kaposi's sarcoma among Haitians in the United States. M.M.W.R. 1982; 31: 353–361

31 Centers for Disease Control. Update on acquired immune deficiency syndrome (AIDS) among patients with haemophilia A. M.M.W.R. 1982; 31: 644–652

32 Gottlieb GJ, Ackerman AB. Kaposi's sarcoma. An extensively disseminated form in young homosexual men. Hum Pathol, 1982; 13: 882–892

33 Brunet JB, Bouvet E, Leibowitch J et al. Acquired immunodeficiency syndrome in France. Lancet, 1983; 1: 700–701

34 Gerstoft J, Malchøw-Moller A, Bygbjerg I et al. Severe acquired immunodeficiency in European homosexual men. Br Med J 1982; 285: 17–19

35 Lissen E, Wichmann I, Jimenez JM, Andreu-Kern F. AIDS in haemophilia patients in Spain. Lancet, 1983; 1: 992–993

36 O'Connor BH, McEvoy MB, Galbraith NS. Acquired immune deficiency syndrome. Br Med J 1983; 286: 1354

37 Ebbesen P, Biggar RJ, Melbye M. AIDS in Europe. Br Med J 1983; 287: 1324–1326

38 Giraldo G, Beth E, Kourilsky FM et al. Antibody patterns to herpesviruses in Kaposi's sarcoma: serological association of European Kaposi's sarcoma with cytomegalovirus. Int J Cancer, 1975; 15: 839–848

39 Giraldo G, Beth E, Henle W et al. Antibody patterns to herpesviruses in Kaposi's sarcoma. II. Serological association of American Kaposi's sarcoma with cytomegalovirus. Int J Cancer, 1978; 22: 126–131

40 Giraldo G, Beth E, Huang ES. Kaposi's sarcoma and its relationship to cytomegalovirus (CMV) III. CMV DNA and CMV early antigens in Kaposi's sarcoma. Int J Cancer, 1980; 26: 23–29

41 Boldogh I, Beth E, Huang E-S, Kyalwazi SK, Giraldo G. Kaposi's sarcoma. IV. Detection of CMV DNA, CMV RNA and CMNA in tumor biopsies. Int J Cancer, 1981; 28: 469–474

42 Fauci AS. The syndrome of Kaposi's sarcoma and opportunistic infections: an epidemiologically restricted disorder of immunoregulation. [Editorial]. Ann Intern Med 1982; 96: 777–779

43 Waterson AP. Acquired immune deficiency syndrome. Br med J 1983; 286: 743–746

44 Gelmann EP, Popovic M, Blayney D et al. Proviral DNA of a retrovirus, human T-cell leukemia virus in two patients with AIDS. Science, 1983; 220: 862–864

45 Friedman-Kien AE, Laubenstein LJ, Rubinstein P et al. Disseminated Kaposi's sarcoma in homosexual men. Ann Intern Med 1982; 96: 693

46 Enlow RW, Roldan AN, LoGalbo P, Mildvan D, Mathur U, Winchester RJ. Increased frequency of HLA-DR5 in lymphadenopathy stage of AIDS. Lancet, 1983; 3: 51–52

47 Clumbeck N, Mascart-Lemone F, de Maubeuge, J, Brenez D, Marcelis L. Acquired immune deficiency syndrome in Black Africans. Lancet, 1983; 1: 642

48 Bygbjerg IC. AIDS in a Danish surgeon. (Zaire, 1976) Lancet, 1983; 1: 925

49 Barre-Sinoussi F, Chermann JC, Rey F et al. Isolation of T-lymphotropic retroviruses from a patient at risk for acquired immune deficiency syndrome. Science 1983; 220: 868–870

50 Brun-Vezinet F, Rouziux C, Barre-Sinoussi F et al. Lymphadenopathy-associated virus in patients with AIDS or lymphadenopathy syndrome. Lancet 1984; i: 1253–1256

51 Gallo RC, Salahuddin SZ, Popovic M et al. Frequent detection and isolation of cytopathic retroviruses (HTLV-III) from patients with AIDS and at risk for AIDS. Science 1984; 234: 500–503

British Medical Bulletin (1984) Vol. 40, No. 4, pp. 359–365

THE GEOGRAPHY OF DIABETES MELLITUS

H KEEN MD FRCP

*Unit for Metabolic Medicine
Department of Medicine
Guy's Hospital Medical School
London*

J M EKOE MD

*NCD/OND Division
WHO Geneva*

1 Geographical variation in diabetes mortality
2 Definitions of diabetes
3 Diabetes in Caucasoid peoples
  a Insulin-dependent diabetes
  b Non-insulin-dependent diabetes
4 Diabetes in developing countries
5 Diabetes in other populations
6 Complications of diabetes
7 Conclusions
  References

Diabetes mellitus (DM), long a major health problem in industrialized countries, has gained increasing recognition in the developing world as the infective and nutritional causes of ill health and death have begun to recede. Over these years, the concept of diabetes itself has undergone revision and change. Once regarded as a single disease entity, a failure of glucose metabolism secondary to inadequate insulin action, with various levels of severity and expression, diabetes mellitus is now seen as a description of a metabolic state resulting from a diversity of aetiologies and with variable clinical manifestation and progression. The unifying feature is the presence (in the untreated state) of persistent hyperglycaemia accompanied by a variety of clinical and bio-chemical phenomena. It is hyperglycaemia which defines diabetes mellitus and the accompaniments which define its subtypes. In the genesis of the well studied subtypes of diabetes in Western countries, the twin features of individual susceptibility, probably inherited, activated by environmental determinants emerge as a major aetiological complex. Many of the other diabetes variants, seen principally in populations of developing countries, probably also involve the interplay of genetic susceptibility and environmental determinants. Ethnic differences and geographically diverse environments are, therefore, likely to give rise to a spectrum of diabetes mechanisms and manifestations.

A justification for retaining the diabetic syndrome as a nosological entity is the characteristic development of a set of long-term sequels. Progressive damage to the eyes, kidneys, nerves and arteries constitute the so-called complications of diabetes and are common (though differing in prevalence and severity) to virtually all the many variants of the diabetic state. Although argued by some to indicate a common underlying cause to the diabetes, this stereotypy of complications seems more likely to point to common pathogenic consequences of the diabetic state, however arrived at.

1 Geographical Variation in Diabetes Mortality

Mortality statistics by causal groupings are notorious for problems of comparability and some of the wide variation in the age-specific mortality rates attributed to diabetes (Table I) is due to diversity of national practices in death certification procedures. West[1] considered the interpretation of data such as these in some detail.

In Britain, Fuller and co-workers[2] attempted to assess the shortfall in the true contribution of diabetes to mortality by analysing death certificates with any mention of diabetes and noting the frequency of accompanying contributing causes also recorded on the certificate. Circulatory diseases were dispropor-tionately more frequently associated with mention of diabetes; deaths in such individuals are most commonly classified to cardiovascular cause without mention of diabetes. In a cohort of about 6000 diabetic patients assembled between 1965 and 1969 by the British Diabetic Association, the standardized mortality ratios for vascular disease and ischaemic heart disease were all in excess of 100, especially in women; women aged 15–44 years on entry into the cohort had an 11-fold greater risk of ischaemic heart disease death than comparably aged non-diabetics. In general, cause-specific mortality rates may greatly underestimate the contribution of diabetes to mortality, a conclusion endorsed by Tokuhata *et al.*[3] and West.[1] The high rates for Malta and Mauritius are notable in Table I. The health departments of both countries have initiated WHO-sponsored enquiries into national diabetes prevalence and its associations and a study of glucose tolerance, nutrition and diabetic complications on an approximately 1% sample of the Maltese adult population has recently been completed.

2 Definitions of Diabetes

Only recently has there been a significant move towards internationally agreed definitions for diabetes (see Appendix). Diabetes mellitus owed its diagnostic origins to a striking *clinical* syndrome of unassuagable thirst, voluminous urination, rapid physical wasting progressing to coma and death, usually occurring in youth or childhood. This is the insulin-dependent diabetes mellitus (IDDM) or Type 1 of the current classification.[4,5] The copious, sugar-laden urine, early recognized as a constant feature, contributed descriptively to the name and, in more recent history, was responsible for drawing a much larger group of clinically rather different people into the diabetic designation. Though

TABLE I. Diabetes mortality by country or area (Rates by age per 100 000 reported between 1973 and 1976)

(Selected from Reference 72)

	Age group				
	35–44	45–54	55–64	65–74	75+
Africa					
Egypt	4.3	15.9	38.9	67.2	67.7
Mauritius	12.6	68.3	158.5	316.9	391.8
America					
El Salvador	3.8	7.9	26.4	58.1	79.4
USA	4.2	10.3	29.3	75.2	174.3
Venezuela	4.8	22.5	72.8	155.6	283.8
Asia					
Hong Kong	1.2	5.6	26.6	56.4	90.5
Japan	2.1	5.5	18.1	54.2	97.0
Singapore	3.5	16.9	64.6	182.7	236.3
Europe					
England and Wales	2.1	3.6	12.0	37.5	93.3
Malta	8.7	28.1	146.4	491.9	1243.9
Norway	2.0	3.6	6.8	23.3	70.3
Sweden	6.1	8.2	17.6	57.8	214.4

sometimes heavily glycosuric, diabetics of this type are usually diagnosed later in life, are often obese, only moderately symptomatic, free of ketosis and spared the progression to coma and death of the classical case. This is non-insulin-dependent diabetes mellitus (NIDDM or Type 2). In the last 50 years, the application of clinical biochemistry and automated technology to large, apparently healthy populations has brought to light large numbers of people with high blood glucose concentrations or glucose 'intolerance' but without signs or symptoms of disease. Depending on the degree of disturbance, such people are diagnosed NIDDM or placed into the new at-risk class of impaired glucose tolerance (IGT) (See Appendix).

This evolution of the concept of diabetes influences estimates of prevalence. Early studies included symptoms or the presence of glycosuria in the diagnostic definition, lowering prevalence estimates compared with those based only upon measurements of blood glucose concentration. Even if case-finding is restricted to blood glucose measurements, prevalence rates vary as much as 10-fold according to the diagnostic glycaemic criteria selected. West has shown that, even among experts, there was little consensus on these.[6] The international propagation of a set of diagnostic values by WHO[5] should achieve a much greater degree of consistency and comparability (Appendix). Estimates of diabetic complications have also lacked standardization, and international agreement on these is only now being achieved. Thus, for all comparisons of prevalence and incidence studies of diabetes conducted until the early 1980s, variability in ascertainment methods, conditions of blood glucose measurement, interpretation of values and levels of confirmation must be allowed for.

3 Diabetes in Caucasoid Peoples

a *Insulin-Dependent Diabetes*

Insulin-dependent diabetes mellitus (IDDM, Type 1) is characteristic of Caucasoid peoples and much less common in, or even absent from, some other ethnic groups. In earlier studies, it has usually been merged in estimates of total diabetes incidence and prevalence. Although IDDM presents clinically throughout life, almost all studies limit themselves to cases diagnosed in childhood (0–14 years, Table II) or before 30 years of age. Methods and levels of ascertainment differ; and variation in these methods may contribute to, but cannot fully explain the distinct differences in prevalence and incidence, even within Europe, which have been reported.

The Scandinavian countries consistently report both incidence and prevalence rates significantly in excess of European averages, particularly in comparison with the countries of Southern Europe (Spain, France, Italy). Even within Finland, prevalence is significantly higher in the East than in the rest of Finland.[9] Some confirmation of the low incidence rates in IDDM in under 17 year olds in France comes from a comparison of juveniles of French compared with non-French (largely British) extraction in Montreal.[16] These regional European differences in prevalence and incidence are unexplained. They may be related to differences in the size of the pool of individuals susceptible to IDDM, a status which has been genetically linked with the DR3 and DR4 antigens of the HLA complex.[17] These specificities, either in heterozygous or homozygous combination and more particularly as the DR3/DR4 heterozygote are found in 90% or more Caucasian subjects with youthful-onset IDDM and appear to be identifiable as (or very closely linked with) the genetic component of IDDM susceptibility. The IDDM link may be with subtypes of the DR antigens, at present more readily identifiable by analysis of the DNA sequence of the MHC coding region of the 6th chromosome than by the conventional methods of HLA typing.[18] The much reduced susceptibility of non-Caucasoid peoples to IDDM has been attributed to the absence of the appropriate HLA antigens from their ethnic repertoire.[19] Variability of allelic frequencies across the peoples of Europe may, in part, explain the IDDM gradients noted above. However, the probable rise in IDDM frequency in Finland[9] and elsewhere[20] since the 1950s directed attention to the environmental determinants of IDDM expression. In only about half the identical twin pairs with IDDM studied by Pyke and colleagues[21] was the condition present in both twins. Viral infections[22] may trigger in immuno-genetically susceptible people a sequence of events resulting in pancreatic B-cell destruction, by way of autoimmune mechanisms.[23] The evidence for viral involvement is largely indirect. Age- and seasonal-peaks of incidence in childhood could coincide with exposure to infection.[24,25] In one celebrated recent-onset case,[26] Coxsackie B4 virus was isolated from the pancreas. It is likely that other as yet unidentified environmental factors play a determining role. From Iceland, Helgason and Jonasson[27] reported a highly significant clustering of birthdates in October of boys with IDDM, diagnosed at 0–14 years of age. They suggested that maternal consumption of smoked mutton, a traditional Christmas/New Year delicacy, at or about the time of conception of these boys might have initiated B-cell damage culminating in ketosis-prone diabetes in childhood. A number of substances (alloxan, streptozotocin, the rodenticide Vacor) are toxic to B cells, sometimes long after repeated low dosage.[28] Even the declining practice of breast feeding has been suggested as a cause of the rising Scandinavian incidence. Socio-economic determinants, suspected in one study,[25] have been unsupported or reversed in effect by others.[16,20,29]

b *Non-Insulin-Dependent Diabetes*

The prevalence of the other major class of DM, the non-insulin-dependent variety (NIDDM) is much the more common type in Caucasoid peoples.[30] It appears to be determined by the prevalence of ill-defined but powerful and probably genetically mediated individual susceptibility factors. Almost 100% of identical twin pairs are concordant for NIDDM[21] by contrast with the 50% discordant for IDDM.

Within large populations, obesity is a predictor of diabetic risk[31] but in Caucasoid peoples there is little information to attribute variation in NIDDM prevalence to differences in the diabetogenic effects of obesity. In West's standardized comparisons of glucose intolerance/diabetes between populations,[32,33] the degree of adiposity was highly significantly correlated with DM rates.

A recent epidemiological study[34] compared the incidence of diabetes newly diagnosed between the ages of 18 and 50 years in nine British towns, selected for upper, medium and lower socio-economic status in three latitudes of England and Wales. There was little, if any, difference in IDDM rates and no influence of latitude on NIDDM rates but more than a two-fold difference in

TABLE II. Prevalence and incidence of IDDM, 0–14 years

Region	Prevalence/10^3	Ref.	Incidence/10^5/yr.	Ref.
Sweden	1.32	7	19.6	7
Norway	1.16	8	17.6	8
Finland	2.23	9	28.6	10
France	0.24	11	3.7	11
Minnesota	1.89	12	19.6	13
Cuba	0.14	14		
Shanghai	<0.09	15		

rates between upper ($10/10^5$/yr age/sex-standardized incidence) and lower ($23/10^5$) socio-economic status towns with medium status towns intermediate ($13/10^5$). The rates standardized for social class composition within the towns remained at 7.5, 10.2 and $19.6/10^5$ (upper, medium and lower towns respectively). There was no evidence for systematic differences in hospital referral patterns, diagnostic standards for NIDDM or body build among the three classes of town.

Systematic application of 75g oral glucose tolerance tests to a large USA population sample in the 1976 to 1980 Health and Nutrition Examination Survey[35] using WHO diagnostic criteria, showed a prevalence of undiagnosed diabetes rising from 1.0% in the 20–44 age group to 8.6% in the 65–74 age group, rates closely comparable to those of known DM. Rates of impaired glucose tolerance (IGT) were three to four times higher. Total (20–74) rate for DM (known and newly diagnosed) was 6.7% and for IGT 11.3%, similar to the rates found in the Bedford Survey of the early 1960s.[36]

4 Diabetes in Developing Countries

The familiar 'Caucasian' patterns of diabetes are modified in non-European peoples, particularly in the populations of developing countries. The most notable 'deviant' type is variously termed tropical, pancreatic, or malnutrition diabetes. It has several distinctive features distributed geographically in such a way as to suggest that they represent several different but overlapping entities. There are two classic descriptive sources. Hugh-Jones[37] described among West Indian people 'many cases in young adults under 40 and even in children . . . [who] . . . persistently require large doses of insulin to control glycosuria and so maintain their weight, are relatively insensitive to its action, and show little or no ketosis if insulin is withheld. Such cases will be called type J.' Insulin requirement ran at 80 or more units daily, contrasting with the 30–50, usual for the Caucasoid IDDM patient. In some, insulin could be withdrawn with no marked relapse of the diabetic state. Type J constituted about 10% of Hugh-Jones' cases, the rest being similar to the IDDM and NIDDM of Caucasians. Hugh-Jones was unable to isolate any local factors provoking J-type diabetes and found no clear dietary or nutritional associations, but he noted the frequency of associated 'complications' in which he included metabolic coma and pyogenic and tuberculous infections as well as the more specific complications of retinopathy, nephropathy, neuropathy, and cataract.

From Indonesia, Zuidema[38] published the first clear description of diabetes associated with pancreatic calcification (Plate 00). Emaciation was severe, high doses of insulin were required for treatment but there was little tendency to ketosis. In all cases, there was a history of protein subnutrition but this was also common in the non-diabetic population. Pancreatic fibrosis without radiologically demonstrable calcification is also associated with a similar type of diabetes. Further reports, in particular those of Geevarghese et al.[39] from India, supported the view that the spectrum of pancreatic fibrosis/calcification with DM represents a single syndrome. Calcific pancreatitis with diabetes has been reported from widely separated tropical areas, from Indonesia, India (particularly the Kerala region), Ceylon, Central Africa, and South America.[40] However, there are regional variations within countries in frequency and manifestation of this form of DM. In New Delhi, Vaishnava et al.[41] found only two instances in 84 youthful-onset diabetics. Kinnear[42] found pancreatic calcification in 75% of young Nigerian diabetics while Seftel[43] found none in diabetic black Africans. Nwokolo and Oli[44] suggested that this variable

frequency of pancreatic diabetes in tropical areas was related to the absence or presence of protein in the largely carbohydrate foods. Even the low (10%) protein content of cereals such as sorghum, millet, maize, and rice could stimulate the flow of pancreatic juice and reduce the stasis, pancreatic duct obstruction, infection, and calcification typical of the syndrome. A further hypothesis investigated by McMillan and Geevarghese,[45] points to the possibility of toxic effects resulting from the cyanogenic glycosides in cassava and other tropical root and leguminous foods. Dietary cyanide is normally detoxicated to thiocyanate at the expense of the sulphur-containing amino acids cysteine and methionine. Under conditions of low protein consumption, pancreatic damage may result either from undetoxicated free cyanide or from the diversion of the limited supply of methionine for which the pancreas has a specific requirement.

Heterogeneity in diabetes in African and Indian patients in South Africa was suggested by the markedly higher frequency of a family history of the disease in the former than the latter.[46] In both groups, there appeared to be clear family links between IDDM and NIDDM forms, not seen in Caucasian populations.[47] Pancreatic damage and diabetes in Africans may follow epidemic infection with hepatitis virus[48] and haemochromatosis associated with pancreatic fibrosis was demonstrated in 7% of a consecutive series of Bantu diabetics aged 40 years or more.[49] All had consumed quantities of home-brewed alcoholic drinks known to be high in iron and also to contain other possibly hepato- and pancreatico-toxic substances.

5 Diabetes in other Populations

Epidemics of diabetes have been described among populations in the Pacific region. High rates were already evident in the 1960s and a relationship with obesity and Westernized life styles was suggested.[50-52] The most striking recent example comes from the population of the Island of Nauru[53] with an estimated per-capita income of US$30000 per annum from the Island's rich phosphate deposit; food intake has risen sharply to about 6000 calories per day and physical activity has declined (with approximately one automobile per adult). The overall diabetes prevalence rate for inhabitants aged more than 20 years and more is 30.3%. Prevalence increases with age but unlike most other populations, blood glucose concentrations are bimodally distributed,[54] suggesting two levels of diabetes susceptibility, probably genetically mediated. In many respects, the Nauruans resemble the Pima Indian tribe[55,56] also grossly obese, relatively inbred, with comparably high diabetes risk and bimodal blood glucose distribution. In both, diabetes is of NIDDM type and IDDM is very uncommon. A comparison of prevalence rates of IGT and DM (using the new WHO definitions) in the three major Pacific population groups is shown in Table III.[57] As elsewhere[30], rates in urban populations usually exceed those in rural communities.

The prevalence of NIDDM is generally considered high in Middle Eastern countries. A recent report from Kuwait,[58] however, suggests that IDDM rates may resemble those in some Caucasoid populations though there is some doubt about their insulin dependency. In 1385 male Saudi Arabs[59] only one was found to be affected under 35 years of age but rates rose rapidly at greater ages.

6 Complications of Diabetes

Comparison of diabetes complication rates has been bedevilled by the absence of agreed definitions and criteria. Encouraged by

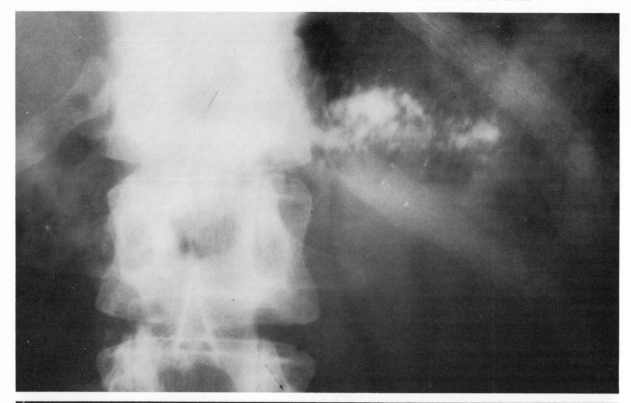

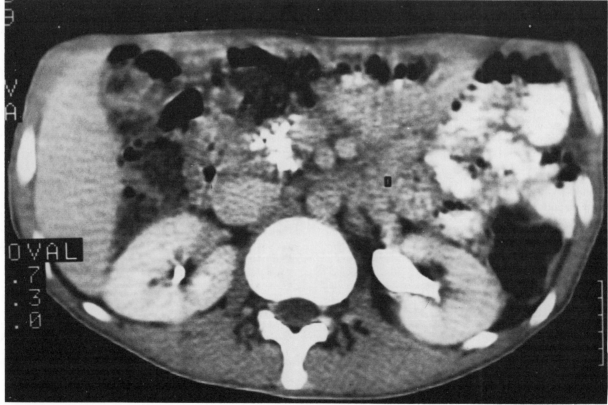

FIG. 1. Calcification in the pancreas is seen in the abdominal x-ray and the computerized tomographic (CT) scan (below) of an Indian patient with 'tropical diabetes'. The CT scan also shows the wasted, scaphoid abdominal contour in section and the absence of intra-abdominal fat depots.

(*Courtesy of Professor M M S Ahuja, New Delhi*)

TABLE III. Prevalence (%) of impaired glucose tolerance (IGT) and diabetes mellitus in some Pacific populations aged > 20 years (crude rates)
(From King *et al.*[58] and other reports of this group)

Population group	Males			Females			Combined sexes		
	No. tested	IGT	DM	No. tested	IGT	DM	No. tested	IGT	DM
Micronesians									
Nauru	217	19.4	30.9	239	25.1	29.7	456	22.4	30.3
Polynesians									
Western Samoa									
Rural	358	4.2	1.7	387	3.6	4.9	745	3.9	3.4
Urban	325	7.7	8.6	419	8.8	8.8	744	8.3	8.7
Tuvalu	189	9.0	1.1	208	17.8	7.2	397	13.6	4.3
New Caledonia									
Ouvea*	164	4.9	6.7	237	10.1	7.2	401	8.0	7.0
Touho rural		4.6			10.6				
urban		5.7			9.1				
Melanesians									
New Caledonia									
Ouvea	228	3.5	0.0	307	6.2	3.9	535	5.0	2.2
Touho	90	6.7	2.2	82	4.9	1.2	172	5.8	1.7

* Including Melanesians.

the success of WHO in creating international standards for cardiovascular disease,[60] a multinational group under WHO sponsorship agreed to a protocol for a standardized study of complications in diabetics.[61] Approximately 500 patients between 35 and 55 years of age were selected from each of 14 national samples, recruited by agreed methods to achieve maximum representativity and stratified for sex, age, and known duration of DM.

A condensed version of the results is presented in Table IV. It shows considerable group-to-group variation in most of the complication indices chosen. Many of the indices were assessed locally so that, despite a 'training' meeting for participating groups, some variation stems from differences between observers. However, all electrocardiograms (ECGs) were read and Minnesota coded[60,61] centrally. The low rate of major ECG changes in Tokyo and Hong Kong diabetics supports earlier reports of the relatively protected status of Oriental diabetics against atherosclerosis,[63,64] which, however, appears to be lost when they move into a more Westernized environment.[65] Only 3 out of 453 Chinese diabetics (0.7%) recruited according to the WHO Study protocol in Beijing had major ECG changes when centrally read (Chi Zhisheng,

personal communication, 1983). Less difference between centres was found in respect of rates of abnormal S-T segment or T-wave items, suggesting their non-ischaemic origin.

The variation in rates of heavy proteinuria and severe retinopathy, specific complications of diabetes, are more difficult to interpret. Part of the three- to five-fold variation is probably real; the Japanese (Tokyo) sample, with its high rates of heavy proteinuria, severe retinopathy and retinopathic blindness appears to be truly more susceptible to diabetic microangiopathy than most of the other groups, corresponding with the relatively high contribution of renal disease to mortality in Japanese diabetics.[66] The Japanese differ as strikingly from the Hong Kong sample in microangiopathy as they resemble them in respect of major ECG changes. The degree of 'control' of the diabetic state is generally accepted as an important determinant of liability to specific diabetic complications,[67] but other non-glycaemic, possibly genetic, factors may play an important part. This first standardized study of diabetic complications suggest that geographical, perhaps ethnic, factors are also involved.

No African (or North American) white or black group was recruited to the WHO Study, but Lester has provided evidence[68]

TABLE IV. Prevalence of complications in diabetics aged 35–55
(From WHO Multinational Study of Vascular Disease in Diabetics)

Centre	Number		Corrected* percent with:				
	Men	Women	Heavy p/u	Severe r/p	r/p blind	ECG prob.	H/t
London	254	243	4.0	6.6	1.9	4.1	25.8
Switzerland	278	256	11.9	7.2	3.6	6.2	36.3
Brussels	236	186	3.3	6.0	2.4	4.4	34.8
Moscow	226	273	13.3	5.2	1.9	2.9	43.2
Warsaw	241	245	12.9	3.5	2.0	2.9	32.3
Berlin	285	275	11.1	6.3	1.1	7.5	37.3
Zagreb	222	180	11.9	11.7	2.7	3.5	42.5
New Delhi	289	266	11.0	5.0	1.7	4.8	29.8
Hong Kong	198	226	2.4	5.4	3.4	0.7	29.3
Tokyo	235	201	17.8	12.3	4.3	1.5	28.2
Havana	258	257	7.2	3.8	2.9	3.6	36.0
Oklahoma	270	383	15.3	9.2	3.0	8.7	35.3
Arizona	87	154	11.6	12.7	2.3	3.2	29.7
Bulgaria	222	251	5.4	11.6	5.2	3.5	33.6

Abbreviations: Heavy p/u: heavy proteinuria; Severe r/p: severe retinopathy (new vessels, vitreous opacity/haemorrhage, large retinal haemorrhages, retinopathic blindness (r/p blind) in either eye); ECG prob.: probable electrocardiographic evidence of myocardial infarction (Minnesota Code Q/QS items items 1.1, 1.2 or 7.1); h/t: hypertension [systolic pressure ≥ 160 mmHg, diastolic pressure (phase 5) ≥ 95 mmHg or receiving antihypertensive treatment].
* In order to allow for deviations from protocol stratification requirements, overall estimates of prevalence rates for heavy p.u, severe r/p and r/p blind were standardized for sex and duration by taking the mean of the six sex/duration (0–6, 7–13, 14 + years × M, F) group means; and for sex and age in respect of ECG prob and h/t overall estimates by taking the mean of the six sex/age (35–41, 42–48, 49–55 × M, F) group means.
Data abstracted from the WHO Report 'Vascular Disease in Diabetics' (NCD/OND/79.4) available on request from WHO, Geneva. Further details of this prevalence study may be obtained from references 62, 63, 70.

that diabetics of relatively long duration observed in Ethiopia are at least as vulnerable to diabetic eye and kidney complications, though they resemble the Oriental diabetics in low rates of coronary heart disease. A summary of the relatively fragmentary data from Uganda, Kenya, Tanzania, Nigeria, Senegal and Ethiopia demonstrates rates of retinal, lens, kidney and nerve disease lying within the WHO Multinational Study prevalence range.[69] Retinopathy and nephropathy in the diabetics of the Pacific region appear to be correlated as elsewhere with severity and duration of hyperglycaemia[70,71] but ethnic differences in susceptibility may also operate.

7 Conclusions

National and regional mortality rates suggest, and systematic population studies confirm, the wide geographical diversity in rates and types of diabetes mellitus. In many groups, ascertainment is far from complete and only recently has there been international consensus on diagnostic standards. In some populations, there is good evidence that the diabetic state results from environmental factors operating in genetically susceptible subjects. However, the relative importance of these two components and their nature probably vary among populations. Their clearer identification is of first importance in respect of planned preventive activities. The retinal and renal complications of diabetes appear to be associated with all forms of the disease although there may be quite large unexplained variation in susceptibility to them; recent studies confirm the very widely diverse susceptibility to atherosclerotic arterial disease, long-suspected and running broadly parallel to differences in non-diabetic populations. Prevention of complications thus appears to

require attention to control of the diabetic state itself as well as of factors, probably dietary, which affect the population as a whole.

APPENDIX: CRITERIA AND CLASSIFICATION OF DIABETES MELLITUS (WHO, 1980)

Glycaemia Criteria. Diagnosis of diabetes mellitus is confirmed by blood glucose measurement. When classical symptoms are present, random venous plasma concentration of 11 mmol (200 mg/dl) or fasting values of 8 mmol/l (140 mg/dl) are diagnostic. If an oral glucose tolerance test (OGTT) is carried out, diagnosis is based on fasting values and/or those 2 hours after 75g oral glucose in solution. DM is present with:

Fasting value	$\geqslant$ 8 mmol/l (140 mg/dl)
and/or 2 hour value	$\geqslant$ 11 mmol/l (200 mg/dl)
Impaired glucose tolerance (IGT):	
Fasting value	$<$ 8 mmol/l (140 mg/dl)
and 2 hour value	$\geqslant$ 8 mmol/l (140 mg/dl)
	$<$ 11 mmol/l (200 mg/dl)

Classification. DM is classified as follows:

Insulin-dependent diabetes mellitus (IDDM, Type 1)
Non insulin-dependent diabetes mellitus (NIDDM, Type 2): (a) non-obese; (b) obese
Other types of diabetes mellitus (of known cause or association)
Gestational diabetes mellitus (first diagnosed in pregnancy)

Two classes of increased risk for diabetes are also recognized in people with normal glucose tolerance, viz. those who have shown 'previous abnormality of glucose tolerance' and those with 'potential abnormality of glucose tolerance'.

For full discussion of criteria and classification, the reader is referred to References 4, 5.

WHO recommended 'rounding off' SI units as indicated. This has not met with agreement and corrected values are preferable, i.e. for 11 mmol/l read 11.1 mmol/l; for 8 mmol/l read 7.8 mmol/l.

REFERENCES

1 West, KM. Epidemiology of diabetes and its vascular lesions. New York: Elsevier, 1978; 159–190
2 Fuller, JH, Elford J, Goldblatt P, Adelstein AM. Diabetes mortality: new light on an underestimated public health problem. Diabetologia 1983; 24: 336–341
3 Tokuhata GK, Miller W, Digon E, Hartman T. Diabetes mellitus: an underestimated public health problem. J Chronic Dis 1975; 28: 23–35
4 National Diabetes Data Group. Classification and diagnosis of diabetes mellitus and other categories of glucose intolerance. Diabetes 1979; 28: 1039–1057
5 WHO Expert Committee on Diabetes Mellitus. Second Report. Geneva: World Health Organization, 1980. (Technical Report Series 646)
6 West KM. Substantial differences in diagnostic criteria used by diabetes experts. Diabetes 1975; 24: 641–644
7 Sterky G, Holmgren G, Gustavson KH, et al. The incidence of diabetes mellitus in Swedish children 1970–1975. Acta Paediatr Scand 1978; 67: 139–143
8 Joner G, Søvik O. Incidence, age at onset and seasonal variation of diabetes mellitus in Norwegian children 1973–77. Acta Paediatr Scand 1981; 70: 329–335
9 Koivisto VA, Åkerblom HK, Wasz-Höckert O. The epidemiology of juvenile diabetes mellitus in Northern Finland. Nord Council Arct Med Res 1976; 15: 58–65
10 Åkerblom, HK, Reunanen A, Käär M-L. The incidence of insulin-dependent diabetes mellitus in 0–4 year-old-children in Finland in 1970–80. Nord Council Arct Med Res Rep 1980; 26: 60–66
11 Lestradet H, Besse J. Prévalence et incidence du diabète juvénile insulino-dépendant en France. Diabete Metab 1977; 3: 229-234
12 Kyllo CJ, Nuttall FQ. Prevalence of diabetes mellitus in school-age children in Minnesota. Diabetes 1978; 27: 57–60
13 Palumbo PJ, Elveback LR, Chu C-P, Connolly DC, Kurland LT. Diabetes mellitus: incidence, prevalence, survivorship and causes of death in Rochester, Minnesota, 1945–1970. Diabetes 1976; 25: 566–573

14 Matteo-de-Acosta O, Amaro S, Díaz O. Diabetes in Cuba. Acta Diabetol Lat 1973; 10: 534–546
15 Shanghai Diabetes Research Cooperative Group. Diabetes mellitus survey in Shanghai. Chin Med J 1980; 93: 663–667
16 Colle E, Siemiatycki J, West R, et al. Incidence of juvenile onset diabetes in Montreal-demonstration of ethnic differences and socio-economic class differences. J Chronic Dis 1981; 34: 611–616
17 Wolf E, Spencer KM, Cudworth AG. The genetic susceptibility to type 1 (insulin-dependent) diabetes: Analysis of the HLA-DR association. Diabetologia: 1983; 24: 224–230
18 Owerbach D, Lernmark A, Platz P, et al. HLA-D region β-chain DNA endonuclease fragments differ between HLA-DR identical healthy and insulin-dependent diabetic individuals. Nature: 1983; 303: 815–817
19 Nerup J, Christy M, Green A, et al. HLA and insulin dependent diabetes—population studies. In: Köbberling J, Tattersall R, eds. The Genetics of Diabetes Mellitus. Proceedings of the Serono Symposia, Vol. 47. London, Academic Press, 1982; 35–42
20 Stewart-Brown S, Haslum M, Butler N. Evidence for increasing prevalence of diabetes mellitus in childhood. Br Med J 1983; 286: 1855–1857
21 Barnett AH, Eff C, Leslie RDG, Pyke DA. Diabetes in identical twins. Diabetologia 1981; 20: 87–93
22 Gamble DR. The epidemiology of insulin dependent diabetes with particular reference to the relationship of virus infection to its etiology. Epidemiol Rev 1980; 2: 49–70
23 Nerup J, Lernmark A. Autoimmunity in insulin-dependent diabetes mellitus. Am J Med 1981; 70: 135–141
24 Larsson Y, Dahlquist G. The epidemiology of Type 1 diabetes. In: Boström H, Ljungstedt N, eds. Recent trends in diabetes research. Skandia International Symposia. Stockholm: Almqvist and Wiksell International, 1982: 41–58
25 Christau B, Kromann H, Ortved Anderson O, et al. Incidence, seasonal and geographical patterns of juvenile-onset insulin-dependent diabetes mellitus in Denmark. Diabetologia 1977; 13: 281–284

26 Yoon J-W, Austin M, Onodera T, Notkins AL. Virus induced diabetes mellitus. N Engl J Med 1979; 300: 1173–1179

27 Helgason T, Jonasson MR. Evidence for a food additive as a cause of ketosis-prone diabetes. Lancet 1981; 2: 716–720

28 Rossini AA, Like AA, Chick WL, Appel MC, Cahill GF Jr. Studies of streptozotocin-induced insulitis and diabetes. Proc Natl Acad Sci USA 1977; 74: 2485–2489

29 Cohen T. Juvenile diabetes in Israel. J Med Sci 1971; 7: 1558–1561

30 Zimmet P. Type 2 (non insulin-dependent) diabetes—an epidemiological overview. Diabetologia 1982; 22: 399–411

31 West KM. Epidemiology of diabetes and its vascular lesions. New York: Elsevier, 1978; 231–248

32 West KM, Kalbfleisch JM. Glucose tolerance, nutrition, and diabetes in Uruguay, Venezuela, Malaya and East Pakistan. Diabetes 1966; 15: 9–18

33 West KM, Kalbfleisch JM. Diabetes in Central America. Diabetes 1970; 19: 656–663

34 Barker DJP, Gardner MJ, Power C. Incidence of diabetes amongst people aged 18–50 years in nine British towns: a collaborative study. Diabetologia 1982; 22: 421–425

35 Harris M. Epidemiologic characteristics of impaired glucose tolerance in the US population. Bethesda, Maryland: National Institutes of Health, National Diabetes Data Group, 1984

36 Keen H, Jarrett RJ, McCartney P. The ten-year follow-up of the Bedford Survey (1962-1972): glucose tolerance and diabetes. Diabetologia 1982; 22: 73-78

37 Hugh-Jones P. Diabetes in Jamaica. Lancet 1955; 2: 891–897

38 Zuidema PJ. Calcification and cirrhosis of the pancreas in patients with deficient nutrient. Doc Med Geogr Trop 1955; 7: 229–251

39 Geevarghese PJ. Pancreatic diabetes. Bombay: Popular Prakasham, 1968

40 West KM. Epidemiology of diabetes and its vascular lesions. New York: Elsevier, 1978: 321–338

41 Vaishnava H, Bashin RC, Gulati PD, *et al*. Diabetes mellitus with onset under 40 years in North India. J. Assoc Physicians India 1974; 22: 879–888

42 Kinnear TWG. The pattern of diabetes mellitus in a Nigerian teaching hospital. East Afr Med J 1963; 40: 288–294

43 Seftel HC, Schultz E. Diabetes mellitus in the urbanised Johannesburg African. S Afr Med J 1971; 35: 66–70

44 Nwokolo C, Oli J. Pathogenesis of juvenile tropical pancreatitis syndrome. Lancet 1980; 1: 456–458

45 McMillan DE, Geevarghese PJ. Dietary cyanide and tropical malnutrition diabetes. Diabetes Care 1979; 2: 202–208

46 Omar MAK, Asmal AC. Family histories of diabetes mellitus in young African and Indian diabetics. Br. Med J 1983; 286: 1786

47 MacDonald MJ. Equal incidence of adult-onset diabetes among ancestors of juvenile diabetics and nondiabetics. Diabetologia 1974; 10: 767–773

48 Oli JM, Nwokolo C. Diabetes after infectious hepatitis: a follow-up study. Br Med J 1979; 1: 926–927

49 Seftel HC, Keeley KJ, Isaacson C, Bothwell TH. Siderosis in the Bantu: the clinical incidence of hemochromatosis in diabetic subjects. J Lab Clin Med. 1961; 58: 837–844

50 Prior AM, Davidson F. The epidemiology of diabetes in Polynesians and Europeans in New Zealand and the Pacific. NZ Med J 1966; 65: 375–383

51 Prior IAM, Beaglehole R, Davidson F, Salmond CE. The relationship of diabetes, blood lipids, and uric acid levels in Polynesians. Adv Metab Disord 1978; 9: 241–261

52 Sloan NR. Ethnic distribution of diabetes in Hawaii. JAMA 1963; 183: 419–424

53 Zimmet P, Taft P, Guinea A, Guthrie W, Thoma K. The high prevalence of diabetes mellitus on a Central Pacific Island. Diabetologia 1977; 13: 111–115

54 Zimmet P, Whitehouse S. Bimodality of fasting and two-hour glucose tolerance distributions in a Micronesian population. Diabetes: 1978; 27: 793-800

55 Bennett PH, Rushforth NB, Miller M, Le Compte PM. Epidemiologic studies of diabetes in the Pima Indians. Recent Prog Horm Res 1976; 32: 333–376

56 Knowler WC, Pettit DJ, Bennett PH, Williams RC. Diabetes mellitus in the Pima Indians: genetic and evolutionary considerations. Am J Phys Anthropol 1983; 62: 107–114

57 King H, Zimmet P, Raper LR, Balkau B. Risk factors for diabetes in three Pacific populations. Am J Epidemiol 1984. In press

58 Taha TH, Moussa MAA, Rashid AR, Fenech FF. Diabetes mellitus in Kuwait. Incidence in the first 29 years of life. Diabetologia 1983; 25: 306–308

59 Bacchus RA, Bell JL, Madkour M, Kilshaw B. The prevalence of diabetes mellitus in male Saudi Arabs. Diabetologia 1982; 23: 330–332

60 Rose GA, Blackburn H. Cardiovascular survey methods. Geneva: World Health Organization, 1968. (WHO Monograph Series No. 56)

61 Jarrett RJ, Keen H, Grabauskas AV. The WHO multinational study of vascular disease in diabetes: 1. General description. Diabetes Care 1979; 2: 175–186

62 Keen H, Jarrett RJ. The WHO multinational study of vascular disease in diabetes: 2. Macrovascular disease prevalence. Diabetes Care 1979; 2: 187–195

63 Goto Y, Sato S-I, Masuda M. Causes of death in 3151 diabetic autopsy cases. Tohoku J Exp Med 1974; 112: 339–346

64 Horiuchi A, Kitamura S, Tanaka G, Niki ZY, Hirose H, Matsuoka K. Angiopathy of diabetes in Japan. In: Tsuji S, Wada M, eds. Diabetes Mellitus in Asia, 1970. Proceedings of a Symposium, Kobe 1970. Amsterdam: Excerpta Medica, 1971; 205–212 (International Congress Series No. 221)

65 Kawate R, Yamakido M, Nishimoto Y, Bennett PH, Hamman RF, Knowler WC. Diabetes mellitus and its vascular complications in Japanese migrants on the Island of Hawaii. Diabetes Care 1979; 2: 161–170

66 Sasaki A, Vehara M, Horiuchi N, Hasagawa K. A long-term follow-up study of Japanese diabetic patients: mortality and causes of death. Diabetologia 1983; 25: 309–312

67 Tchobroutsky G. Relation of diabetic control to development of microvascular complications. Diabetologia 1978; 15: 143–152

68 Lester FT. Long-standing diabetes mellitus in Ethiopia: a survey of 105 patients. Diabetologia 1983; 25: 222–225

69 Jarrett RJ, Keen H. The WHO multinational study of vascular disease in diabetes: 3. Microvascular disease. Diabetes Care 1979; 2: 196–201

70 Zimmet P, Taylor R, Bennett PH. Diabetic microangiopathy in Pacific populations. Igaku Kenkyū Shinkō Zaidan 1982; 20: 355–364

71 King H, Balkau B, Zimmet P *et al*. Diabetic retinopathy in Nauruans. Am J. Epidemiol 1982; 117: 659–667

72 World Health Organization. World health statistics annual 1978. Vol. 1. Vital statistics and causes of death. Geneva: WHO, 1978

British Medical Bulletin (1984) Vol. 40, No. 4, pp. 366–373

GEOGRAPHIC VARIATIONS IN CARDIOVASCULAR MORTALITY IN GREAT BRITAIN

A G SHAPER FRCP FRCPath FFCM

Department of Clinical Epidemiology and General Practice
Royal Free Hospital School of Medicine
London

For more than a century, the regional variations in cardiovascular disease in Great Britain have aroused considerable interest and have been described, mapped and debated.[1-3] The aims have been fairly constant, 'to determine . . . if the mortality from this cause showed any notable variation in different parts of the country, if the districts with high and low rates of mortality were distributed in any special manner, and if the geographical distribution of heart disease had any . . . association with special features, or industrial conditions'.[2] There have been some changes over the century, with myocardial degeneration 'disappearing'[4] and with the focus of attention moving from rheumatic heart disease to ischaemic heart disease. There has also been a growing interest in those factors controlled by society and the individual rather than those determined by the climatic and physical characteristics of the regions, particularly those which we may be able to modify in attempts to reduce morbidity and mortality from cardiovascular disease, e.g. diet, cigarette smoking, high blood pressure and psycho-social stress.

But the essential geographic question has persisted: why a line drawn from the Severn Estuary to the estuary of the Humber divides the country into a northern half with high mortality from cardiovascular disease and a southern half with low mortality.[5]

1   The Water Story

Modern examination of the regional variations in cardiovascular disease in Great Britain is closely related to studies of the association between cardiovascular mortality and the hardness of drinking water. The initial stimulus came from Japan, where a close association between death rates from apoplexy (cerebrovascular accidents) and the acidity of the river water used for drinking was reported.[6] The more acid the water, the higher the death rates from apoplexy. Schroeder examined the data and found 'a fairly good correlation between deaths from apoplexy and acidity of river water and a better one between death rates from heart disease and water'.[7]

The nature of the 'heart disease' is uncertain, but it seems extremely unlikely that it included any appreciable amount of ischaemic heart disease, which at that time (1950) was rare in Japan.

Schroeder made it clear that 'There were no significant correlations of death rates from heart disease or cerebrovascular accidents by districts *with hardness* or with any other common constituent of water, except for the sulphate-bicarbonate ratios (acidity)'.[8] He went on to examine the relationships between cardiovascular mortality and treated water supplies in the United States and found significant negative correlations between water hardness and all cardiovascular diseases and to a lesser extent with coronary heart disease and strokes.[9-11]

a   *Statistical Studies*

Morris and Crawford and their colleagues in the MRC Social Medicine Unit in London set out to see whether there was a case for investigating the 'Water Story' in Great Britain, using mortality data for 1948–1954 from the 83 county boroughs of England and Wales.[12] They found striking negative correlations between water hardness and total cardiovascular mortality and substantial negative correlations for deaths from cerebrovascular disease and myocardial degeneration for males and females aged 45–64 and 65–74. For coronary heart disease, the correlation was significant for men aged 45–64 but not for older men or for women. The negative correlation with bronchitis was also consistently significant.

Correlations between water hardness and a wide variety of local environmental and socio-economic indices failed to reveal any confounding variables likely to explain the relationship between water hardness and cardiovascular mortality.

A further statistical study was carried out using improved water data and mortality data for 1958–1964, for the 61 county boroughs of England and Wales with a total population of 80000 or more at the 1961 Census.[13] The findings were similar to the earlier study except that now the negative correlations between water hardness and coronary heart disease were significant for men and women in both age groups; this probably reflects the transfer of 'myocardial degeneration' into 'coronary heart disease'.[4] Multiple regression analysis showed that the contribution of socio-economic factors to the differences in cardiovascular mortality between the towns was small and that latitude had some slight effect. A more detailed examination of the 1948–1954 and the 1958–1964 mortality data was later made using five independent variables in a multiple regression analysis: a social factor score, domestic air pollution, latitude, water calcium and rainfall.[14] Analysis showed that rainfall, latitude and water calcium all made significant independent contributions to the explanation of the variance in total cardiovascular mortality between the 61 county boroughs, with broadly similar associations for coronary heart disease and for cerebrovascular disease.

b   *Pathological Studies*

A comparison was then made of cardiac lesions at necropsy in men in Glasgow (high cardiovascular mortality, very soft water) and London (low cardiovascular mortality, hard water).[15] The men had died either in accidents (88) or suddenly from ischaemic heart disease (194). The prevalence of confluent atheroma was much the same in the accident cases from the two cities; more healed infarcts were present in the Glasgow series. In the ischaemic heart disease subjects, the Glasgow men showed less confluent atheroma and less stenosis than the London subjects. The authors concluded that myocardial disease seemed more likely to develop in men in Glasgow than in London, given the same amount of coronary atheroma and suggested that the myocardium was more susceptible to minor degrees of ischaemia in Glasgow (soft water) than in London (hard water). The implication was that the increased cardiovascular mortality in Glasgow was related to the lack of calcium and magnesium in the drinking water.

c *Changes in Water Hardness*

Morris and his colleagues then tried to determine whether a change in the hardness of water supply would affect cardiovascular mortality. Their study was based on a comparison of the changes in death rates of towns which had increased water hardness (n = 5), decreased water hardness (n = 6) or remain unchanged (n = 72) over the 30 or so years up to 1960.[16] The results showed that in general, changes in cardiovascular death rates between 1951 and 1961 showed a favourable effect in the towns where the water had become harder and an unfavourable effect in the towns where water had become softer; non-cardiovascular death rates were not affected. The findings were consistent for men aged 45–64 and 65–74 and for women aged 45–64; women aged 65–74 years behaved in an anomalous and unexplained manner (see Reference 31). The overall statistical significance of these differences, based on the combination of results from the four age–sex classes, was high (p < 0.02). The authors considered that the study had produced evidence of a direct relationship between cardiovascular death-rates and water hardness.

d *Clinical Studies*

The MRC Social Medicine Unit also carried out a clinical study in twelve towns in England and Wales, six with hard water and six with soft water, to investigate the clinical and biochemical characteristics of populations with differing water supplies.[17] The soft-water towns all had very soft water (<40 ppm total hardness) and all were high-mortality towns for cardiovascular disease. The hard-water towns were all low in mortality for cardiovascular disease and all had very hard water (>250 ppm total hardness). The selection of towns is commented upon because any findings might well be regarded as reflecting the differences between high-cardiovascular-mortality and low-cardiovascular-mortality towns rather than between towns with very soft and very hard drinking water.

The subjects examined in 1972 were male executive-grade Civil Servants aged 40–65 years who had completed a questionnaire in a national study of leisure activity and health in 1968–70. The response rate in the earlier study was 86% and on this occasion 77% of men (n = 489) agreed to participate, i.e. 66% of those originally eligible to participate were examined. Smoking habits were similar in the two groups, and there were no significant differences in the prevalence of existing ischaemic heart disease as determined by chest pain questionnaire or by 12-lead electrocardiogram. Plasma total cholesterol concentrations were slightly but not consistently, higher in the soft-water towns (p < 0.05) and mean casual diastolic blood pressure was higher in the soft water towns. Men in the soft-water (high cardiovascular mortality) towns showed an increase in diastolic blood pressure with age; men in the

hard-water (low cardiovascular mortality) towns showed no such increase.

e *Sudden Death*

A study was made to assess the contribution made by sudden death to cardiovascular mortality in hard and soft water towns in England and Wales, using the same 12 towns described in the clinical study.[18] Death certificates were obtained on a weekly basis for the calendar year 1970 for men and women aged 30–59 years and further information was obtained from the certifying doctor in all deaths attributed to or associated with cardiovascular disease. Sudden death was defined as death within 1 hour of the onset of acute symptoms. Sudden death made up a greater proportion of male ischaemic heart disease deaths in the soft than in the hard water towns, but at a low level of statistical significance.

2 Other Explanations for Regional Variations

Although some of those working on the water story felt that the evidence was such that 'the technical problems of increasing the hardness of soft water should now be explored',[16] others felt less confident. In South Wales, water hardness was more strongly associated negatively with total mortality, bronchitis and perinatal mortality than with coronary heart disease mortality.[19] Hart was sceptical about the association of water hardness with 'such a wide and apparently unconnected variety of mortality', all having high correlations with poverty and social class.

a *Climate*

Roberts and Lloyd[20] presented data on the association between rainfall and ischaemic heart disease mortality in 50 local authority areas in South Wales and 58 county boroughs in England and Wales. They focused their attention on rainfall because Gardner *et al.*[14] had shown rainfall, water calcium, latitude and domestic air pollution—in that order of decreasing statistical significance—to account for most of the variance in cardiovascular mortality in males aged 45–64 years for 1958–64. A high correlation (r = 0.6) between rainfall and water calcium had also been noted. They concluded that the negative association between hardness and IHD was probably *entirely* dependent on the association of hardness with rainfall: they made no examination of total cardiovascular mortality.

The climatic aspect was further examined by West, Lloyd and Roberts in a study of death rates from IHD (1968–1970) in 114 boroughs of England and Wales and an analysis of their dependence on rainfall, temperature and water calcium.[21] Temperature emerged as most strongly correlated (negatively) with IHD mortality; rainfall (positive) and water calcium (negative) were apparently far less closely related. The authors concluded that climate is the primary factor accounting for differences in inter-town mortality from IHD in England and Wales, and that the mechanism is 'by way of a low temperature/high rainfall interaction precipitating death in a pre-initiated disease'. They point to the evidence for there being widespread coronary atheroma in the UK[22] and consider that 'the factor which distinguishes high from low IHD mortality towns is one which precipitates death rather than one which initiates disease'. While accepting that water calcium is associated with IHD mortality, they suggested that it owed this association almost entirely to its own association with both temperature and rainfall.

b *Age, Sex and Specificity*

Fulton and her colleagues examined regional variations in mortality from all causes, ischaemic heart disease, cerebrovascular disease and lung cancer for men and women aged 35–64 years during 1969–73 for nine standard regions of England and Wales and for five regions in Scotland.[23]

The highest rates for ischaemic heart disease and cerebrovascular mortality were in the north and west of Great Britain, with west central Scotland having the highest mortality. The regional effects were not explained by random variation or annual fluctuations and age and sex had more effect than region. The regional effect was not more pronounced for any of the age groups, contrary to the view of West[24] who used standardized proportional mortality to suggest that regional variations in mortality were 'largely differences in age at death, irrespective of cause of death'. The authors noted that regional variations were only marginally changed when considering men compared with women or the younger with the older age groups. Ischaemic heart disease and cerebrovascular disease had a very similar pattern of variation while lung cancer showed a different pattern, indicating that the regional effect is different for at least some diseases.

c *Dietary Factors*

Knox analysed the relationship between standardized mortality rates for ischaemic heart disease (1964–1969) and the dietary intakes of a number of nutrients for eight standard regions of England and Wales.[25] The dietary data were derived from the National Food Survey. Fully aware that correlation analysis by large region and using such survey data is a crude technique, he considered it justified only because of the prior hypothesis that calcium intake was related to IHD mortality through the 'water story'. Calcium intakes showed a strong negative correlation, consistent with the variations between IHD mortalities in hard and soft water areas.

After the effects of calcium had been excluded, fat and vitamin D intakes both showed positive associations with the residual variation in the mortality rates. However, examination of the correlations between different nutrients and SMRs for deaths from a range of other diseases (stomach cancer, diabetes, bronchitis, etc.), showed a consistent pattern which was not at all specific for ischaemic heart disease. 'The pattern suggests an overriding set of determinants, not specific for any individual disease but influencing all forms of mortality. It probably represents a long-established regional gradient of life style and social circumstances, associated only in a secondary way with a variety of causes of death'. Knox observed, with more poetry than point, that 'for ischaemic heart disease, almost all of the high SMRs . . . are located north-west of a frontier passing through the Roman legionary fortresses of York, Chester and Caerleon-on-Usk'.

Armstrong *et al.*[26] investigated temporal changes in male and female (35–64 years) IHD mortality and in commodity consumption (food and tobacco) in England and Wales for 1950–1967. They also compared these results with a cross-sectional study of nine standard regions in England, Wales and Scotland for 1969. From the welter of data and statistical analyses, a few findings emerged, albeit not very clearly. In the examination of temporal changes in England and Wales, coffee (positively) and flour (negatively) were most strongly related to IHD mortality. The analyses of the nine standard regions showed the strongest association to be a negative relationship with the consumption of total fresh green vegetables. Both IHD mortality and total fresh green vegetable consumption show a strong north–south gradient in Great Britain, and the authors accept that this correlation could readily be confounded by any other variable showing this gradient.

d *Cigarette Smoking*

In a recent review of the Decennial Supplement on Area Mortality 1969–73, the pattern of mortality from circulatory diseases in 10 standard regions of England and Wales is presented.[3] The well-established pattern is described and it is noted that there is no urban–rural gradient for either ischaemic heart disease or cerebrovascular disease. The age-standardized percentage of current smokers in 1952 derived from the General Household Survey showed a clear correlation ($r = 0.84$) with the SMRs for ischaemic heart disease for males by region.

e *Social Class*

The relative stability of regional variations in overall mortality over time suggests a geographic influence on mortality patterns over and above the influence of factors measured by social class. In recent decennial supplements produced by OPCS, occupation (social class) and geography have been considered separately to see if these two factors have independent effects on mortality patterns.[27]

When the overall SMR (all causes) for men aged 15–64 years is examined on a regional basis, there are higher rates in the north and west and lower rates in the south and east. The social class gradient, with lower SMRs in social classes I and II and higher SMRs in IV and V, persist throughout the regions and for cause-specific mortality; for bronchitis and lung cancer the gradients are consistently steeper than those for ischaemic heart disease. When the SMRs for all causes of death in the 10 regions of England and Wales are standardized for age and social class, to take account of the differences in population distribution between age groups and social classes in the different regions, this procedure has virtually no effect on the SMR for the regions. This suggests that the regional and social class variations which are observed represent two separate factors affecting mortality rates, and that these two factors are more or less independent for adult mortality. For example, the SMRs by social class in the north-west region range from 113 to 118, in the south-east region from 89 to 96 and in the south-west region from 90 to 96. Such small variations between the social classes within regions compared with the major variations between the same social class in different regions, clearly demonstrate the independence of social class and geography with respect to adult male mortality differences.

3 The British Regional Heart Study

The British Regional Heart Study (RHS) was established to assess the role of water quality in determining regional variations in cardiovascular mortality and to determine the extent to which other risk factors could account for regional variations. The critical feature of the RHS was the decision to study individuals on a prospective basis in order to provide fundamental information about the causes of cardiovascular disease, both environmental and personal. The study falls into three main phases, each of which has been described in detail in various publications; only brief outlines of the findings will be given in this review.

a *Statistical Studies*

In this statistical study of 253 British towns, the possible contributions of drinking water, climate, air pollution, blood groups, and socio-economic factors were evaluated.[28] A two-fold range in mortality from cardiovascular disease was apparent, the highest mortality being in the west of Scotland and the lowest in south-east England. Figure 1 shows the standardized mortality ratios (SMRs) for cardiovascular disease for men and women aged 35–74 years, the rate for all towns in Britain being taken as 100. This combined SMR has a two-fold range from 69 in the London suburbs of Chigwell and Esher to 147 in the Glasgow suburbs of Hamilton and Dumbarton. Figure 2 shows the association between the SMR and the total hardness for 234 of these towns. Towns with soft water tend to have higher cardiovascular mortality than towns with hard water, with notable exceptions, and there is a wide range of mortality present at any given level of water hardness.

Although the data show a significant association between cardiovascular mortality and water hardness, the relation does not allow for the effects of other factors. Indeed, the study noted 24 factors, each of which had a marked association (r > ±0.5) with cardiovascular mortality, including water quality, climate, latitude/longitude, socio-economic factors, blood groups and air pollution. The influence of climate was especially relevent since

high rainfall and areas with soft water tended to coincide (r = 0.70).

Viewing the data made it evident that water hardness was merely one of the many factors which might influence cardiovascular mortality. In addition, water hardness was not the only water measurement associated with cardiovascular mortality; there was a high degree of negative correlation between total hardness and calcium, carbonate hardness, conductivity, nitrate, silica and the Langelier index (a measure of corrosiveness). The percentage upland water was positively correlated with cardiovascular mortality. Two other water measurements of interest, magnesium and sodium, had no association with cardiovascular mortality in this study. In passing, one might note that the percentage water derived from upland sources correlated (positively) with the SMRs for cardiovascular disease as strongly as total hardness or calcium (both negatively). Rainfall (positive), temperature (negative) and latitude (positive) all had higher correlation coefficients with cardiovascular mortality than water hardness.

The extent to which all these factors might simultaneously explain the variations between towns in cardiovascular mortality was examined in a *multiple regression model*. After testing many different models, it was concluded that there were five variables that collectively had a highly significant relationship with the SMR: namely, water hardness (negative), percentage of days with measurable rain (positive), mean daily maximum temperature (negative), percentage of manual workers (positive), and percentage car ownership (negative). Each variable was shown to make a *separate* and *important* contribution to explaining regional variations in cardiovascular mortality, which could not be attributed to its association with other variables in the study. In particular, the effect of water hardness could not be explained away by its correlation with rainfall.

Further investigation showed that the effect of water hardness was non-linear, being much greater in the range from very soft to medium-hard water than from medium-hard to very hard water. Figure 3 shows the geometric mean SMR for cardiovascular disease for towns grouped according to water hardness, both with and without adjustment for the effects of the climatic and socio-economic variables. Adjusting for climatic and socio-economic differences considerably reduced the apparent magnitude of the effect of water hardness. A better-fitting regression model was therefore obtained by considering the effects of hardness on the SMR in two separate intervals, above and below 1.7 mmol/l (170 mg/l calcium carbonate equivalent).

Table I shows the standardized regression effects (percentage

FIG. 1. Standardized mortality ratios for cardiovascular disease in men and women aged 35–74 years for 1969–1973

(from Pocock et al.[28])

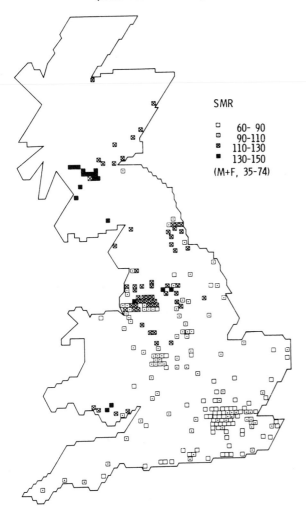

SMR

☐	60– 90
⊡	90–110
⊠	110–130
■	130–150

(M+F, 35–74)

TABLE I. The effect of five key variables on SMRs for cardiovascular disease, stroke, ischaemic heart disease and non-cardiovascular disease in men and women aged 35–74

(from Pocock et al.[28])

Variable	Standardized regression effects			
	CVD	Stroke	IHD	non-CVD
Water hardness:				
Up to 1.7 mmol/l	−7.8	−6.8	−8.2	−0.1
Over 1.7 mmol/l	−0.8	−3.0	+0.0	+0.0
Rain	+4.1	+4.2	+4.3	+1.8
Maximum temperature	−3.0	−7.5	−2.1	−0.4
Per cent manual workers	+5.1	+6.1	+5.0	+3.5
Car ownership	−2.9	−2.2	−3.2	−6.5

FIG. 2. Water hardness plotted against the SMR for cardiovascular disease for men and women aged 35–74 years for 234 towns

(from Pocock *et al.*[28])
Water hardness: 1 mmol/l = calcium carbonate equivalent 100 mg/l

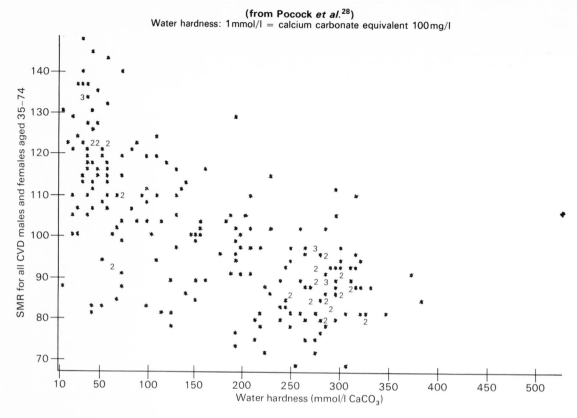

change in SMR for a 1 SD increase in each variable, keeping all other variables constant) which give some idea of the relative importance of the variables. It can be seen that the climatic and socio-economic variables have roughly similar effects, although the percentage of manual workers and rainfall seem somewhat more important than the other two measures. Water hardness below 1.7 mmol/l (very soft to medium-hard water) had the greatest standardized regression effect; water which was harder than this had virtually no effect at all on cardiovascular mortality. It can be estimated that the maximal effect of water hardness on cardiovascular mortality lies principally between very soft and medium-hard water and may be of the order of 10–15% of cardiovascular mortality.

Conventional use of multiple regression in this context makes no allowances for towns being of unequal population size, and for towns close to one another having similar mortality patterns. A method of extending multiple regression to allow for these problems of weighting and spatial correlation has been described.[29] When this method is applied to the findings described above, there is a reduction in the statistical significance of each of the five factors in Table I but the overall conclusions are confirmed.

Specificity of relations. It has been suggested that the apparent effect of water hardness on cardiovascular mortality is part of a general effect on mortality. The five-variable regression on the SMR was computed for non-cardiovascular mortality and no significant effect of water hardness was seen.

Socio-economic effects were of paramount importance in explaining geographic variations in non-cardiovascular mortality,

whereas the effect of climate was much reduced. The effect of water hardness remained significant and of similar magnitude for both stroke and ischaemic heart disease. The association between mortality and maximum temperature was greater for stroke than for ischaemic heart disease. Further regression analyses showed that the effect of water hardness on geographic variations in cardiovascular mortality was of the same order of magnitude for men and women and for the age ranges 35–64 and 65–74 years.

Rainfall and temperature. There has been considerable speculation as to why rainfall and temperature should be related to cardiovascular mortality. Cold weather might enhance the spread of infections or directly affect body temperature, either of which might precipitate cardiovascular events, and wet conditions might accentuate these effects. Cold and wet weather predispose to physical inactivity and it is of some interest that the percentage of days with rain correlates better with the SMR than does total rainfall. Any cold-weather conditions may lead to exceptionally demanding physical activity in those unaccustomed to exercise, and might precipitate major coronary heart disease events in susceptible subjects.

Socio-economic factors. The finding that towns containing predominantly manual workers had higher SMRs is consistent with the higher cardiovascular mortality rates in manual workers shown in the 1971 occupational mortality data. Car ownership is a measure of the relative prosperity of different urban areas, and a low car ownership in a town together with a high proportion of manual workers may reflect a lack of prosperity, possibly deprivation, and life-styles which may be conducive to ill-health.

FIG. 3. Mean SMRs (for men and women aged 35–74 years) for towns grouped according to the hardness of their water supply

(from Pocock *et al.*[28])

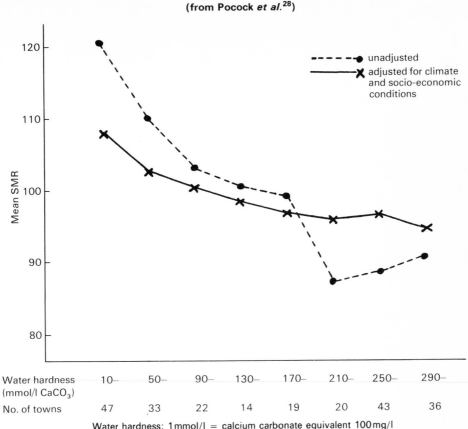

Water hardness (mmol/l CaCO₃)	10–	50–	90–	130–	170–	210–	250–	290–
No. of towns	47	33	22	14	19	20	43	36

Water hardness: 1 mmol/l = calcium carbonate equivalent 100 mg/l

Blood-group distribution. Differences in blood-group distribution between towns was the only other factor to show a possible association with cardiovascular mortality; the O-gene frequency correlated significantly with the SMR for cardiovascular disease after adjusting for the five variables in the regression model (r = +0.21). Applying this finding to individuals in this study would imply that blood group O has more than twice the cardiovascular mortality risk of blood group A. This is contradictory to published studies of individuals with ischaemic heart disease which show that type O individuals are at *lesser* risk than type A. For these reasons, blood groups were not included in the regression model. This blood group finding has previously been demonstrated by Mitchell,[30] who felt that not enough account was taken 'of what people are, as well as what they do'. The concurrence of higher frequencies of the O gene in Scotland and the north of England with higher rates of cardiovascular mortality may have some causal associations. It is more likely, however, that the higher cardiovascular mortality in the north will be explained by other factors, e.g. cigarette smoking, which are linked with occupation (socio-economic status), and thus with the geography of industry.

Dietary factors. Regional information on diet for 1969–73 was obtained from national food surveys and gave no support to the suggestion that the high cardiovascular mortality in Scotland was related to current total fat consumption. This does not refute the possible role of a high fat intake in the development of coronary heart disease but suggests that it does not account for the regional differences in cardiovascular disease. The most noticeable

differences in the Scottish diet was a marked reduction in the intake of fresh fruit and green vegetables compared with south-east England. This finding might be associated with a deficiency of linoleic and linolenic acids which occur in high concentrations in fresh fruit and vegetables.

Conclusion. After allowing for climatic and socio-economic conditions, a significant negative association remains between water hardness and cardiovascular mortality in British towns. The effect is specific for cardiovascular disease (stroke and ischaemic heart disease) and is not present for non-cardiovascular disease. The relation is non-linear and the study estimates a 10–15% excess of all cardiovascular deaths in areas with *very* soft water compared with areas of medium hardness. This degree of excess mortality must be measured against the effect of risk factors such as cigarette smoking, which produces at least a two-fold (200%) increase in coronary heart disease mortality. Whether the 'water factor' actually is a component of water or whether it represents a confounding variable whose distribution closely resembles water hardness has not been determined, though not for want of looking!

It must also be remembered that both temperature and rainfall also affect mortality from cardiovascular disease significantly and independently.

Changes in water supply. A further study has been carried out based on the changes that have taken place in water hardness and in cardiovascular death rates between 1961 and 1971.[31] It indicates a significant trend for men, in the direction of decreasing cardiovascular mortality with increasing hardness, but no trend for women. The trend for male mortality appears to be specific for cardiovascular disease. The results are similar to the earlier study and support the hypothesis of a *weak* casual relationship between the hardness of drinking water and mortality from cardiovascular disease.

b *Clinical Studies in Twenty-Four Towns*

The second phase of the Regional Heart Study relates to 7735 men aged 40–59 years drawn at random from age–sex registers of one general practice in each of 24 British towns. The criteria for selecting the towns, the general practices and the subjects, as well as the methods of data collection have been reported in detail.[32]

Risk factors. In the initial report on the prevalence of risk factors in the 24 towns, a comparison was made between the SMRs for *all* cardiovascular disease in men aged 35–64 years for the years 1969–1973 and a number of variables measured at the examination of the men.[32] *On a town basis*, cardiovascular mortality was associated with mean systolic blood pressure (r = 0.55), the prevalence of heavy cigarette smoking (r = 0.50) and heavy alcohol consumption (r = 0.67). No such associations were seen for mean body mass index, or mean serum total cholesterol or high density lipoprotein-cholesterol concentration. It was emphasized that the absence of an association did not imply that the particular factor was not important in the development of cardiovascular disease, but merely that it did not apparently contribute to inter-town variation in cardiovascular mortality. The role of alcohol is at present uncertain and the strong association may merely reflect its close correlation with cigarette smoking.

Prevalence of CHD. All men had an electrocardiogram and completed an administered questionnaire enquiring into chest pain suggestive of myocardial infarction or angina.[33] The overall prevalence of ischaemic heart disease was 25%, with 14% having possible myocardial infarction and/or angina on questionnaire and 14.5% having electrocardiographic evidence of myocardial infarction or ischaemia. There was thus a moderate degree of overlap between questionnaire and electrocardiograph evidence, the frequency of overlap i.e., both questionnaire and ECG evidence of IHD concurrently present, increasing three-fold over the age-range studied.

The prevalence of IHD, based on the chest pain questionnaire and electrocardiogram, ranged from 17% in Lowestoft to 30% in Merthyr Tydfil, an almost two-fold difference. The standardized mortality ratios for IHD for men aged 35–64 years for the years 1979–1982, ranged from 71 in Ipswich to 135 in Ayr, a similar two-fold difference (A G Shaper *et al*, in preparation). There is a strong correlation between these two measures (r = 0.74), indicating that the routinely collected mortality data for ischaemic heart disease is strongly related to the prevalence of IHD in these towns, and that the difference in mortality between towns is not merely a reflection of differences in case-fatality.

Prevalence and risk factors. The prevalence data for ischaemic heart disease in the men in the 24 towns have been compared with the mean levels of risk factors in the same men measured at the same time. When this is done, the findings in our initial report[32] are confirmed and, in some cases, strengthened (A G Shaper *et al*, in preparation). The only difference of note from the earlier report is that mean diastolic blood pressure correlates significantly with the prevalence of IHD, whereas it did not correlate with the SMR for all cardiovascular disease 1969–1973. Alcohol ('heavy' drinking) is more strongly correlated and cigarette smoking slightly less strongly correlated than in the earlier report and the relationship with social class (per cent manual workers) remains unchanged.

Those variables which were *not* associated with the SMRs for all cardiovascular disease (1969–1973) showed no association with the percentage prevalence of IHD in the towns i.e., serum total cholesterol, HDL-cholesterol and body mass index. Again, one cannot emphasize too strongly that this lack of association on a *town* basis does not preclude the possibility of important relationships in *individuals* between these variables and ischaemic heart disease. This caution refers in particular to serum total cholesterol concentration, which may well be the most important risk factor for ischaemic heart disease in individuals.

Conclusion. Mean blood pressure (systolic and diastolic) and cigarette smoking are strongly correlated with the prevalence of ischaemic heart disease in these 24 British towns. It seems likely that these variables account to a considerable extent for the regional variations in ischaemic heart disease in Great Britain.

4 Conclusions

Water hardness, temperature, and rainfall each play an independent role in determining cardiovascular mortality in Great Britain. The magnitude of their effects, however, would seem to be relatively small, compared with the effects of other risk factors such as cigarette smoking and blood pressure. While direct modifications are feasible but costly, their effectiveness in relation to cardiovascular disease cannot be estimated. At present, recommendations to harden very soft water cannot be justified on the basis of possible effects on cardiovascular disease.[34]

The Regional Heart Study shows that the regional variations in ischaemic heart disease mortality are reflected in similar variations in the prevalence of ischaemic heart disease. Variations in mean blood pressure levels and in the prevalence of heavy cigarette smoking in British towns are closely associated with town variations in ischaemic heart disease prevalence and mortality. It is suggested that these factors determine to a major extent the regional variations in cardiovascular disease. Other factors, including blood lipid concentrations, probably play a more fundamental role in the development of atherosclerosis and its complications, but in a country with a high level of cardiovascular disease—such as Great Britain—they do not appear to be responsible for regional variations in cardiovascular mortality.

There are major dangers in geographic studies of this kind and 'here be dragons' might well be the marking on the map. A significant association between a variable and the disease is greeted with enthusiasm and often accepted with uncritical fervour—particularly if the variable seems capable of modification. Plausible mechanisms are sought or devised and possible confounding variables left undisturbed and unprovoked, lest they become destructive. Lack of association is likely to spell total neglect for some poor variable that fails to differ between the geographic areas being examined. The possibility that it is an important (necessary) aetological factor in the disease process may pass unnoticed, for when the prevalence of a disease is high, observers become accustomed to above-threshold levels; all are equally at high risk and there is no longer 'a difference' to arouse attention. In the search for causes, it is reasonable to draw inferences from both positive and negative findings in geographic comparisons and to pursue them further. To attribute causality to association requires far more searching criteria to be fulfilled, and rarely can this be achieved without prospective studies based on individuals. And this is why we go beyond the maps and among the people.

ACKNOWLEDGEMENTS

The British Regional Heart Study is supported by a programme grant from the Medical Research Council. The Water Research Centre, Medmenham and the Wolfson Research Laboratories, Birmingham are major collaborators in this Study. I am grateful to all those involved for their contributions to the Study and their constructive comments on this review.

REFERENCES

1 Haviland A. The geographical distribution of heart disease and dropsy in England and Wales. London: Churchill, 1871
2 Young M. The geographical distribution of heart disease in England and Wales, and its relation to that of acute rheumatism and to some other factors. Lancet 1925; 2: 590–593
3 Chilvers C, Adelstein AM. Interpreting patterns of mortality from circulatory disease in the regions of England and Wales: results from the Decennial Supplement on Area Mortality, 1969–73. Health Trends 1981; 13: 28–31
4 Clayton DG, Taylor D, Shaper AG. Trends in heart disease in England and Wales 1950–1973. Health Trends 1977; 9: 1–6
5 Howe GM. Man, environment and disease in Britain. A medical geography of Britain through the ages. Harmondsworth: Penguin, 1976; 233
6 Kobayashi J. On geochemical relationship between the chemical nature of river water and death-rate from apoplexy. Ber Ohara Inst landwirtschaft Biologie 1957; 11: 12–21
7 Schroeder HA. Degenerative cardiovascular disease in the Orient. II. Hypertension. J. Chron Dis. 1958; 8: 312–333
8 Schroeder HA. Hardness of local water-supplies and mortality from cardiovascular disease. Lancet 1961; 1: 1171
9 Schroeder HA. Relation between mortality from cardiovascular disease and treated water supplies. Variations in states and 163 largest municipalities of the United States. JAMA 1960; 172: 1902–1908
10 Schroeder HA. Municipal drinking water and cardiovascular death rates. JAMA 1966; 195: 81–85
11 Schroeder HA, Kraemer LA. Cardiovascular mortality, municipal water, and corrosion. Arch Environ Health 1974; 28: 303–311
12 Morris JN, Crawford MD, Heady JA. Hardness of local water-supplies and mortality from cardiovascular disease in the county boroughs of England and Wales. Lancet 1961; 1: 860–862
13 Crawford MD, Gardner, MJ, Morris JN. Mortality and hardness of local water supplies. Lancet 1968; 1: 827–831
14 Gardner MJ, Crawford MD, Morris JN. Patterns of mortality in middle and early old age in the county boroughs of England and Wales. Br J Prev Soc Med 1969; 23: 33–140
15 Crawford T, Crawford MD. Prevalence and pathological changes of ischaemic heart-disease in a hard-water and in a soft-water area. Lancet 1967; 1: 229–232
16 Crawford MD, Gardner MJ, Morris JN. Changes in water hardness and local death-rates. Lancet 1971; 2: 327–329
17 Stitt FW, Clayton DG, Crawford MD, Morris JN. Clinical and biochemical indicators of cardiovascular disease among men living in hard and soft water areas. Lancet 1973; 1: 122–126
18 Crawford MD, Clayton DG, Stanley F, Shaper AG. An epidemiological study of sudden death in hard and soft water areas. J Chron Dis 1977; 30: 69–80
19 Hart JT. The distribution of mortality from coronary heart disease in South Wales. J R Coll Gen Pract 1970; 19: 258–268
20 Roberts CJ, Lloyd S. Association between mortality from ischaemic heart-disease and rainfall in South Wales and in the county boroughs of England and Wales. Lancet 1972; 1: 1091–1093
21 West RR, Lloyd S, Roberts CJ. Mortality from ischaemic heart disease-association with weather. Br J Prev Soc Med 1973; 27: 36–40
22 Morris JN, Crawford MD. Coronary heart disease and physical activity of work. Evidence of a national necropsy survey. Br Med J 1958; 2: 1485–1496
23 Fulton M, Adams W, Lutz W, Oliver MF. Regional variations in mortality from ischaemic heart and cerebrovascular disease in Britain. Br Heart J 1978; 40: 563–568
24 West RR. Geographical variation in mortality from ischaemic heart disease in England and Wales. Br J Prev Soc Med 1977; 31: 245–250
25 Knox EG. Ischaemic-heart-disease mortality and dietary intake of calcium. Lancet 1973; 1: 1465–1467
26 Armstrong BK, Mann JI, Adelstein AM, Eskin F. Commodity consumption and ischaemic heart disease mortality, with special reference to dietary practices. J Chron Dis 1975; 28: 455–469
27 Office of Population Censuses and Surveys. Occupational mortality. The Registrar General's decennial supplement for England and Wales, 1970–1972. London, HMSO. 1978. (Series DS No 1)
28 Pocock, SJ, Shaper AG, Cook DG. et al. British Regional Heart Study: geographic variations in cardiovascular mortality, and the role of water quality. Br Med J 1980; 280: 1243–1249
29 Pocock SJ, Cook DG, Shaper AG. Analysing geographic variation in cardiovascular mortality: methods and results. J R Statist Soc A 1982; 145 (Part 3): 313–341
30 Mitchell JRA. An association between ABO blood-group distribution and geographical differences in death-rates. Lancet 1977; 1: 295–297
31 Lacey RF, Shaper AG. Changes in water hardness and cardiovascular death-rates. Int J Epidemiol 1984; 13: 18–24
32 Shaper AG, Pocock SJ, Walker M, Cohen NM, Wale CJ, Thomson AG. British Regional Heart Study: cardiovascular risk factors in middle-aged men in 24 towns. Br Med J 1981; 283: 179–186
33 Shaper AG, Cook DG, Walker, M, Macfarlane PW. The prevalence of ischaemic heart disease in middle-aged British men. Br Heart J 1984; 51: 595–605
34 Shaper AG, Pocock SJ, Packham RF, Lacey RF, Powell P. Softness of drinking water and cardiovascular disease—practical implications of recent research. Health Trends 1983; 15: 22–24

Additional Reference

US National Committee for Geochemistry. Panel on the Geochemistry of Water in Relation to Cardiovascular Disease. Geochemistry of water in relation to cardiovascular disease. Washington, DC; National Academy of Sciences, 1979

British Medical Bulletin (1984) Vol. 40, No. 4, pp. 374–379

EUROPEAN REGIONAL VARIATION IN CARDIOVASCULAR MORTALITY

W CAIRNS SMITH MB MPH MFCM

HUGH TUNSTALL-PEDOE MD FRCP FFCM

Cardiovascular Epidemiology Unit
Ninewells Hospital and Medical School
Dundee, Scotland

1   Definition
2   Diagnostic biases
3   Do mortality rates reflect differing incidence or case fatality?
4   International differences and trends
5   Regional variation within countries
6   International studies of variation
7   Conclusions
    References

1   Definition

Cardiovascular disease constitutes Chapter VII (Diseases of the Circulatory System) of the International Classification of Diseases. European countries adopted the Eighth Revision in 1968 or 1969 and most changed to the Ninth Revision in 1979 but the Eighth is still in use in Scandinavia and Switzerland. However, the few changes are small. The constituent sections and rubrics in the Ninth Revision are given below with the total numbers of deaths (both sexes) in England and Wales in 1982 (differences in Eighth Revision in brackets).[1-3]

Diseases of the circulatory system 390–459 (390–458)	284246 (100%)
Acute rheumatic fever 390–392	4 (0%)
Chronic rheumatic heart disease 393–398	2904 (1%)
Hypertensive disease 401–405 (400–404)	5160 (2%)
Ischaemic heart disease 410–414	154605 (54%)
Diseases of pulmonary circulation 415–417 (new section)	4270 (2%)
Other forms of heart disease 420–429	27989 (10%)
Cerebrovascular disease 430–438	69028 (24%)
Diseases of arteries, arterioles and capillaries 440–448	15786 (6%)
Diseases of veins and lymphatics, and other diseases of circulatory system 451–459 (450–458)	4500 (6%)

Although the constituent disease groups are numerous, some of them are minor causes of death and in the UK and most other European countries ischaemic (or coronary) heart disease and cerebrovascular disease or stroke account for most of the deaths. However, one pathological disease process, atheroma, accounts for almost all the ischaemic heart disease, a large part of the cerebrovascular disease (excepting haemorrhage) and also most of the deaths from arterial disease (which includes the codes for atherosclerosis and for abdominal aneurysms). There is a potential drift of cases between the diagnoses of arterial disease, ischaemic heart disease, heart failure and arteriosclerotic heart disease which are coded to 'other forms of heart disease'. While it is possible to examine all the cardiovascular deaths together (Table I), most studies of aetiology and natural history have been concerned with more specific sub-categories, such as ischaemic heart disease and stroke.

2   Diagnostic Biases

Different varieties of cardiovascular disease create different diagnostic problems and potential biases. The prevalence of manifestations of all chronic diseases increases with age so that the choice of cause of death in an elderly person with several potential diagnoses will depend on the training of the certifying doctor. Coronary heart disease is diagnosed in life by the presence of typical chest pain, electrocardiographic findings, and raised serum enzymes. However, the majority of victims of coronary heart attacks die too suddenly to have the diagnostic tests done on them. Although half have a suggestive previous history, the evidence for the certifying doctor's diagnosis will depend on the medico-legal practices of the country concerned; in some Scandinavian countries necropsy rates are very high, England and Wales is intermediate, whereas the Scottish medico-legal system is different and necropsies are uncommon. Where necropsies are done there is no international standard for how much coronary artery stenosis can cause death. As almost everybody has some coronary atheroma, as pathologists are under pressure to make a diagnosis, and as death from coronary disease is socially acceptable with no attendant stigma for either the patient or the doctors concerned, it can be a diagnosis of convenience, with or without a necropsy, and in the presence or absence of other disease. From the viewpoint of international comparison, this means that local medical and medico-legal practices may cause systematic biases between one place and another and also over time. However, where coronary disease is common, it is such a predominant cause of death, that systematic drift in diagnosis in or out of this category should be revealed by changes in the competing diagnoses.[4,5]

Stroke, unlike coronary heart disease, is less likely to kill its victims extremely rapidly, and the diagnosis is made on the basis of an acute neurological deficit preceding death. While the clinical diagnosis of individual pathologies for stroke is often erroneous, the overall diagnosis is fairly reliable.[6]

3   Do Mortality Rates Reflect Differing Incidence or Case Fatality?

The natural history of ischaemic, or coronary heart disease is very variable in individuals. Deaths may occur in the first episode, or after a long history of disease. There is not therefore a straightforward relationship between mortality from the disease and incidence. The same is also true to some extent of cerebrovascular disease. Studies of differences in mortality rates have therefore been concerned with two different questions:

(1) Is the natural history of the disease the same or different? Is the case fatality of acute attacks the same and the proportion of deaths that are sudden constant? Does the prevalence rate of manifestations of ischaemic heart disease (positive responses to an angina questionnaire or electrocardiographic abnormalities) correlate with mortality rates or not?

(2) If the differences in mortality reflect incidence, do they correlate with known disease risk factors? (e.g. blood-pressure, cigarette smoking, serum cholesterol, diet or environmental factors).

These are the recurrent themes in the papers discussed subsequently.

TABLE I. Age-standardized mortality rates per 100000 for men and women aged 40–69 in 1978 (Czechoslovakia 1975) for all cardiovascular disease, IHD, stroke and all cardiovascular disease except stroke
(data supplied by World Health Organization)

Country	All Causes		All Cardiovascular disease		Ischaemic heart disease		Cerebrovascular disease		All Cardiovascular less cerebrovascular	
	Men	Women	Men	Women	Men	Women	Men	Women	Men	Women
Austria	1388	657	570	229	316	87	114	64	457	165
Belgium	1355	653	504	202	294	78	81	56	423	146
Bulgaria	1316	757	620	388	270	119	242	185	378	203
Czechoslovakia	1611	769	707	326	410	129	183	117	524	209
Denmark	1175	659	530	186	403	109	62	41	468	145
Finland	1609	575	872	259	649	138	122	72	749	188
France	1278	522	341	121	144	32	82	40	258	81
Germany (FRG)	1323	646	530	201	326	81	92	53	439	148
Greece	936	511	349	166	186	46	92	72	257	94
Hungary	1710	889	768	382	398	140	185	112	583	270
Ireland	1377	784	698	305	514	169	100	77	598	228
Italy	1227	561	463	205	236	63	110	66	353	138
Netherlands	1122	521	479	161	353	85	61	41	419	120
Norway	1060	502	515	167	386	88	61	46	454	121
Poland	1616	722	677	290	263	65	92	65	585	225
Portugal	1356	643	512	271	164	55	217	131	295	140
Romania	1394	804	624	403	186	80	170	136	454	267
Spain	1087	527	390	188	153	37	103	68	286	120
Sweden	1030	507	504	159	381	92	66	38	439	120
Switzerland	1055	507	403	147	228	53	58	30	346	118
UK England and Wales	1325	711	686	271	503	142	92	69	594	202
UK Northern Ireland	1497	792	841	372	643	208	108	96	733	276
UK Scotland	1621	924	839	391	628	219	124	103	715	288
Yugoslavia	1374	755	537	325	181	71	120	90	410	235

4 International Differences and Trends

The Table shows the age-standardized mortality rates for all causes and for cardiovascular deaths for different countries in Europe (data courtesy of World Health Organization Geneva). The year 1978 has been chosen because all countries were using the same (eighth) Revision of the International Classification of Diseases. The rates for men and women aged 40–69 have been age-standardized using a formula from Pisa and Uemura*.[7] The Table shows that Finland, Northern Ireland, and Scotland have the highest cardiovascular and ischaemic heart disease mortality rates in Europe. On the other hand, rates in France and countries in the Eastern Mediterranean are low. Stroke mortality does not correlate with that from ischaemic heart disease with high rates in Bulgaria, Hungary, Czechoslovakia and Romania and low rates in the Netherlands, Norway and Switzerland.

In the last decade, differences in the trends of mortality rates over time have generated as much interest as the absolute levels did previously. Comparison of these figures for 1978 with those for 1969, the first year when the Eighth Revision of the ICD was in general use shows that there has been some movement in the international league table for Europe. Belgium, Denmark, Finland and Norway show decreases in standardized male rates of more than 30 per 100000 per year, while Bulgaria, Greece, Hungary, Ireland, Poland, Romania, Spain, Sweden, Northern Ireland and Yugoslavia show increases of this size. In male deaths from cerebrovascular disease, on the other hand, while there has been a general decline in rates, this has been most prominent in Belgium, Finland, France and Ireland, but there has been a notable increase in Bulgaria, Hungary and Poland. Female death rates tend to follow the same pattern. The subject of varying trends is discussed in more detail by Pisa and Uemura[7] and by Marmot.[8]

5 Regional Variation Within Countries

Problems of studying variations in mortality between countries are reduced when looking at variations within one country or state. There should be a uniform system of death certification and registration, one disease classification and information on denominators should be consistent. Although doctors trained in different medical schools may adopt different patterns of diagnosis which may be reflected in apparent regional variations of disease within a country, regional variations within a country are generally more likely to be valid than those between countries. Nevertheless, they can be almost as large.

Once regional variation of a disease within a country has been established, the next step is to look for possible explanations. These may include regional geophysical differences as well as those in ethnic group distribution, genetic factors, social class composition, and diet and other behavioural factors. Differential migration between regions of a country, usually related to employment, needs to be taken into account. Large foreign immigrant populations may distort numbers at risk, as for example, in Switzerland.[9]

There is a large literature on within country variation in cardiovascular disease in the European region. The following is a selective review for certain countries only, based in part on the authors' knowledge of the work and in part on its availability in international journals. Research has been patchy and related to local expertise and facilities, the perceived importance of cardiovascular disease, and stimulants such as obvious heterogeneities within the country, or participation in international projects.

Belgium. Most studies of regional variation in cardiovascular mortality have divided Belgium into four areas: two Dutch-speaking areas in the north (Campine and Flanders), Wallonia, the French-speaking area in the south, with Brussels in the middle; others have used the nine Belgian provinces. Despite the language differences, the population has been considered homogeneous in terms of the health care system and socio-economic status.

* Weighting of the six five-year age groups from 40–69 was 7/36, 7/36, 7/36, 6/36, 5/36 and 4/36 to total 36/36 in all.

Coronary heart diseases mortality is higher in the south compared with the Dutch-speaking north. Studies of prevalence using ECG and angina questionnaires have shown a similar regional difference. The mean serum cholesterol level is higher in the south. Only small differences in blood pressure, body weight and cigarette smoking have been found between north and south Belgium, if anything smoking was more prevalent in the north.[10] The difference in serum cholesterol has been related to dietary differences between north and south Belgium.[11] Health education advice to lower saturated fat and increase polyunsaturates in the diet in the Dutch-speaking north has not filtered through to the French-speaking south until comparatively recently.[12] Surveys have reflected this difference with the Dutch areas consuming more margarine and less butter. Cardiovascular mortality has been correlated with butter consumption for the nine Belgium provinces. Thus the regional variations in coronary heart disease in Belgium have been largely attributed to regional differences in serum cholesterol and consumption of fats.

Federal Republic of Germany. The cardiovascular death rates in Germany rose dramatically between 1950 and 1970 and then levelled off; coronary death rates were responsible. The standardized mortality rates for ischaemic heart disease in both men and women for the year 1975 have been calculated on a regional basis. The regional pattern shows a general south-to-north trend with the rates in the north being higher. The lowest rate for men was in Bayern in the south. Saarland in the west is an exception to the general trend and has the highest rates for both men and women. Bremen in the north also appears to be an exception to the general trend as its ischaemic heart disease rates for men and women are lower than those in other northern regions.[13]

Finland. Finland has had the highest coronary heart disease mortality rates in the world. Extensive investigations have included that of the regional variations which led to the community intervention project in North Karelia. The 12 Finnish counties are used as the geographical units.[14] These show increasing ischaemic heart disease mortality from south-west to north-east, both for males and females. The most easterly county, Pohjois-Karjala (North Karelia) shows the highest rates and the Ahvenanmaa (Aland) Islands the lowest. The regional trend is also seen in the rural and urban municipalities, with the urban rates usually higher than the rural rates. East–west comparisons in all causes mortality show that the excess mortality in eastern Finland is almost entirely caused by the high cardiovascular disease mortality, especially that from ischaemic heart disease.

Regional studies of ischaemic heart disease prevalence show a similar pattern to that of mortality. Variations in history of chest pain are marked but those for prevalence of ECG findings are quite small. The regional differences in cigarette smoking behaviour have changed over time and while studies in the 1950s showed the prevalence of cigarette smoking in men to be much higher in the east, more recent studies show the east–west difference to be rather small. Regional differences in the prevalence of high blood pressure (higher in the east than the west) also seem less marked now and improved control of hypertension has been suggested as a possible explanation.[15] Finnish serum cholesterol levels are high and increase from west to east but laboratory problems have caused difficulty in interpreting some studies.[16]

The regional variation in coronary heart disease in Finland has been the basis of the community project in North Karelia and one of the neighbouring counties; Kuopio has been used as a control. Risk factor surveys at 5 years have demonstrated a mean net reduction of 17% among men and 12% among women in estimated coronary heart disease risk in North Karelia.[17] At 10 years there was a 28% reduction in smoking, 3% in mean serum cholesterol and 3% in mean systolic blood pressure among middle aged men.[18] The project area showed a decline in coronary heart disease mortality over the 10 year period; however a similar trend was also observed in the control area and the rest of Finland. Over the 11 year period, 1969–1979, a reduction of 12% for men and 26% for women took place in the standardized coronary heart disease mortality rate for the 35–64-year age group in the whole of Finland.[19] A decline has been observed in all the Finnish countries apart from one, Turku which initially had the lowest rate of the 11 mainland counties. North Karelia, which had the highest rate initially showed the greatest decline, 24% for men and 51% for women.

France. The outstanding feature of coronary heart disease mortality in France is its extremely low rate compared with its immediate neighbours. Misclassification had been proposed as an explanation of the low mortality rate but joining other cardiovascular disease rubrics shows the maximum estimated mortality rate to be still relatively low. Morbidity studies have confirmed these low rates. Risk factor levels appear to be low, but not sufficiently so to account for French rates. Thus, although smoking, serum cholesterol and blood pressure levels discriminate high and low risk groups in French prospective studies, the rates are nonetheless lower than would be expected in a North American population with similar risk factor levels.[20] Mortality rates in France are higher in the north than the south but results of coronary registers show similar incidence rates in the north and south. Alcohol consumption in France has been suggested as an explanation for the low mortality rates but a positive correlation has been observed among the French regions between alcohol consumption and coronary heart disease mortality. Alcohol consumption is high in areas such as Normandy in the north which have higher mortality rates.[21]

Italy. Regional variations in cardiovascular mortality rates in Italy are based on crude death rates because age- and sex-specific mortality data are not yet available at regional level. There are also differences in the age structure between the Italian regions due to differing trends in birth rate, mortality rate from infectious disease and internal migration. Attempts have been made to adjust mortality rates for age; these lead to a more even geographical distribution than the crude rates for acute ischaemic heart disease. Nonetheless, there is a very distinct south–north gradient in acute ischaemic heart disease mortality rates with the higher rates in northern Italy.[22] Epidemiological studies of coronary heart disease in Italy are few and are not comparable because of differing methods and criteria. Many of the studies have been published in local Italian journals and these have recently been reviewed.[23] Serum cholesterol levels decrease from north to south and are lower than in the USA while blood pressure levels appear similar and 60% of middle-aged men smoke.

Norway. There has been a rapid increase in coronary heart disease mortality in Norway between 1951–70. Age- and cause-specific mortality rates at county level were first analysed for the 1959–62 period when the most northerly county, Finmark showed the highest rate. Later analysis in 1964–67 showed increasing rates, the greatest being in the three northern counties of Nordland, Troms and Finmark. Review in 1969–72 showed that the rate of increase was less.[24] The blood pressure levels in the high-mortality counties were similar to the rest of Norway but cigarette consumption and serum cholesterol appeared to be higher. A study in 1965 looked at serum cholesterol in three areas with widely differing ischaemic heart disease mortality rates. This study found the heart disease rates to be related to serum cholesterol but that cholesterol alone could not fully explain the mortality differences.[25]

Poland. Mortality rates from cardiovascular diseases and ischaemic heart disease in Poland have steadily increased in both men and women and in both urban and rural areas over the period 1961–79. Differences between urban and rural communities in Poland have been extensively studied.[26] Incidence of myocardial infarction is higher in larger cities compared with smaller ones and also in the south than in the north of Poland. The prevalence of ischaemic heart disease in Warsaw has also been shown to be higher than in the south. Risk factor studies show higher levels in the urban, highly industrialized regions of Poland. The mean body weight, blood pressure and cholesterol levels are higher in Warsaw compared with southern Poland but the proportion of smokers is higher in the south.[27]

Soviet Union. A large increase in all causes mortality is reported for the Soviet Union between 1960–77. Heart disease has been responsible for 95% of this observed increase. An increasing trend has occurred in all the Soviet Republics except Armenia and Azerbaijan. An autopsy study of geographic variation in atherosclerosis demonstrated that the Russian Soviet Federated Socialist Republic and the Baltic regions had rates far in excess of those in Siberia, Central Asia and the Caucasus. Death rates in the less populous regions of the Soviet Union have either continued to fall or have risen very slightly.[28]

United Kingdom. Regional variation in the United Kingdom (which led to the establishment of the Cardiovascular Epidemiology Unit in Dundee in Scotland) is not included in this review as it is the subject of a separate paper in this volume (pp. 366–373).

Yugoslavia. The Yugoslavia Cardiovascular Disease Study has examined two different communities with regard to cardiovascular disease. One community resided in a mountainous area and was largely Moslem, while the second area was a suburb of Zagreb with a mainly Roman Catholic population and a life-style more like that of Western Europe. There were no significant differences between the two areas in the prevalence of ECG findings nor in the disease incidence rates. The number of cases was very small so that the power of the study to detect differences was weak.[29]

6 International Studies of Variation

International agencies collect data on the trade, commodity consumption and economic activity of different countries and it is possible to correlate these with mortality statistics.[30–32] Results of such studies suggest that there is no simple unitary explanation for regional differences in cardiovascular mortality. However, the data are crude, unvalidated and indirectly related to the personal risk factors shown to be powerful predictors in prospective studies. While such 'armchair epidemiology' is useful and necessary, it has to be supplemented by international fieldwork which is more difficult to organize, fund, and execute than studies within one country. Credit should be given to the World Health Organization European Office and to the Cardiovascular Diseases Unit in Geneva for stimulating some such studies, and also to various organizations in the United States of America which have organized and funded others. Some of the studies described below have both European and outside elements but European participation has predominated. The list is illustrative and not comprehensive. Participation is illustrated in Fig. 1.

Prevalence study in European civil servants. Six groups of subjects from five countries totalling 4522 subjects were examined to see how the prevalence of indicators of ischaemic heart disease

FIG. 1. European centres participating in certain collaborative projects

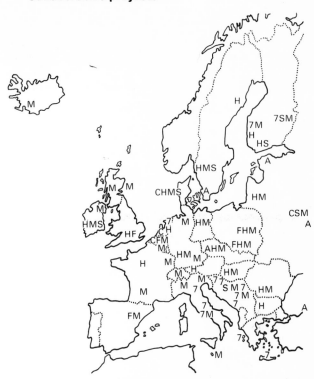

Key: 7: Seven countries study;[38] A: Atheroma study;[37] C: Civil servant study;[33] H: Heart attack register;[34] F: Factory study;[42] M: MONICA centre;[45] S: Stroke register[35]

correlated with national cardiovascular mortality. No good correlation was found.[33]

Heart attack and stroke registers. Following experience gained in Scotland and elsewhere, the European Office of the World Health Organization stimulated the establishment first of heart attack and then of stroke registers in different countries. Suspected cases were notified to a central office, where the circumstances and diagnostic criteria of the attack were recorded and evaluated. The heart-attack registers served a number of different functions and there were some methodological problems, but it appeared from the overall results that the attack rates correlated well with national mortality statistics. This suggests that mortality rates can be used as a crude indicator of incidence, and that case fatality does not show any systematic correlation with mortality rates.[34] However, heart attack registers are better able to identify false-positive cases than false negatives. Hopelessly missed, misdiagnosed and uninvestigated cases will not be detected.[5] A similar study was done on strokes although there was no stroke analogue for the electrocardiogram and serum enzymes at that time.[35]

Atheroma studies. Oslo was the only European centre to participate in the International Atherosclerosis project which took place mainly in the western hemisphere,[36] but five European centres participated in an autopsy study of the World Health Organization, three in the USSR plus one in Sweden and one in Czechoslovakia. This study showed interesting similarities and differences in the distribution of atheroma in different sites; in general towns with more atherosclerotic deaths had more atheroma.[37]

Seven-countries study. This study is a classic of cardiovascular epidemiology; it included five European countries, Japan, and the USA. Groups of several hundred men, usually two from contrasting parts of each country, were screened for evidence of ischaemic heart disease and for coronary risk factors; dietary analyses were done including some central analysis of homogenized, deep-frozen diet replicates and the men were followed for 5 and then for 10 years. The result was a major triumph for the dietary-fat story. Incidence rates supported national mortality statistics and correlated better with mean serum cholesterol levels than with other risk factors and the serum cholesterol correlated well with saturated fat in the diet.[38] However, there was also some correlation with systolic blood pressure; a recent finding suggesting that saturated fat raises blood pressure as well as serum cholesterol may be relevant.[39]

Two two-centre studies. The Edinburgh–Stockholm study makes an interesting contrast with the last study in that mean cholesterol levels in Sweden and Scotland are similar although coronary death rates are very different. A painstaking series of metabolic comparisons revealed a number of interesting differences in body build, smoking, blood pressure, polyunsaturated fat intake, lipid fractions, and metabolism between men aged 40 in the two cities. Because the study was bilateral, however, every difference that was found may or may not be significant and would have to be tested elsewhere.[40] A bilateral comparison has been made between French and Scottish farmers. Their dietary fatty acid intake was shown to be different and to correlate with tests of platelet function performed in the field.[41]

European factory study. This was designed as a trial of multifactorial coronary heart disease prevention but it involved risk factor screening in five European countries and follow-up of incidence. Although factory workers were used, the nature of the industries recruited was not standardized between countries. The results do not suggest that there is a good correlation between the study's incidence rates for national groups, the predicted incidence rates based on risk-factor screening, the prevalence rate of ischaemic findings or national mortality rates.[42–44] While selection pressures in employment and retirement could be responsible, some such correlations would have been useful and their absence leaves a potential gap for non-established risk factors.

MONICA and ERICA studies. Some of the difficulties in explaining regional variation in cardiovascular mortality in Europe may be overcome by these two large studies. The World Health Organization MONICA project is concerned with 'Multinational monitoring of trends and determinants in cardiovascular disease'. Some 30 or 40 centres, mostly in Europe, are attempting to measure the numbers of validated fatal and non-fatal coronary events in men and women under 65 years of age over 10 years in defined communities in which risk-factor levels and medical care will be followed over the same period.[45] Many centres are also monitoring strokes. Diagnostic criteria are similar to those in the register studies of a previous decade but have been developed further. The ERICA project is a 'European Risk and Incidence Co-ordinated Analysis' and seeks to pool the results of the major European prospective studies of risk factors and coronary heart disease incidence initiated in the 1970s.[46]

7 Conclusion

Cardiovascular disease is one of the major areas of interest of contemporary epidemiology. Regional variation in mortality within Europe has been one of the stimulants to both national and international studies. While further data are in process of being collected, it does appear that real differences do exist in mortality rates and that these reflect large differences in incidence rates rather than being the result only of differences in case-fatality. No single factor has been found to explain all regional differences; serum cholesterol explains some but fails to explain some others. However, as coronary heart disease risk in individuals is known to be multifactorial, it is not surprising that group differences follow the same pattern. Research is currently in progress on specific polyunsaturated fatty acids in the diet, on vitamins C and E, and on selenium as well as established factors. A better ability to explain regional differences and time trends in cardiovascular mortality by quantifying the contribution of different factors would be a great help in planning prevention. Some nations however have already looked at their data and their trends and drawn their own conclusions.[47]

REFERENCES

1 World Health Organization. Manual of the international statistical classification of diseases, injuries and causes of death: Eighth revision. Geneva: World Health Organization, 1967
2 World Health Organization. Manual of the international statistical classification of diseases, injuries and causes of death: Ninth revision. Geneva: World Health Organization, 1977
3 Office of Population Censuses and Surveys. Mortality statistics: cause England and Wales 1982. London: HMSO, 1983 DH2 No. 9
4 Tunstall-Pedoe, H. Coronary heart disease. In: Miller DL, Farmer RDT, eds. Epidemiology of diseases. Oxford: Blackwell Scientific, 1982: 103–121
5 Tunstall-Pedoe H. Uses of coronary heart attack registers. Br Heart J 1978; 40: 510–515
6 Tunstall-Pedoe H. Stroke. In: Miller DL, Farmer RDT, eds. Epidemiology of diseases. Oxford: Blackwell Scientific, 1982: 136–145
7 Pisa Z, Uemura K. Trends of mortality from ischaemic heart disease and other cardiovascular diseases in 27 countries 1968–77. World Health Stat 1982; 35: 11–47
8 Marmot MG. Life style and national and international trends in coronary heart disease mortality. Postgrad Med J 1984; 60: 3–8
9 Alexander J, Junod B. Coronary heart mortality is still increasing in Switzerland. Lancet 1980; 1: 598
10 Kornitzer M, DeBacker G, Dramaix M, Thilly C. Regional differences in risk factor distributions, food habits and coronary heart disease mortality and morbidity in Belgium. Int J Epidemiol 1979; 8: 23–31
11 Joossens JV, Vuylsteek K, Brems-Heyns E et al. The pattern of food and mortality in Belgium. Lancet 1977; 1: 1069–1072
12 Joossens JV. Epidemiology of coronary heart disease: lessons from North and South Belgium. Postgrad Med J 1980; 56: 548–556
13 Blohmke M, Koschorreck B. Ermittlung und Darstellung des zeitlichen Verlaufs und der regionalen Verteilung der kardiovaskularen Mortalität in der Bundesrepublik Deutschland und Berlin (West). Eine Auswertung der amtlichen Todesursachen-statistiken. Heidelberg, October 1980
14 Pyorala K, Valkonen T. The high ischaemic heart disease mortality in Finland. In Medical aspects of mortality statistics symposium, September 23–25, 1980. Stockholm: Skandia International Symposia, 1981: 37–57
15 Karvonen MJ, Blomquist G, Kallio V et al. Epidemiological studies related to coronary heart disease: characteristics of men aged 40–59 in seven countries. Acta Med Scand 1967; 181 (Suppl 460): 169–190
16 Reunanen A, Aromaa A, Pyorala K, Punsar S, Maatela J, Knekt P. The social insurance institution's coronary heart disease study. Baseline data and 5-year mortality experience. Acta Med Scand 1983, Suppl 673

17 Puska P, Tuomilehto J, Salonen J *et al*. Changes in coronary risk factors during comprehensive five year community programme to control cardiovascular diseases. (North Karelia project) Br Med J 1979; 2: 1173–1182

18 Puska P, Salonen JT, Nissinen A *et al*. Change in risk factors for coronary heart disease during 10 years of a community intervention programme. (North Karelia project) Br Med J 1983; 2: 1840–1844

19 Salonen JT, Puska P, Kottke TE, Tuomilehto J, Nissinen A. Decline in mortality from coronary heart disease in Finland from 1969 to 1979. Br Med J 1983; 1: 1857–1860

20 Ducimetiere P, Richard JL, Cambieu F, Rakotovao R, Claude JR. Coronary heart disease in middle-aged Frenchmen. Lancet 1980; 1: 1346–1350

21 Richard JL. Peculiarities of coronary heart diseases in the French population. Atherosclerosis 1983; 6: 821–825

22 Vetere C. General trends in death rates and current health information system in Italy. Atherosclerosis Reviews 1980; 7: 25–31

23 Menotti A, Farchi G. Epidemiology of coronary heart disease in Italy: a review. Atherosclerosis Reviews 1980; 7: 97–122

24 Thelle DS, Forde OH, Try K, Lehmann EH. The Tromso Heart Study. Acta Med Scand 1976; 200: 107–118

25 Jervel A, Meyer K, Westlund K. Coronary heart disease and serum cholesterol in males in different parts of Norway. Acta Med Scand 1965; 117: 13–23

26 Rywik S, Wagrowska H. Changes in the rates of mortality due to cardiovascular diseases with particular reference to ischaemic heart disease and hypertension in the years 1971–1977. Przegl Lek 1979; 36: 699–706

27 Rywik S, Sznajd J. Epidemiology of ischaemic heart disease in Poland. In: Levy RI, Rywik S, eds. USA–Poland Symposium: Ischaemic heart disease. US Department of Health and Human Services, National Institutes of Health, 1982; Publication No. 82–1273: 9–27

28 Cooper R. Rising death rates in the Soviet Union. The impact of coronary heart disease. N Engl J Med 1981; 304: 1259–1265

29 Kozarevic D, Pirc B, Dawber TR, Kahn HA, Zukel WJ. Prevalence and incidence of coronary disease in a population study. The Yugoslavia Cardiovascular Disease Study. J Chron Dis 1971; 24: 495–505

30 Armstrong BK, Mann JI, Adelstein AM, Eskin F. Commodity consumption and ischaemic heart disease mortality with special reference to dietary practices. J Chron Dis 1975; 28: 455–469.

31 Knox EG. Foods and disease. Brit J Prev Soc Med 1977; 31: 71–80

32 Cox H, Marks L. Sales trends and survey findings: a study of smoking in 15 OECD countries. Health Trends 1983; 15: 48–52

33 Rose GA, Ahmeteli M, Checcacci L, Fidanza *et al*. Ischaemic heart disease in middle-aged men. Bull WHO 1968; 38: 885–895

34 World Health Organization Regional Office for Europe. Myocardial infarction community registers. Copenhagen 1976 (Public Health in Europe No. 5)

35 Aho H, Harmsen P, Hatano S, Marquardsen J, Smirnov VE, Strasser T. Cerebrovascular disease in the community; results of a WHO collaborative study. Bull WHO 1980; 58: 113–130

36 Tejada C, Strong, JP, Montenegro MR, Restrepo C, Solberg LA. Distribution of coronary and aortic atherosclerosis by geographic location, race and sex. Lab Invest 1968; 18: 509–526

37 Kagan AR, Sternby NH, Uemura K *et al*. Atherosclerosis of the aorta and coronary arteries in five towns. Bull WHO 1976; 53: 485–645

38 Keys A. Seven countries: a multivariate analysis of death and coronary heart disease. Cambridge Mass: Harvard University Press, 1980

39 Puska P, Iacono JM, Nissinen A *et al*. Controlled randomised trial of the effect of dietary fat on blood pressure. Lancet 1983; 1: 1–5

40 Logan RL, Riemersma RA, Thomson M *et al*. Risk factors for ischaemic heart disease in normal men aged 40: Edinburgh–Stockholm Study. Lancet 1978; 1: 949–956

41 Renaud S, Dumont E, Godsey F, Marazain R, Thevenon C, Ortchanian E. Dietary fats and platelet function in French and Scottish farmers. Nutr Metab 1980; 24 (Suppl 1): 90–104

42 World Health Organization European Collaborative Group. An international controlled trial in the multifactorial prevention of coronary heart disease. Int J Epidemiol 1974; 3: 219–224

43 World Health Organization Collaborative Group. Multifactorial trial in the prevention of coronary heart disease: 1. Recruitment and initial findings. Eur Heart J 1980; 1: 73–80

44 World Health Organization Collaborative Group. Multifactorial trial in the prevention of coronary heart disease: 3. Incidence and mortality results. Eur Heart J 1983; 4: 141–147

45 World Health Organization. Proposal for the multinational monitoring of trends and determinants in cardiovascular disease and protocol (MONICA Project). Geneva 1983 (WHO/MNC/82.1)

46 ERICA Project. Unpublished document from WHO Collaborating Centre for research and training in cardiovascular disease. Klinikum der Universitat Heidelberg

47 World Health Organization Expert Committee. Prevention of coronary heart disease. WHO Tech Rep Ser 1982; 678

British Medical Bulletin (1984) Vol. 40, No. 4, pp. 380–386

GEOGRAPHY OF BLOOD PRESSURE AND HYPERTENSION

M G MARMOT MB BS PhD MPH

Department of Epidemiology
London School of Hygiene and Tropical Medicine
London

1 Definition and measurement
2 Genes versus environment
3 International studies of blood pressure
   a Rise of blood pressure with age
   b Low-blood-pressure populations
   c Acculturation and blood pressure
   d Urban–rural differences
4 Migrants
   a 'Cross-sectional' studies
   b Longitudinal migrant studies
5 Diet and geographical variations
   a Correlational studies of salt
   b Potassium
   c Acculturation and dietary change
   d Regional variations in Japan
   e Other factors
6 Psycho-social changes and blood pressure
7 Conclusions
   References

Geographical studies have profoundly influenced our understanding of blood pressure: its nature, its determinants, and its relation to subsequent pathology. By studying the distribution of blood pressure in different populations, we gain perspective on the arbitrariness of the labels 'normal' and 'abnormal'; the relative importance of genes versus environment; variation in the rise of blood pressure with age; changes with migration; the possible roles of diet and other aetiological factors; and the relation of blood pressure to ischaemic heart disease and stroke. All but the last of these will be considered.

1   Definition and Measurement

Blood pressure is a continuously distributed variable. During the 1960s there was a debate, led respectively by Platt and Pickering, as to whether the blood pressure distribution in populations had two peaks or one, i.e. whether there were two populations, normal and hypertensive, or only one. Inspection of blood pressure distributions from a number of populations supports the Pickering position that 'essential hypertension represents a type of disease . . . in which the deviation from the norm is quantitative not qualitative'[1] (see Section 2).

At what level of pressure should the label 'hypertension' then apply?[2] It could be applied with reference to, say, two standard deviations above the mean, but this tells us what is uncommon, not what is abnormal, pathologically. Such a definition of hypertension would constrain prevalence always to be 2.5% and would be of little use in geographical epidemiology, where the aim is to compare frequencies in different populations. A clinical definition is also not appropriate, as there is no clearly defined clinical picture associated with elevations of pressure.

The importance of elevated blood pressure is in the vascular and renal complications consequent upon it. Hence a more promising approach to the definition of 'hypertension' might be the level of pressure above which there is an increased risk of complications. Even this approach does not solve the problem, as there is a graded relationship between level of pressure and risk of vascular disease, and the absolute level of risk varies between populations depending on the degree of exposure to other aetiological factors.

Within a population, the definition of hypertension is best made on a pragmatic basis: the level of pressure at which action is warranted, weighing up the risks and benefits. For comparisons between populations it is better to compare levels and distributions of blood pressure rather than prevalence of hypertension.

This quantitative approach to comparisons avoids the problems of international differences in definition, but brings in its train a different problem: differences in the way blood pressure is recorded. Unless attention is paid to training the observers and standardizing the conditions and frequency of blood pressure measurement, comparisons of levels of pressure should be treated with caution. This caution applies to much of the attempts (discussed in Section 5) to compare figures from studies conducted by different investigators. Less susceptible to the effects of variation in methods is the rise of blood pressure with age. This can be compared within and between populations.

2   Genes Versus Environment

The relative contribution of nature and nurture in setting blood pressure levels is an open question, but its importance should not be overemphasized. Most students of the subject would agree that both heredity and environment play a role. The relative importance of each varies according to circumstances. In a population where exposure to environmental determinants of high blood pressure is uniformly high, genetic differences between *individuals* will assume prominence. By contrast, in comparisons between *populations*, environmental differences are likely to be more important.

This has important implications. The results of a study comparing individuals *within* a population may not necessarily be extrapolated to comparisons between populations. The reverse is also true. Thus, for example, a twin study from the USA estimated that 60% of observed variability in blood pressure within a population was due to genetic variation.[3] This assumes that the greater similarity between monozygotic than dizygotic twins is due to greater similarity of genes rather than of shared environment. Even if we accept this, it would be wrong to conclude from a study in a relatively homogeneous environment, that 60% of variability of blood pressure between populations is due to genetic variability. Conversely, if it were shown convincingly that geographical variations in blood pressure were related to differences in consumption of sodium and potassium, one could not conclude that differences in blood pressure between individuals within a homogeneous population could be explained on the same basis.

In discussing this issue, Pickering's working hypotheses included the following:[1]

(a) arterial pressure is inherited polygenically—regardless of level of pressure; (b) the rate of rise of pressure with age does not seem to be inherited, but is presumably related to environmental exposure; and (c) in determining pressures in middle age and beyond, environment is more important than inheritance.

Support for these hypotheses comes from studies of the geography of blood pressure.

3 International Studies of Blood Pressure

a *Rise of Blood Pressure with Age*

Blood pressure levels, means, and distributions, vary widely between countries and between areas within countries. In general, differences are more marked at older ages, reflecting variation in speed of rise of pressure with age. Epstein and Eckoff reviewed data from 34 population studies in different parts of the world and showed that the mean rise of systolic blood pressure varied between populations from 0 mm Hg to an estimated 40 mm Hg over the age span 10–70 years.[4]

b *Low-Blood-Pressure Populations*

Several populations have now been identified where mean blood pressure does not rise with age. These include New Guinea highland and lowland populations, Kalahari bushmen, Congo pygmies, Polynesians and Melanesians in the Pacific islands, and Brazilian and Guatemalan Indians.[5,6] These groups have in common their isolation and lack of contact with urban, Western culture, and are not necessarily typical of developing countries. Fig. 1 illustrates this. It shows mean blood pressures by age recorded from two groups of Polynesians living in the Cook Islands. The more isolated remote group, dwelling on the coral atoll Pukapuka, has lower mean pressures that rise less with age. The group living on the larger volcanic island Raratonga, the administrative capital and involved in the cash economy, has higher mean pressures and a steeper rise with age, seen most clearly for systolic pressure.[7]. The rise with age of pressure, seen in Raratonga, is the more usual situation in developing countries, as it is in industrialized countries. With blood pressure, we thus have the remarkable situation that what is usual is not necessarily 'normal', in the sense of healthy.

Where pressures are low and do not rise with age, it is unlikely that racial/genetic characteristics alone are responsible, as the variety of such populations is wide. They have been observed in Africa, Asia, Australasia, the Americas, and Pacific Islands. It is possible that the burden of parasites and infectious disease in these communities keeps blood pressures low. There is, however, no real evidence that this can happen, apart perhaps from one study in New Guinea which showed a tendency to lower pressures in people with enlarged spleens—presumably the result of malaria.[8]

Conclusions that pressures do not rise with age, in general, have not been based on following individuals prospectively, and the flat age curve could be an artefact of cross-sectional studies. If individuals destined to have increased pressures as they aged were selectively removed from the populations, by death or migration, theoretically a 'flat' age curve could result. However, this would imply (a) an association between tendency of pressure to rise and mortality from the diseases common in low blood pressure populations, viz., infectious disease, and (b) removal by death of large numbers of people in young to middle age, as studies in Western countries have shown that an increase of pressure with age occurs in most, although not all, individuals.[9] There is no evidence for (a), and (b) would, more or less, rule out selective mortality as an explanation. It is more likely that, in some communities, blood pressures do not rise with age.

c *Acculturation and Blood Pressure*

'Acculturation' is the change that takes place when cultures come in contact. In practice, it usually refers to the changes that occur with what may be called modernization, westernization, urbanization or industrialization. Studies of similar ethnic groups living under different degrees of acculturation provide strong evidence against a simple genetic explanation for immunity to hypertension. Such studies have been of three types: studies of societies undergoing modernization, comparisons at one time of groups varying in degree of acculturation, and studies of migrants from a less to a more urbanized setting (migration is rarely the other way).[10]

Perhaps the best known of the reports of societies undergoing modernization is that from East Africa.[5] Trowell links his own experience to published reports from Uganda and Kenya over 40 years.[11] In 1929 Donnison reported low blood pressures in Africans living on the shores of Lake Victoria that actually fell in men aged more than 60.[12] In the 1960s a survey of Ugandans in a rural community near the capital showed a European/American picture: higher blood pressures rising steeply with age.[13] These studies were in similar but not identical groups and the mode of selection of the populations differed, which raises doubts about their direct comparability.[5] Different methods of measurement could also result in differences in levels of blood pressure in studies 30 years apart, but it is unlikely that this could account for the markedly different age patterns.

These African studies suggest that blood pressure patterns can change. Studies of Micronesians on Ponape show that this does not happen inevitably with acculturation. Cassel[10] reports that studies on Ponape in 1947 and 1950 showed the persistence of traditional cultural patterns and little rise of blood pressure with age. The social and cultural changes brought to Ponape by becoming part of the US Trust Territory had little effect on blood pressures. In 1971, the rise with age hardly differed from the earlier picture.[10] What changed in East Africa that did not in Ponape? The discrepancy between the East African and the Ponape experience points to the need for further specification of what changes acculturation entails (see Section 5).

A second type of acculturation study is the comparison at one time of similar ethnic groups living under different degrees of contact with urban culture. Henry and Cassel collected reports of a large number of blood pressure studies and classified them by ethnic group.[14] It appeared that, for each ethnic group, there was a relationship between degree of acculturation and rise of blood pressure with age. But the studies varied widely in methodology and the degree of acculturation was inferred rather than measured directly.

FIG. 1. Mean blood pressure of 2 groups of Cook Island Polynesians living in a more remote (○) and more urbanized (●) setting

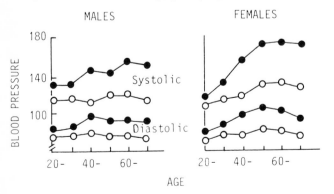

FIG. 2. Prevalence of hypertension (160+ and/or 95+) among different groups of men in Japan[20]

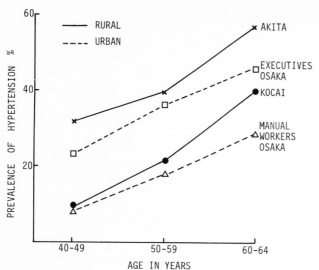

Their hypothesis is borne out more convincingly by the type of study shown in Fig. 1. The same investigators measured the blood pressures in both groups of Polynesian islanders, reducing the possible sources of error.[7] These, and other studies in New Guinea,[15] Palau (Micronesia),[16] South Africa,[17] and Chile[18] provide evidence of a changed age-pattern of blood pressure in more urban settings.

d *Urban–Rural Differences*

The many words used to describe this culture change are vague. Without knowing what dietary, environmental, and/or psycho-social processes are in operation, one cannot assume 'urban equals bad'. In Ponape, for example, there was no consistent difference in blood pressures between the zones of the island with different degrees of urbanization. In Japan the urban/rural gradient is reversed. In national surveys, inhabitants of agricultural, forestry or fishing areas have higher blood pressures than populations in big cities.[19] Komachi *et al.* confirmed this in seven different groups in Japan. Fig. 2 shows the prevalence of hypertension in four of these.[20] The highest prevalence (and highest mean pressure) is in rural Akita in north-east Japan. In urban Osaka the blood pressures in men rise with social status, which is the reverse of the pattern in England and Wales.[21]

In Yugoslavia, the urban/rural gradient varies by region.[22] In Catholic Remetinec, a suburb of Zagreb (the capital of Croatia), pressures in rural inhabitants are higher than in urban. The reverse is true in Tuzla, a Turkish area in the mountains of Bosnia.

Rural inhabitants of Japan and Yugoslavia are not isolated and 'pre-modern' like atoll-dwelling Polynesians or pastoralists in East Africa. In Japan and Yugoslavia, all groups studied show a rise of blood pressure with age and the lack of, or reversed, urban/rural gradient emphasizes the need for more specific aetiological hypotheses.

4 Migrants

a *'Cross-Sectional' Studies*

The third type of study showing the influence of cultural and geographic change on blood pressure is a comparison of migrants with the native-born in their place of destination and with their compatriots in the place of origin who have not migrated. The migration may take place within a country. For example, Shaper *et al.* compared nomadic Samburu warriors who had entered the Kenyan army with controls who had not.[5] Table I shows that weight increased within 6 months of entering the army. Blood pressures did not increase in that time, but an increase was apparent at 2 years and sustained at 6 years after entering the army.

International studies of migrants from a low to a high blood pressure population similarly show increases in blood pressure.[10] Of interest are blood pressures in people of African origin. There are rural communities in East Africa and South Africa[17], and the Gambia in West Africa[23] where blood pressures are low and do not rise with age. This contrasts with higher pressures which rise with age in urban Nigeria,[23] South Africa[17] and East Africa,[11] and in people of African origin in Jamaica,[24] elsewhere in the Caribbean,[25] and in the United States.[26] In the United States, blacks have commonly been found to have higher blood pressures than whites, and an increased risk of hypertensive disease.[27] Limited data from England suggest higher blood pressures in adult blacks than whites, after controlling for social class[28] but not in children.[29] Certainly, mortality from hypertensive and cerebrovascular disease is high in Caribbean and African immigrants to England and Wales (Table II).[30] If the mortality of relatively recent immigrants is high, we may infer that the mortality from these causes is likely to be high in the subgroups of the population in the home (old) country from which the immigrants come.

The high blood pressures of people of African origin in many parts of the world might suggest a genetic basis[27] although the low pressures of rural unaccultured Africans make this unlikely. A

TABLE I. Weight, skinfold thickness and blood pressure in Nomadic Samburu warriors at varying periods after entering the Kenyan army, compared with controls who did not[5]

Time in army	N	Weight (kg)	Skinfold* (mm)	Blood Pressure (mm Hg)
6 months	15	61.7†	13.4‡	113/67
controls	15	52.6	11.2	116/72
2 years	29	57.6§	12.1	122/70‡
controls	29	54.4	11.1	114/71
6 years	30	60.8†	13.5*	124/75†
controls	30	54.9	11.0	112/71

* Sum of triceps and subscapular
† P < 0.001
‡ P < 0.01
§ P < 0.005

TABLE II. Standardized mortality ratios (England and Wales = 100) of immigrants to England and Wales from the Caribbean and Africa, with comparison to SMRs in Trinidad and Tobago*

Country of birth		Hypertensive disease		Cerebrovascular disease	
		Migrants	'Home'*	Migrants	'Home'
Caribbean	M	343	357	178	174
	F	430	690	157	223
Africa	M	447		165	
	F	235		124	

* 'Home' country rates were available for Trinidad and Tobago. These have been standardized taking England and Wales = 100

parallel may perhaps be drawn with tuberculosis in the United States at an earlier period. Blacks had higher mortality rates than whites, and there was speculation as to whether there may be a genetic component to their apparent greater susceptibility. However, as tuberculosis mortality declined, presumably as a result of nutritional and socio-environmental improvements as well as medical and public health efforts, it declined in blacks as well as whites. If there were a genetic component to TB susceptibility, there was clearly a major environmental one as well. A similar argument may be applied to high blood pressure in people of African origin. If there is a genetic susceptibility, it is at most a genetic susceptibility to environmental influences.[31]

b *Longitudinal Migrant Studies*

Cassel has suggested that the ideal migrant study '. . . should be able to identify migrants before migration, compare them with non-migrants from the same population (to test for selection factors), follow the migrants over time in their new environment (to ensure that the age relationship of blood pressure is not being produced by selective mortality . . .), and also follow the non-migrants over the same period of time (to control for secular changes common to both groups)'.[10]

The Tokelau Island migrant study approaches this ideal.[32] Polynesians dwelling on these Pacific atolls were studied before and after migration to New Zealand, and people remaining on the islands were followed. The systolic blood pressures are shown in Fig. 3. Mean blood pressures of the migrants prior to migration were actually lower than those of non-migrants. At the second survey, blood pressures of the migrants to New Zealand had risen, but not of the non-migrants.

These migrant figures may shed light on a dilemma.[25] One view of the rise of blood pressure with age has been that factors acting early in life lead to differences in blood pressure; there is then a vicious circle, i.e. high blood pressures cause blood pressure to rise further. An alternate view holds that the rise of blood pressure with age reflects the cumulative effects of exposure or decreased ability of older persons to adapt to a 'hypertension' environment. The data in Fig. 3 are more compatible with the second. In most

migrant studies, age is confounded with length of stay, as migration usually occurs in the third decade of life. In this study, people of different ages have presumably been in New Zealand for the same length of time. The greater change in blood pressure in older compared with younger migrants suggests that older people are less able to adapt to whatever it is in the New Zealand environment that is responsible for higher blood pressures.

5 Diet and Geographical Variations

The preceding evidence suggests that, in determining blood pressure differences between populations, environmental rather than genetic factors are likely to be paramount. Two types of explanation have been proposed for the changes in blood pressure with acculturation: changes in diet, including the development of obesity and psycho-social changes. If the focus is broadened beyond acculturation studies to look more generally at geographical variations within and between countries, there is some support for dietary hypotheses; less for psycho-social ones, in large part because of the difficulty of translating hypotheses about such factors into specific testable form.

a *Correlational Studies of Salt*

Dahl, who bred rats that, when given a high salt diet, developed hypertension, made famous a graph (Fig. 4) that showed a straight line correlation between mean intake of sodium chloride and prevalence of hypertension, among five populations.[33] The previously stated doubts about comparability of measurement apply to this study, as to the later review by Gleibermann of published reports from 27 studies[34] (Fig. 5). As is usual, sodium intake was estimated from urinary excretion. From the regression lines (somewhat mysteriously, the equation is given in linear form but plotted on a log scale) one can estimate that a difference of 1 g NaCl in daily excretion corresponds to a difference in blood

FIG. 3. Mean systolic blood pressure by age of Tokelauan men comparing non-migrants at two surveys with migrants before and after migration to New Zealand

(after Prior[32])

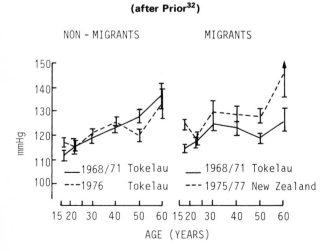

FIG. 4. Correlation of average daily salt (NaCl) intake with prevalence of hypertension in different geographic areas

(after Dahl[33])

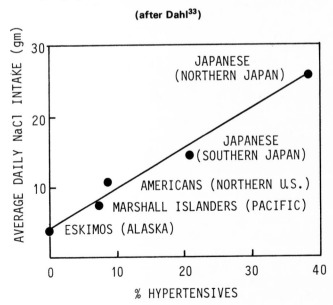

FIG. 5. Correlation of blood pressure with salt intake in 27 populations

(after Gleibermann[34])

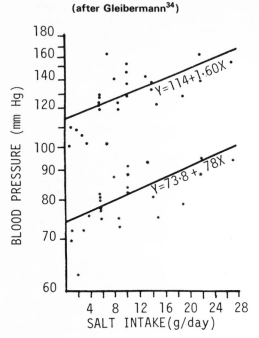

Systolic pressure is shown by dots, diastolic pressure by stars

pressure of 1.6 mm Hg systolic and 0.8 mm Hg diastolic. However, in addition to the worry about comparability of measurement in published reports, several of the reports did not have adequate data on sodium intake/excretion.

Joossens, in more qualitative fashion, points to the pattern of low salt intake (<1 g NaCl/day), low blood pressure; moderate salt intake (8–12 g NaCl/day), intermediate prevalence of hypertension and stroke; high salt intake (≥15 g NaCl/day), such as in parts of Japan, Korea, Portugal, and Eastern Europe, high prevalence of hypertension and stroke.[35] Joossens and Geboers also observed a strong correlation between stroke mortality and gastric cancer mortality between countries and over time.[36] They postulated that a high intake of sodium chloride is a common factor and suggest that the decline in stroke and stomach cancer in many countries can be attributed to increased use of refrigeration and consequent decreased use of salt as a preservative.

b *Potassium*

The above work suggests that high intake of sodium is harmful, but does not consider the possibility that high intake of potassium is protective. Reviewing studies from many countries, Froment showed a high-order correlation between populations, of urinary sodium/potassium ratio with blood pressure.[37] From these figures one cannot distinguish between three hypotheses: sodium bad, potassium good, high ratio of sodium to potassium bad.

c *Acculturation and Dietary Change*

Several of the studies of acculturation and blood pressure suggest that an increase in salt intake is responsible for the increase in blood pressure and changed age pattern.[38] Trowell points to

increased salt intake in East Africa at the time that higher blood pressures were found,[11] and Shaper reports that when Samburu warriors entered the Kenyan army, their diet changed from milk, meat and blood to a diet high in carbohydrate with an increased intake of salt.[5] In the study of Polynesians on the Cook Islands (Fig. 1) the more acculturated group had higher mean sodium excretion, although lower intake of fat.[7] The Tokelau study showed higher sodium concentrations in early-morning urine specimens in Tokelauans in New Zealand than on Tokelau, and lower potassium concentrations.[40] Either or both could be important in the higher blood pressures in New Zealand.

Page studied six communities of Melanesians in the Solomon Islands, all at a low level of acculturation.[40] There was no consistent relationship between degree of acculturation and level of blood pressure, but only in the three most acculturated communities (and only in women) was systolic blood pressure positively correlated with age. It was estimated that salt intake was higher in the three more acculturated groups, but salt consumption data were imprecise as timed urinary collections could not be obtained. Nevertheless, highest blood pressures were obtained in the one fishing community that boiled vegetables in sea water, and had the highest estimated salt intake. Potassium intake was not reported.

Increase in obesity competes with increase in salt as a potential explanation for changes in blood pressure with acculturation, although the data are somewhat less consistent, as for example in Table I on Samburu entering the Kenyan army. Given the consistent relationship found in Western countries between obesity and blood pressure, it is likely that increases in body weight must play some role, even if only a contributory one.

d *Regional Variations in Japan*

As shown in Fig. 2, there are marked regional, and social, variations in blood pressure in Japan, and concomitant variations in stroke mortality.[19] These show no correlation with regional variations in obesity. In Akita, in the cold north-east of Japan, salt intake had been estimated at over 30 g/day in 1935.[41] By 1965, it was still high at 23 g/day. By contrast, in Osaka where blood pressures were lower, salt intake was estimated at 14 g/day.[41] In eight populations studied by Komachi *et al.*, sodium chloride intake varied from <10 g to >20 g/day and there was a positive correlation with 'prevalence of hypertension'.[41]

Sasaki also working in north-east Japan found lower blood pressures in Aomori prefecture than in neighbouring Akita. Intake of sodium did not appear to differ appreciably between the two areas, and the lower blood pressure in apple-producing Aomori was ascribed to a high potassium intake from apples.[18] Attempts to reduce salt intake in both areas have been accompanied by decreases in blood pressure.[42]

e *Other Factors*

Diets of 'low-salt' populations may differ from 'high-salt' diets in other ways. Studies in vegetarians in Western countries and in omnivorous people asked to eat a vegetarian diet show lower blood pressures, compared with an omnivorous diet, that cannot be explained by differences in sodium or potassium.[43]

Previous studies had ascribed Japanese regional variations in hypertension and stroke to variations in temperature.[44] Blood pressures in the cold north-east were shown to be higher during the severe winters than in summer and room temperature rather than outside temperature was shown to be critical. However, a small-scale intervention study on the effects of introducing stoves in a farming village failed to reduce blood pressures.[19]

6 Psycho-Social Changes and Blood Pressure

In reviewing the data on low-blood pressure populations, Cassel hypothesized that 'low pressures occur in societies with a coherent value system which remains relatively unchallenged during the lifetime of the oldest inhabitants. Migration to a society with different value systems leads to situations in which previously sanctioned behaviour, especially those the individual acquired during critical learning periods, can no longer be used to express normal behavioural urges. This, in turn, creates repeated autonomic system arousal', which leads eventually to sustained elevations of pressure.[10]

Eyer, similarly, looks on hypertension as a disease of modern society, two particular features of which may be responsible: community disruption and work pressure. He suggests that stress leads to increased sodium retention thereby interacting with a high salt diet.[45]

If the data on dietary change as an explanation of blood pressure change with acculturation are incomplete, the data on the psycho-social hypothesis are even more so. A major difficulty is that, unlike salt intake, the meaning of a psycho-social measure varies with the context in which it is found. Two examples may serve to illustrate both the promise and the problems of the psycho-social approach.

In the study of Zulus in South Africa, Scotch found blood pressures higher in the urban than the rural area.[17] Within the urban area, hypertensives were more likely to retain traditional cultural practices, suggesting an inability to adapt successfully to the demands of urban living. The Tokelau Island migrant study found the opposite.[46] Tokelauans in New Zealand who retained traditional styles of social interaction, thereby gaining social support, had lower blood pressures than more acculturated Tokelauans.

The problem is that both findings may be true. Urban South Africa is different politically and culturally from urban New Zealand. In addition, the measures of tradition were greatly different in the two studies, hence a difference in results is not unexpected. The comparison does, however, point to the difficulty of testing the psycho-social hypothesis in international studies.

7 Conclusions

International and regional comparisons make it clear that blood pressure levels and prevalence of hypertension vary and that a rise of blood pressure with age is not a fixed human attribute. The variety of low-blood-pressure populations that have been described and the changes that occur in migrants make a simple genetic explanation unlikely. At most, there may be a genetic predisposition to environmental stimuli.

The salt hypothesis remains in doubt (see e.g., Reference 47) for several reasons. With a few exceptions, international comparisons have been based on unstandardized measurements of uncertain comparability; a high sodium hypothesis has not been compared with a low potassium, or a high Na/K ratio hypothesis; there has not been a concerted attempt to control for confounding variables, in particular body weight; within populations a relationship in individuals of salt intake to blood pressure level is usually not observed. This last may be the result of difficulty in accurately characterizing individual levels of blood pressure or salt excretion.[48] It may also relate to the notion formulated in Section 2. Within a population, homogeneous with respect to diet, other factors, including possibly genes, may be more important in setting individual blood pressure levels. Between populations, environmental factors are likely to be more important.

Data such as those collected in South Africa[17] and among Tokelauan migrants provide some support for a psycho-social explanation of blood pressure changes with acculturation. The hypothesis may be correct but it will prove difficult to test internationally until valid methods for the assessment of stress cross-culturally are developed. Evidence is more likely to come from studies within a single cultural/ethnic group.

REFERENCES

1 Pickering G. The inheritance of arterial pressure. Proceedings of an international symposium, Chicago, 1964. In: Stamler J, Stamler R, Pullman TN, eds. The epidemiology of hypertension. New York: Grune & Stratton, 1967; 18–25

2 Barker DJP, Rose G. Epidemiology in medical practice. 3rd edition. Edinburgh: Churchill Livingstone, 1984

3 Feinleib M, Garrison R, Borhani N, Rosenman R, Christian J. Studies of hypertension in twins. In: Paul O, ed. Epidemiology and control of hypertension. Papers and discussions from the Second International Symposium on the Epidemiology of Hypertension . . . 1974, [etc.]. New York: Stratton Intercontinental Medical Book Corporation, 1975; 3–20

4 Epstein FH, Eckoff RD. The epidemiology of high blood pressure—geographic distributions and etiological factors. In: Stamler J et al. op. cit; 155–166*

5 Shaper AG. Cardiovascular disease in the tropics III, blood pressure and hypertension. Br Med J 1972; iii: 805–807

6 Vaughan JP. A review of cardiovascular diseases in developing countries. Ann Trop Med Parasitol 1978; 72: 101–109

7 Prior IAM, Evans JG, Harvey HPB, Davidson F, Lindsey M. Sodium intake and blood pressure in two Polynesian populations. New Engl J Med 1968; 279: 515–520

8 Maddocks I, Vines AP. The influence of chronic infection on blood pressure in New Guinea males. Lancet 1966; ii: 262–264

9 Kannel WB. Host and environmental determinants of hypertension: perspective from the Framingham Study. In: Kesteloot H, Joossens V, eds. Epidemiology of arterial blood pressure. Developments in Cardiovascular Medicine 8. The Hague: Martinus Nijhoff, 1980; 265–295

10 Cassel JC. Studies of hypertension in migrants. In: Paul O. op. cit; 41–61†

11 Trowell H. Hypertension, obesity, diabetes mellitus and coronary heart disease. In: Trowell HC, Burkitt DP, eds. Western diseases: their emergence and prevention. London: Edward Arnold, 1981; 3–32

12 Donnison CP. Blood pressure in the African native. Lancet 1929; i: 6–7

13 Shaper AG, Saxton GA. Blood pressure and body build in a rural community in Uganda. East Afr Med J 1969; 46: 228–245

14 Henry JP, Cassel JC. Psychosocial factors in essential hypertension. Recent epidemiologic and animal experimental evidence. Am J Epidemiol 1969; 90: 171–200

15 Maddocks I. Blood pressures in Melanesians. Med J Aust 1967; 1: 1123–1126

16 Labarthe D, Reed D, Brody J, Stallones R. Health effects of modernization in Palau. Am J Epidemiol 1973; 98: 161–174

17 Scotch NA. Sociocultural factors in the epidemiology of Zulu hypertension. Am J Public Health 1963; 53: 1205–1213

18 Cruz-Coke R, Donoso H, Barrera R. Genetic ecology of hypertension. Clin Sci 1973; 45: 55s–56s

19 Hatano S. Hypertension in Japan: a review. In: Paul O. op. cit; 63–99†

* For full bibliographical details see Reference 1.
† For full bibliographical details see Reference 3.

20 Komachi Y, Shimamoto T. Regional difference of blood pressure and its nutritional background in several Japanese populations. In: Kesteloot H, Joossens JC. op. cit; 379–394‡

21 Marmot MG, Rose G, Shipley M, Hamilton PJS. Employment grade and coronary heart disease in British civil servants. J Epidemiol Community Health 1978; 32: 244–249

22 Kozarevic Dj, McGee D. Epidemiology of essential hypertension in Yugoslavia: the Yugoslavia cardiovascular disease study. In: Kesteloot H, Joossens JV. op. cit; 207–216‡

23 Vaughan JP. A brief review of cardiovascular disease in Africa. Trans R Soc Trop Med Hyg 1977; 71: 226–231

24 Miall WE, Kass EH, Ling J, Stuart KL. Factors influencing arterial pressure in the general population in Jamaica. Br Med J 1962; 2: 497–506

25 Marmot MG, Khaw K-T. Implications for population studies of the age trend in blood pressure. In: Bahlmann J, Leibau H, eds. Stress and hypertension. Contributions to Nephrology 30. Basel: Karger, 1982; 101–107

26 Stamler J, Berkson DM, Lindberg HA, Miller WA, Stamler R, Collette P. Socioeconomic factors in the epidemiology of hypertensive disease. In: Stamler J et al. op. cit; 289–320*

27 McDonough JR, Garrison GE, Hames CG. Blood pressure and hypertensive disease among Negroes and Whites in Evans County, Georgia. In: Stamler J et al. op. cit; 167–187*

28 Marmot MG, Rose G. Epidemiology of hypertension. In: Sleight P, Vann Jones J, eds. Scientific Foundations of Cardiology. London: Heinemann, 1984

29 Khaw K-T, Marmot MG. Blood pressure in 15- to 16-year old adolescents of different ethnic groups in two London schools. Postgrad Med J 1983; 59: 630

30 Marmot MG, Adelstein AM, Bulusu L. Mortality of immigrants to England and Wales. OPCS. Studies on medical and population subjects. London: HMSO, In press

31 Oliver WJ. Sodium homeostasis and low blood pressure populations. In: Kesteloot H, Joossens JV. op. cit; 229–242‡

32 Prior IAM. Isolated groups, particular populations and their contributions. In: Hayase S, Murao S, eds. Cardiology. Proceedings of the VIII World Congress of Cardiology, Tokyo. . . 1978. Amsterdam: Excerpta Medica, 1979; 131–136. (International Congress Series 470)

33 Dahl LK. Salt intake and hypertension. In: Genest J, Koiw E, Kurchel O, eds. Hypertension: physiopathology and treatment. New York: McGraw-Hill, 1977; 548–559

34 Gleibermann L. Blood pressure and dietary salt in human populations. Ecology Food Nutri 1973; 2: 143–56

35 Joossens JC, Geboers J. Salt and hypertension. Prev Med 1983; 12: 53–59

36 Joossens JV, Geboers J. Nutrition and gastric cancer. Nutr Cancer 1981; 2: 250–261

37 Froment A, Milon H, Gravier Ch. Relation entre consommation sodée et hypertension arterielle. Contribution de l'épidémiologie géographique. Rev Epidemiol Santé Publique 1979; 27: 437–454

38 Freis ED. Salt, volume and the prevention of hypertension. Circulation 1976; 53: 589–595

39 Prior IAM, Stanhope JM. Blood pressure patterns, salt use and migration in the Pacific. In: Kesteloot H, Joossens JV. op. cit; 243–262‡

40 Page LB, Damon A, Moellering RC Jr. Antecedents of cardiovascular disease in six Solomon Islands societies. Circulation 1974; 49: 1132–46

41 Komachi Y, Shimamoto T. Salt intake and its relationship to blood pressure in Japan: present and past. In: Kesteloot H, Joossens JV. op. cit; 395–400‡

42 Sasaki N. Epidemiological studies on hypertension in Northeast Japan. In: Kesteloot H, Joossens JV. op. cit; 367–377‡

43 Rouse IL, Armstrong BK, Beilin LJ, Vandongen R. Blood-pressure-lowering effect of a vegetarian diet: controlled trial in normotensive subjects. Lancet 1983; i: 5–9

44 Takahashi E, Sasaki N, Takeda J, Ito H. The geographic distribution of cerebral hemorrhage and hypertension in Japan. Hum Biol 1957; 29: 139–166

45 Eyer J. Hypertension as a disease of modern society. Int J Health Serv 1975; 5: 539–558

46 Beaglehole R, Salmond CE, Hooper A et al. Blood pressure and social interaction in Tokelauan migrants in New Zealand. J Chron Dis 1977; 30: 803–812

47 Swales JD. Dietary salt and hypertension. Lancet 1980; i: 1177–1179

48 Liu K, Cooper R, McKeever J, et al. Assessment of the association between habitual salt intake and high blood pressure: methodological problems. Am J Epidemiol 1979; 110: 219–226

---

* For full bibliographical details see Reference 1.
† For full bibliographical details see Reference 3.
‡ For full bibliographical details see Reference 9.

British Medical Bulletin (1984) Vol. 40, No. 4, pp. 387–389

NON-INFECTIVE DISEASE OF THE LARGE BOWEL

D P BURKITT CMG MD FRCS (Ed) FRS

The Old House
Bussage
Stroud, Gloucestershire

1 Volvulus
2 Appendicitis
   a Geographical and socio-economic distribution
   b Postulated causative factors
3 Haemorrhoids
   a Nature and distribution
   b Postulated causative factors
4 Cancer and polyps
   a Geographical, cultural and socio-economic distribution
   b Changes following immigration
   c Sub-groups within a general culture
   d Postulated causative and protective factors
5 Diverticular disease of the colon
6 Ulcerative colitis
7 Crohn's disease
   References

The distribution of infective bowel diseases like amoebiasis and schistosomiasis can be explained on the basis of the presence of both causative organisms and their vectors, and cholera epidemics which come and go relate to sewage disposal and purity of drinking water. It is the non-infective diseases of the large bowel that exhibit distinctive patterns of geographical, and sometimes socio-economic, distribution and these only will be considered. All of those to be considered except the purely mechanical problem of volvulus have been shown to be characteristic of the life-style that is associated with modern Western culture, and none of them has been observed to be other than rare in communities still living in a traditional environment, and in particular persisting in the dietary customs to which they have become adapted. Volvulus is often more frequently observed in Third World communities than in the West, so this condition will be considered first and the others will be dealt with in the order in which they have been observed to emerge or increase in frequency in Third World communities following impact with Western culture.

1 Volvulus

Volvulus, or twisting of a loop of gut on its mesentery, most commonly affects the pelvic or sigmoid colon but sometimes involves portions of the small bowel. Rarely the caecum may be involved. Only vulvulus of the pelvic colon will be considered. This is much more frequently observed in developing than in more industrialized countries, but in the former its distribution is very patchy.

Sigmoid volvulus is a common cause of intestinal obstruction in certain regions, but by no means in all, of Africa. It accounts for about 20% of cases of intestinal obstruction in Bulawayo (Zimbabwe) and in Kampala (Uganda). In the north and south-west of Uganda, however, this disorder is rare. It has been reported to be common at least in parts of South Africa, Ethiopia, Eritrea, and Zambia. In Western Kenya, however, only 5 of over 1000 major operations performed in a 5-year period were for pelvic colon volvulus. Only one in over 400 cases of intestinal obstruction seen at Ibadan, Nigeria was caused by volvulus. Sixty-six of 73 cases observed during a 4-year period in Kampala, Uganda belonged to the Baganda tribe and all were males. The vast majority of patients are males.

Postulated Causative Factors

Certain types of bulky, fibre-rich diets almost certainly contribute to the causation of sigmoid volvulus, but the enormous male proponderance and patchy distribution in Africa indicate other contributory causes.[1]

2 Appendicitis

a *Geographical and Socio-economic Distribution*

This is the commonest indication for emergency abdominal surgery in most Western countries but the condition is invariably rare in rural communities in the Third World.[2] It is one of the first of characteristically Western diseases to emerge following impact with Western culture. During both World Wars, its prevalence fell in German occupied countries in association with severe food restrictions[3] and it was almost unknown in concentration camps. In Africa and Asia, appendicitis is more common in urban and otherwise westernized communities than in rural populations.

Reports from India half a century and more ago indicate that appendicitis was observed in army officers but not amongst other ranks, and in the more prosperous but not in the poor. In former days when African students were sent to European countries for further education, appendicitis would appear amongst them within a year.[2] So rare is the condition among Malaysian Aborigines that the only cases in a hospital caring for this group occurred in members of staff. Black and white Americans are equally affected today. Fifty years ago, blacks were much less affected than whites and the ancestors of the former must have been as free from the disease as are rural Africans today. In Western countries, the disease most commonly affects young people.

b *Postulated Causative Factors*

Appendicitis is a disease almost invariably restricted to a portion of the appendix between the tip and a more proximal line of more or less distinct demarcation between normal and diseased tissue. In view of this and the clinical symptomatology, the initial lesion is believed to be an obstructive phenomenon. The only concept of causation which is consistent with the epidemiological features is increased viscosity of the faecal content resultant of fibre-depletion of the diet.[4] The lymphoid follicles in the appendix which can, in the presence of infection, swell and narrow the lumen, begin to atrophy in adolescence and this could explain the preponderance of the disease in the young.

3 Haemorrhoids

a *Nature and Distribution*

The nature of haemorrhoids has until recently been misunderstood. They were formerly and wrongly believed to be varicosities of haemorrhoidal veins comparable to varicose veins in the legs, or in the lower oesophagus consequent on portal cirrhosis. Largely as a result of the work of Thomson,[5] they are now recognized to be normal cushions or sponges having the express purpose of ensuring rectal continence of both flatus and fluid when squeezed by the encircling sphincter muscle. They have in fact been compared to the lips which fulfil a similar function when forced together by contraction of the orbicularis-oris muscle.[6] Only the complications of haemorrhoids, bleeding, prolapse or thrombosis, can be viewed as pathological, and these are so common in Western communities that it has been estimated that one in two people over the age of 50 suffers at some time from them. Complications are rare in Third World communities. Monthly replies received over a period of 2 years from over 150 rural hospitals in Africa seeking evidence of patients with bleeding, prolapsed or thrombosed piles, indicated a frequency of under two cases per hospital per year.[7]

b *Postulated Causative Factors*

Straining to evacuate hard faecal masses causes venous engorgement of these cushions. This renders them more susceptible to the trauma imposed by hard faecal masses being forced through the anal canal. This can be abrasive, causing haemorrhage, and can disrupt the attachments of the cushions to the sphincter, leading to prolapse, or can initiate thrombosis.

The fundamental cause is believed to be depletion in dietary fibre which increases firmness and reduces volume of faeces.

Consequently a change to fibre-rich diets is increasingly being viewed as the basis of initial treatment.

4 Cancer and Polyps

a *Geographical, Cultural and Socio-Economic Distribution*

The prevalence of both malignant and benign tumours of the large bowel has been shown to be more closely related to economic development than that of any other neoplasms. The geographical distribution of both lesions is similar, although the contrasts between the prevalence of polyps in poorer and in richer nations is even more striking than the demonstrated differences in cancer rates. The former are estimated to be present in about 20% of adults in Western countries yet are extremely rare in Third World populations, being found in under 0.1% of subjects in carefully performed autopsy examinations.[8] Rates of colon and rectal cancer are usually together high or low in different populations, which suggests that they share common aetiological factors. In the few situations where this is not so, for example the relatively higher rates of rectal cancer in Japan, it must be assumed that additional factors act selectively on this gut segment.

In general bowel cancer rates increase progressively in relation to contact with Western culture. Minimal rates are found in rural communities in Africa, the Pacific, and other similar situations, intermediate rates in South America, Eastern Europe and more developed parts of Asia, and maximum rates in Western Europe, Australia and New Zealand and North America, in which continent rates in the black and white populations are closely similar.[9] Two generations ago the tumour was much less prevalent among blacks[10] and their ancestors on first arrival in the New World must have experienced rates at least as low as those of rural Africans today.

b *Changes Following Immigration*

Bowel cancer rates have been low in Japan but are beginning to rise following the changes in dietary habits which occurred after the Second World War. Rates in second and subsequent generations of Japanese immigrants to Hawaii and California are comparable to those of Americans from other ethnic groups.[11] The descendants of Jews who immigrated from the Yemen and North Africa to the new state of Israel have rates approaching those of European descent.

Eskimos who have adapted to a Western life-style in Alaska have subsequently experienced a rise in bowel cancer rates.

c *Sub-Groups Within a General Culture*

In the United States, both Seventh Day Adventists[12] and Mormons[13] experience about a third less bowel cancer than do other Americans. The majority of the former are vegetarians, with a diet having a higher fibre and lower fat content than other Americans.

The latter are not vegetarian but commonly consume bread made from home ground meal with its full fibre content.

Rural Finns have little over a quarter of the colon cancer rate of urban Danes.[14] Rates steadily decline from urban Danes through rural Danes and urban Finns to rural Finns. The component of food shown to be inversely related to this decline has been the pentose fraction of fibre found most abundantly in cereals and, in this case, in the abundant consumption of rye bread.

d *Postulated Causative and Protective Factors*

The main differences that characterize the diets of populations with high and with low rates of bowel tumours are the high fat and low fibre content of the former and the reverse in the latter.

Excessive fat intake is considered to be a risk factor for bowel cancer.[15] Not only does this increase bile acid content in the gut, but it fosters the growth of certain clostridia which have the capacity to degrade cholesterol and bile acids to potentially carcinogenic substances.

On the other hand, a high content of fibre in the diet, and in particular of the fibre of cereal foods which is rich in pentosans, is believed to be protective against the development of bowel cancer.[16, 17] The mechanisms whereby fibre is believed to operate include the following:[18]

1. Fibre raises faecal pH and bacterial degradation of bile acids is greatly enhanced in a less acid medium.
2. The stool-bulking capacity of fibre dilutes any potential carcinogens in the gut.
3. Since fibre shortens intestinal transit times, it presumably reduces duration of contact between faecal carcinogens and bowel mucosa.
4. The bacterial proliferation resultant in adequate fibre intake uses up available ammonia, thus reducing in the faeces the ammonia which can predispose to malignant transformation in mucosal cells.
5. Fibre increases the fatty acid butyrate which has been shown experimentally to protect cells against malignant transformation.

These concepts are consistent with the epidemiological features of the disease, and can explain the increased frequency with growing affluence, the changes following emigration and the existence of low-risk groups within Western communities including the Finns, Adventists, and Mormons.

5 Diverticular Disease of the Colon

This is a condition in which raised intracolonic pressures force the bowel mucosa out through weak spots in the overlying muscle wall to form sacular protrusions or diverticula. On barium x-ray examinations, these appear like berries attached to the surface of the colon.

This is one of the last of Western diseases to emerge in developing countries, usually over a generation after they have become influenced by Western dietary customs. The term 'diverticulitis' is applied when the diverticula become infected.

This condition is present in an estimated one third of Western populations over the age of 60 years and in one in two of those over 70. In contrast it is almost unknown in Africa and rare in Asia. Even in Western countries this disorder used to be so rare before the First World War, even in Britain and North America, that individual cases were presented as curiosities at clinico-pathological meetings.[19]

Numerous radiological series and autopsy studies have confirmed the rarity of diverticular disease throughout Asia and Africa and its high frequency in Western communities. Its frequency is apparently identical today in both black and white Americans although, like bowel cancer, it was, a generation and more ago, much less common in the black community. Again, as in the case of bowel cancer, the incidence has risen in Japanese immigrants to the USA to a figure comparable to that for other ethnic groups.

This disease has been shown to be less than half as common in vegetarians as in omnivores in Britain.[20] The former have approximately twice the dietary fibre intake of the latter.

Diverticular disease has been associated with hiatus hernia and gall-stones in Saint's Triad. All three are diseases of Western culture and adequate fibre intake has been postulated to confer protection against each.[21]

Postulated Causative Factors

Diverticular disease was, with the exception of constipation the first of the characteristically Western diseases to be generally believed to result from a deficiency in dietary fibre.[22]

Fibre-depleted diets result in the presence of an unnaturally small and firm faecal content in the colon. In attempting to propel these resistant masses forwards the bowel contracts and within segments closed at either end by circular muscle spasm, pressures can build up and force out the pouches of mucosa mentioned above.[19]

The new understanding of the pathogenesis of this disorder has completely reversed the therapeutic approach to the disease, a high-fibre diet now being universally recommended to replace the low-fibre diet formerly prescribed. This change in approach has not only been highly effective in relieving symptoms, but has also greatly reduced the rate of complications.

6 Ulcerative Colitis

This is a chronic ulcerative process that can spread widely to involve the whole of the colon. It is occasionally complicated by liver disease, skin involvement, and lesions in the eyes and joints. Adenocarcinoma is liable to develop in long-standing cases, in which the risk of developing bowel cancer is multiplied many-fold.

In the USA, the condition is most prevalent amongst Jews. Black Americans are affected less frequently than white Americans, but much more often than Africans, amongst whom the disease remains very rare.[23]

Postulated Causative Factors

All epidemiological evidence points to this disease being related to some aspects of modern Western culture. Diet is most likely to be incriminated but what specific items of diet are responsible remains obscure.

7 Chrohn's Disease

This is a transmural chronic inflammation usually involving the small bowel, but the large bowel can also be affected. It was first described in 1932 and since that time its prevalence has apparently been increasing in most Western countries.

The highest prevalence rates have been observed in Sweden, where they reach 750 per 100 000 population. In the USA, the prevalence is significantly higher in whites than in blacks, but it has been increasing in the latter, who have a much higher prevalence than sub-Saharan Africans, among whom the disease is extremely rare. Rates are similar in Australia and New Zealand to those in Northern and Western European countries. The disease is less common in southern Europe.

In Isreal, the disease is commoner in Jews born in Europe than in those born in Asia and Africa. It is rare in Arabs and Indians and in populations in Malaysia and Singapore. It is also rare in Japan.

Although Crohn's disease is primarily an intestinal lesion it is occasionally complicated by arthritis, and an eye complaint, uveitis. The aetiology of the disease remains obscure.

REFERENCES

1 Burkitt DP. No relation of sigmoid volvulus to fibre content of African diet. New Engl J Med 1981; 304: 914

2 Burkitt DP. Appendicitis in refined carbohydrate foods and disease. Some implications in dietary fibre. In: Burkitt DP, Trowell HC, eds. London: Academic Press, 1975; 87–97

3 Walker ARP. Gastrointestinal diseases and fiber intake with special reference to South African populations. In Spiller GA, Amen, RJ eds. New York: Plenum Press, 1976; 241–261

4 Burkitt DP. The protective properties of dietary fiber. N C Med J 1981; 42: 467–471

5 Thomson WHF. The nature of haemorrhoids. Br J Surg 1975; 62: 542–552

6 Alexander-Williams J. The nature of piles. Br Med J 1982; 2: 1064–1065

7 Burkitt DP. Hemorrhoids, varicose veins and deep vein thrombosis: epidemiologic features and suggested causative factors. Can J Surg 1975; 18: 483–488

8 Templeton AC. Tumours in a Tropical Country. A survey of Uganda 1964–1968. London: Heinemann, 1973; 52

9 Waterhouse J, Muir C, Shanmugaratnam IC, Powell J, eds. Cancer incidence in five continents. Lyon: IARC, 1982; Vol IV. (IARC Scientific Publications No. 42)

10 Steiner PE. Cancer race and geography. Baltimore: Williams & Wilkins, 1954; 75

11 Wynder EL, Shigematsu TH. Environmental factors of cancer of the colon and rectum. Cancer 1967; 20: 1520–1561

12 Phillips, RL, Garfinkel L, Kuzma JW, Beeson WL, Lotz T, Brin B. Mortality among California Seventh-Day Adventists for selected sites. J Natl Cancer Inst 1980; 65: 1097–1107

13 Lyon JL, Kleuber MR, Gardner JW, Smart CR. Cancer incidence in Mormons and non-Mormons in Utah, 1966–1970. New Engl Med J 1975; 294: 129–133

14 McLennan R, Jensen OM, Mosbech J et al. Dietary fibre, transit time, faecal bacteria, steroids and colon cancer in two Scandinavian populations. Lancet 1977; 2: 207–211

15 Wynder EL, Reddy BS. Dietary Fat and Colon Cancer. J Natl Cancer Inst 1975; 54: 7–10

16 Burkitt DP. Epidemiology of Cancer of the Colon and Rectum. Cancer 1971; 28: 3–13

17 Walker ARP, Burkitt DP. Colonic cancer—hypothesis of causation, dietary prophylaxis, and future research. Am J Digest Dis 1976; 21: 910–917

18 Cummings JH, Branch WH. Postulated mechanisms whereby fibre may protect against large bowel cancer. In: Vahouny, G. and Kritchevsky, D, eds. Dietary fiber in health and disease. New York: Plenum Press, 1982; 313–325

19 Painter NS. Diverticular disease of the colon. London: Heinemann, 1975

20 Gear JS, Ware A, Fursdon P et al. Symptomless diverticular disease and intake of dietary fibre. Lancet 1979; 1: 511–514

21 Burkitt DP, Walker ARP. Saint's triad: confirmation and explanation. S Afr Med J 1976; 50: 2136–2138

22 Painter NS Burkitt DP. Diverticular disease of the colon. A deficiency disease of Western civilization. Br Med J 1971; 2: 450–454

23 Segal I, Tim LO, Hamilton DG, Walker ARP. The rarity of ulcerative colitis in South African Blacks. Am J Gastroenterol 1980; 74: 332–336

British Medical Bulletin (1984) Vol. 40, No. 4, pp. 390–395

THE GEOGRAPHICAL DISTRIBUTION OF NEURAL TUBE DEFECTS AND ORAL CLEFTS

IAN LECK MB PhD DSc FFCM

Department of Community Medicine
University of Manchester

1   Oral clefts
    a Cleft lip (with or without cleft palate)
    b Cleft palate (without cleft lip)
2   Neural tube defects
    a Variations among Caucasoids
    b Variations between primary races
    c Other findings
3   Conclusion
    References

Except for neural tube defects and oral clefts, studies of geographical variations in frequency have so far contributed relatively little to our understanding of congenital malformations. The other types of major defects are either less common or less readily diagnosed at birth, and few workers have surveyed enough births to obtain reliable figures for the former or used methods capable of ascertaining all cases of the latter.

For these reasons, neural tube defects (NTDs) and oral clefts are the only malformations considered here. Even in these conditions, some of the available data, especially for places in the developing countries, are flawed by being based only on hospital births—among which some defects, especially anencephaly (An), tend to be over-represented because of their associations with obstetric problems. In the absence of this bias, some of the figures reported from developing countries might be lower by one third.[1] However, although such a bias would be serious in some contexts, it is small in relation to the range of variation in prevalence between different countries. It therefore seems legitimate to use data for hospital births as well as for whole communities to explore the geographical distribution of oral clefts and NTDs.

1 Oral Clefts

Among the common oral clefts, both cleft lip and palate combined (CL + P) and cleft lip alone (CL) affect more males than females and are commoner than average among the relatives of patients with either, whilst cleft palate (CP) is more common in females and runs in other families.[2] Cleft lip with or without cleft palate (CL $\pm$ P) is therefore best considered as one entity and CP as another. There is also a strong case for treating cases of CL $\pm$ P with other major defects (about one fifth of all CL $\pm$ P cases) as a separate group, since they appear to differ from the remainder in exhibiting a female excess, a marked association with high maternal age, and little difference in prevalence between black and white Americans;[3–5] but it is not feasible to break down in this way the data considered below.

The birth prevalence of oral clefts in 29 series from 19 countries is plotted in Fig. 1. These series were selected because each

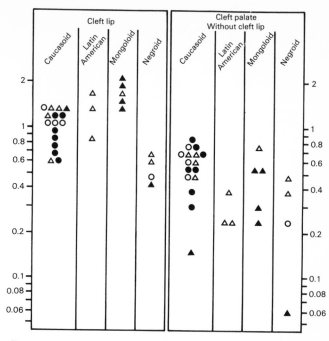

FIG. 1. **Prevalence of oral clefts per 1000 total births (log. scale) in series of over 15000 individuals (including stillbirths) of relatively uniform racial origin[5–20]**

The alignment of the point plotted for each estimate of prevalence shows the predominant primary race of the population concerned, and the type of point shows its location ($\bigcirc$ = British Isles; $\triangle$ = the Americas (including Hawaii); $\bullet$ = mainland Europe; $\blacktriangle$ = other continents)

included more than 15000 individuals who could all or nearly all be inferred to belong to one broad ethnic group, and who had been screened by methods which should at least have ascertained almost all cases of CL $\pm$ P, including those associated with stillbirth or with other malformations. The two southern Nigerian series[13,16] among the 29 have been pooled, because they included too few CP cases to yield satisfactory separate estimates of prevalence. For each series, the type of point plotted indicates region of residence, and the vertical alignment shows the primary race that predominated in the ancestry of the study population. Latin Americans described as Mestizo or European have been grouped separately since they are of mixed Caucasoid and Amerindian ancestry.

a Cleft Lip (With or Without Cleft Palate)

Among the series shown, the prevalence of CL $\pm$ P varies from 2.1/1000 in Japan[15] to 0.4/1000 in Nigeria.[13,16] Live birth statistics indicate that prevalence is even higher in some North American Indian populations.[21,22]

Most of the geographical variation shown in Fig. 1 seems to be secondary to ethnic differences, prevalence being high in Mongoloids, low in Negroids and intermediate in Caucasoids. Among the Caucasoid populations, those with a prevalence of less than 1.0/1000 were all either from mainland European countries (ranging from Spain to Finland) or from Hawaii, whilst rather higher rates were reported from Hungary, Sweden, the United Kingdom, mainland North America, and India.

When Negroid and Mongoloid communities in the United Kingdom and United States are compared on the one hand with

TABLE I. Birth prevalence of cleft lip (per 1000 total births) by place: communities of West African, European and Western Pacific ancestry

Country of birth	Ancestral origin					
	West African		European		Western Pacific	
	Prevalence	Births at risk	Prevalence	Births at risk	Prevalence	Births at risk
Nigeria						
Lagos[13]	0.30	16720	–	–	–	–
Various cities[16]	0.52	17203	–	–	–	–
United Kingdom[11]	0.46	19636	1.17	174446	–	–
United States						
Atlanta[5]	0.62	48700	1.14	121900	–	–
Various cities[9]	0.67	24030	1.36	22811	1.71	45013 (Japanese)
					1.36	11801 (Filipino)
Hawaii[14]	–	–	0.62	40221	2.14	64570
Japan[15]	–	–	–	–	1.43	29134
Philippines[19]	–	–	–	–		

their Caucasoid neighbours and on the other hand with natives of the areas where most of their ancestors originated (Table I), the ethnic differences in CL $\pm$ P prevalence are found largely to persist after migration. The only qualifications required by this statement are firstly that rather higher figures were observed in the United States than elsewhere among people of West African origin (perhaps reflecting the part-Caucasoid descent of the American black population), and secondly that in Hawaii European and Japanese figures were both lower although no less different than elsewhere.

Except for suggesting that prevalence is reduced by residence in Hawaii, this geographical pattern provides no evidence that environmental factors associated with place cause CL $\pm$ P, but points strongly to the involvement of race-related genetic factors such as those influencing face shape (which apparently tends to be less convex in the parents of children with CL $\pm$ P than in others of the same race[23]).

These conclusions are broadly reinforced by studies of the frequency of CL $\pm$ P in relation to attributes such as urbanization, birth order, and time. Such studies have revealed hardly any variations that suggest environmental causes, except for an association with maternal anticonvulsant therapy[24] and possible tendencies for births affected by CL (a minority of those with CL $\pm$ P) to be commoner in towns than in rural areas and to cluster in time.[25]

Despite providing evidence that the genotype strongly influences the prevalence of CL $\pm$ P, geographical and ethnic comparisons have been less enlightening as to how this influence operates. Most of the patterns observed in family studies of CL $\pm$ P appear to fulfil broadly the predictions of the 'multi-factorial threshold model', which pictures the effects on the embryo of many genes and perhaps other factors as combining to produce a score which has only to exceed a threshold for the defects to occur. However, one prediction of this model is that the Japanese, whose population prevalence is high, should also have a higher familial prevalence than Caucasoid populations,[26] whereas in fact the reverse seems to be true.[15,20,25,27,28]

b Cleft Palate (Without Cleft Lip)

The highest figure for CP shown in Fig. 1 (0.86/1000) occurred in Finland,[17] but two small series from Hawaii, one of Filipino and the other of Polynesian and part-Polynesian children, yielded even higher figures (1.1 and 1.0/1000).[14] The lowest figure (0.06/1000) occurred in Nigeria,[13,16] but this is one of a number of estimates based exclusively on observations made soon after birth, when CP

is much more likely than CL $\pm$ P to be overlooked. Among series that included cases ascertained later, the lowest CP figures were 0.38 per 1000 births in Budapest, Hungary,[7] and 0.25 per 1000 offspring of West Indian immigrants to Birmingham.[11]

Unlike CL $\pm$ P, CP shows no coherent pattern of variation between races: in particular, its prevalence did not vary significantly between black and white infants in one English and two United States series[5,9,11] or between infants of Japanese and European origin in Hawaii (although the difference between Europeans and Filipinos in Hawaii was just significant at the 5% level).[14] Hardly any aetiological clues have been discerned either here or in the variations in CP prevalence between populations that are racially more similar but inhabit different places, although there is one report suggesting that an increase in prevalence from the west to the east of Finland may be linked to a tendency for head width relative to length to be greater in the east.[17]

It may be a reflection of greater aetiological heterogeneity that CP shows a less coherent geographical and racial pattern than CL $\pm$ P. Family studies are consistent with this view, suggesting that a purely multifactorial threshold model fits CP less well than CL $\pm$ P and that a more plausible model for CP is that some cases have a polygenic background whilst others are related to single genes.[29,30]

2 Neural Tube Defects

Unlike CL $\pm$ P and CP, the common NTDs—anencephaly and spina bifida cystica—are best discussed simultaneously, since they have many epidemiological features in common, including a high prevalence of each among the relatives of cases of either. Another difference from oral clefts is that the prevalence of NTDs tends to vary markedly over time. In particular, prevalence at birth has declined markedly during the last decade, especially in the United Kingdom. One reason for this decline and for the geographical variations in its magnitude is the introduction and growth of antenatal screening and induced abortion for NTDs, particularly in high-risk areas.[31,32]

To avoid confusing differences in prevalence that reflect induced-abortion rates with differences that could be of aetiological significance, this review will consider mainly the geographical and racial pattern before the introduction of screening. The review follows the widespread convention of placing all NTDs in only two categories—anencephaly (An) which includes craniorrhachischisis, and spina bifida (SB) which comprises meningocele, myelocele and encephalocele. Most published studies relate only to these two categories, except that some give separate figures for encephalo-

FIG. 2. Prevalence of neural tube defects per 1000 total births (log. scale) in series of over 10000 individuals (including stillbirths) of relatively uniform racial origin[5,11,13,16,34,35]

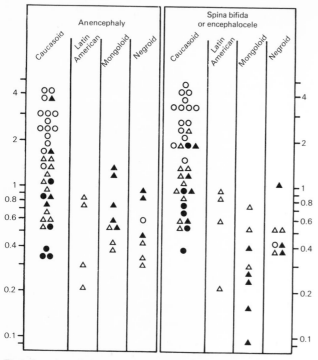

The alignment of the point plotted for each estimate of prevalence shows the predominant primary race of the population concerned, and the type of point shows its location (○ = British Isles; △ = the Americas (including Hawaii); ● = mainland Europe; ▲ = other continents)

cele. The latter series suggest that over most of the world, encephalocele occurs mainly at the occiput and is much less common than true spina bifida, which English data suggest that it resembles closely in other epidemiological respects.[11,19] There are, however, parts of south-east Asia where both true spina bifida and occipital encephalocele occur very seldom, and where fronto-ethmoid encephalocele may be more common than either.[19,33]

The birth prevalence of An and SB in 53 series from 24 countries is plotted in Fig. 2. Each series was selected on the basis of having included over 10000 infants (including stillbirths) who could almost all be assumed to have belonged to a single broad racial group. Forty-six of the 53 were drawn from two previous compilations[11,34] and the remainder were added because the previous compilations included very few Negroid data.

a Variations among Caucasoids

Among the predominantly Caucasoid series in Fig. 2, the lowest figures for each defect (0.32/1000 for An and 0.38 for SB) occurred in Finland[36] and the highest (4.45/1000 for An and 4.50 for SB) in Belfast, Northern Ireland.[19,37] The figures occupying the upper part of this range are mostly from Great Britain and Ireland, whilst most of the results from North America and mainland Europe are clustered towards the centre and the lower end of the range respectively.

Marked variations have, however, been observed within as well as between these regions. In the United Kingdom, the prevalence of each defect during the 1960s was only about one third as high in London as in Belfast and some of the coal-mining valleys of South Wales,[38] with a fairly regular gradient between these extremes.[39] For mainland Europe, the limited data available do not reveal any regular geographical pattern; but for each defect Hungary has the highest reported figures, which are more than double those observed in the neighbouring countries of Czechoslovakia and Yugoslavia.

In continental North America, prevalence rose at least twofold from west to east. This is particularly well established for the Canadian provinces,[34] but more limited data appear to reveal a trend of comparable magnitude between the west and the south-east of the United States.[5,35,40,41]

Among the four Caucasoid populations outside Europe and America that are represented in Fig. 2, there are two with figures below 1.0 for each defect and two with higher figures, especially for An. The first two are white South African and Australian populations descended mainly from European emigrants. The others are Indian and Egyptian hospital populations. Other hospital data[42-45] also suggest that a belt of high prevalence may extend from the Eastern Mediterranean to India, and that An accounts for about two thirds of the NTDs that occur there—an unusually high proportion. In North India the figures for An reached 5/1000, which would seem unlikely to occur even with selective hospital admission policies unless the true prevalence of An was at least as high as in the United Kingdom. One exception to the tendency for NTDs to be relatively common in the Middle East is the Jewish population of Israel, in which An only occurs in 0.86/1000 births and SB in 0.60/1000.[46] The risks there are particularly low among Ashkenazim (Jews of European origin), for whom lower risks than for other Caucasoids have also been reported from the United States.[47]

Although the risks among the Ashkenazim may be relatively stable, a more usual finding when Caucasoids have migrated between areas of high and low prevalence of NTDs is that prevalence tends to shift from the level seen in the migrants' ancestral homelands toward that found in other residents of the places to which they have come. Thus, the children of migrants from Ireland and North India to Birmingham, England, were closer to the Birmingham-born children of British parents than to Irish and North Indian populations in respect of the prevalence of NTDs, although with one exception the migrant figures deviated from the British in the direction of those for the migrants' countries of origin (Table II). From studies of the descendants of migrants from France, Great Britain, and Ireland to Canada,[34] from Ireland to the United States,[47] and from various Middle Eastern countries to Israel,[46] it seems that the prevalence of NTDs in the second and later generations born after migration moves even closer to the norm for the country of birth.

Turning now to variations in the prevalence of NTDs over short distances, observations made throughout the United Kingdom and Quebec, mainly during the 1960s, suggest that both An and SB tend to be more common in industrialized communities than elsewhere in the same areas.[39,48-51] This, however, may not be true of all times and places. Thus, the figures for Greater London and the less urbanized parts of south-eastern England during the 1960s appear similar when differences in ascertainment are taken into account;[39,52] the prevalence of An (although not of SB) was apparently equally high in town and country during the 1950s in Scotland[53] and more recently in Japan;[54] and higher rural than urban figures for An have been reported from the Netherlands.[55] Several studies suggest that within urban areas, the more deprived districts have the higher prevalence of NTDs.[48,56,57]

TABLE II. Birth prevalence of neural tube defects (per 1000 total births) by place: communities of Irish, British, and North Indian, Pakistani or Bangladeshi ancestry

Place of birth	Ancestral origin								
	Irish			British			North Indian, Pakistani or Bangladeshi		
	Prevalence		Births at risk	Prevalence		Births at risk	Prevalence		Births at risk
	An	SB*		An	SB*		An	SB*	
Belfast, UK[37]	3.96†	4.50	41351	–	–	–	–	–	–
Birmingham, UK[11]	2.37	2.85	14733	1.59	1.84	92464	2.37	1.50	10258
North Indian cities[45]	–	–	–	–	–	–	5.08	2.55	58445

* Figures do not include cases described only as encephalocele or cranial meningocele
† The figure originally published—4.20—included encephalocele and has therefore been reduced by 0.24 (the prevalence of encephalocele in another Belfast series[19])

Several of the above findings, including the variations over short distances and the marked reductions in the prevalence differences between ethnic groups that occur when they become neighbours, suggest that environmental factors associated with place influence the prevalence of NTDs. These factors may include the sources of the oft-reported association between prevalence and low socio-economic status,[38] since differences in affluence also match several of the geographical variations—e.g. between more and less salubrious urban areas, between the south-east and the north and west of the United Kingdom, between the west and the south-east of the United States, and between Israeli Jews and other Middle Eastern communities. However, this association breaks down when we consider the downward prevalence gradient from Britain to central Europe. Possibly the latter gradient is related to genetic differences.

Another hint that genetic factors may contribute to the geographical variations in prevalence among Caucasoids is given by family studies. These suggest that heritability is at least as high in areas of high frequency as of low,[38] whereas one might expect it to be less in the former areas if these owed their high prevalence to environmental factors alone.

b *Variations Between Primary Races*

The figures shown in Fig. 2 for non-Caucasoid populations are distributed over much the same range as those reported from mainland Europe, except that spina bifida tends to occur much less among Mongoloids; it was less than half as common as An in every Mongoloid series other than those from the United States. In the cities in England and the United States where data for more than one primary race have been collected (Table III), infants of predominantly Negroid or Mongoloid ancestry tended to be at lower risk of both An and SB than their Caucasoid neighbours, but different patterns for An and SB emerge when prevalence in the former infants and in their ancestral homelands is compared. In the case of SB, which seems to be much less common in these ancestral homelands (West Africa and the Western Pacific) than in the Caucasoid neighbours of the migrants' descendants, some of the figures given for these migrants' descendants are similar to the figures for their ancestral homelands, while others lie between these and the figures for the Caucasoid neighbours. In the case of An there is less difference in prevalence between the Caucasoid neighbours and the residents of the migrants' main regions of origin; and the migrants' descendants tend to be at lower risk than either, although this trend is not statistically significant for infants of Western Pacific ancestral origin.

Presumably the factors responsible for NTDs being less common in Mongoloids and Negroids than in Caucasoids in the same places are mainly genetic; any environmental differences, at least within places with substantial Caucasoid and Negroid populations, would be expected to make the Caucasoid figures the lower, given the inverse association between affluence and the prevalence of NTDs. However, the differences in prevalence between migrants

TABLE III. Birth prevalence of neural tube defects (per 1000 total births) by place: communities of West African, European and Western Pacific ancestry

Country of birth	Ancestral origin									
	West African			European			Western Pacific			
	Prevalence		Births at risk	Prevalence		Births at risk	Prevalence		Births at risk	
	An	SB*		An	SB*		An	SB*		
Nigeria										
Lagos[13]	0.84	0.30	16720	–	–	–	–	–	–	
Various cities[16]	0.99	0.35	17203	–	–	–	–	–	–	
United Kingdom[11]	0.59	0.36	19636	1.83	1.94	174446	–	–	–	
United States										
Atlanta[5]	0.35	0.53	48700	1.07	1.33	121900	–	–	–	
Various cities[58]	0.24	0.68	25126	0.99	0.66	24153	–	–	–	
Los Angeles[35]	0.31	0.38	124112	0.56	0.54	707221	0.38	0.19	10451	(Japanese)
Hawaii[14]	–	–	–	0.62	1.02	40221	0.56	0.64	45013	(Japanese)
							0.42	0.34	11801	(Filipino)
Japan[15]	–	–	–	–	–	–	0.63	0.20	65570	
Philippines[19]	–	–	–	–	–	–	0.51	0.07	29134	

* Figures do not include cases described only as encephalocele or cranial meningocele

and the populations of their ancestral homelands—notably the apparent reductions for An among Negroids and increases for SB among some Mongoloids after migration—provide further evidence of environmental influences.

Such influences may modify birth prevalence by affecting both incidence and miscarriage rates. English, Irish, and Japanese studies suggest that the prevalence trends for An between all three countries, and for SB between south-eastern England and Northern Ireland, are much the same in late embryos as at birth, but that the main reason for SB being less common in Japan than in Britain may be that fewer Japanese than British cases survive.[38] A fall in the miscarriage rate among Mongoloids after migration could therefore explain the evidence that their birth prevalence of SB then increases, whereas a more attractive explanation for American and English Negroids having a lower birth prevalence of An than West Africans is that affluence reduces incidence.

An alternative suggestion is that it is the mixed ancestry of the black minorities of England and the United States that makes them less prone to An than the white and West African populations with whom they have been compared. This mixed ancestry would be likely to reduce incidence if being heterozygous at a high proportion of gene loci was protective or if the defects were not related to the same genetic systems in Negroids and Caucasoids.[15]

c *Other Findings*

The concept that environmental as well as genetic factors participate in the aetiology of neural tube defects is supported not only by the above findings but also by the many reports of NTDs changing in prevalence over periods of several years and being particularly common among females, spring conceptions, firstborn infants, and the offspring of highly fertile women (i.e. those whose ultimate family size is high).[34,38]

The associations with spring conception, primiparity and (in the case of An) the female sex seem to occur predominantly in places where NTDs are relatively common. Particularly marked excesses of female and firstborn infants (although not of spring conceptions) among cases have also sometimes been observed during years when overall prevalence was high.[34] It follows that the causes of some variations in prevalence over space and time may be factors to which firstborn and female offspring are especially susceptible; but this lead has not been pursued much, although the tendency for the female excess in An to increase with overall prevalence fits Knox's hypothesis that NTDs can occur when the tissues of two zygotes meet in the uterus and interact.[59]

More attention has been paid to exploring possible associations between the geographical distribution of NTDs and of various nutrients and electrolytes. Among electrolytes, a recent review suggested that the only one with even the scantiest evidence worth noting was zinc. This evidence included reports of zinc deficiency in the high-prevalence areas of the Middle East, and of relatively low zinc levels in the drinking water, serum and red cells of mothers of affected infants and possibly in the serum of the infants themselves.[38] More recently a report of relatively high nitrate levels in the water drunk by cases' mothers[60] has recalled the finding several years ago of parallel variations over space and time in the prevalence of An and the consumption of cured meats (which contain nitrate).[61]

Interest in the possible effects of nutrients on the prevalence of NTDs was aroused by evidence that NTDs and other malformations can be produced in humans by the folate antagonist aminopterin and in rodents by deficiencies of several vitamins (including folate), and by the epidemiological evidence that birth prevalence is reduced by affluence and reaches a peak among conceptions in spring, when the body's reserves of some nutrients may be minimal. These observations have led on to several analytic and intervention studies in the United Kingdom. All this work has been extensively reviewed and evaluated elsewhere.[62] Its most striking results have come from tests of a multivitamin preparation and iron in women who had previously borne an affected child and who wished to become pregnant again. Six per 1000 offspring of fully supplemented women and 45/1000 controls were found to have NTDs. Unfortunately, these two groups were selected non-randomly, the fully supplemented having accepted treatment before conception and the controls having declined or already conceived. Despite the resulting uncertainty (which the randomized trials recently launched in Great Britain and Ireland may be unable to resolve[31]), all this work strongly suggests that aspects of nutrition play an important role among the many factors, genetic and environmental, that probably contribute to the aetiology of NTDs and thereby affect their geographical distribution.

3 Conclusion

Cleft lip and neural tube defects differ markedly in distribution by place and race. For cleft lip, the main variations are between primary races and withstand changes in environment. For neural tube defects there is more variation between populations of the same primary race, and migrant studies suggest that this variation is largely of environmental origin. Studies of the influence of time and personal attributes on prevalence are consistent with the foregoing in suggesting that aspects of the environment such as nutrition play an important part in the causation of neural tube defects, but that cleft lip could be due almost entirely to genetic factors, perhaps supplemented by random accidents during embryogenesis. The data for cleft palate are less revealing, perhaps because of under-ascertainment and aetiological heterogeneity.

REFERENCES

1 Master-Notani P, Kolah PJ, Sanghvi LD. Congenital malformations in the new born in Bombay. Part I. Acta Genet 1968; 18: 97–108

2 Fogh-Andersen P. Inheritance of harelip and cleft palate. Copenhagen: Busck, 1942

3 Hay S. Incidence of clefts and parental age. Cleft Palate J 1967; 4: 205–213

4 Emanuel I, Culver BH, Erickson JD, Guthrie B. Schuldberg D. The further epidemiological differentiation of cleft lip and palate: a population study of clefts in King County, Washington 1956–1965. Teratology 1973; 7: 271–282

5 Erickson JD. Racial variations in the incidence of congenital malformations. Ann Hum Genet 1976; 39: 315–320

6 Bonaiti C, Briard ML, Feingold J et al. An epidemiological and genetic study of facial clefting in France. I Epidemiology and frequency in relatives. J Med Genet 1982; 19: 8–15

7 Czeizel A, Tusnády G. An epidemiologic study of cleft lip with or without cleft palate and posterior cleft palate in Hungary. Hum Hered 1971; 21: 17–38

8 Emanuel I, Huang S-W, Gutman LT, Yu F-C, Lin C-C. The incidence of congenital malformations in a Chinese population: the Taipei collaborative study. Teratology 1972; 5: 159–169

9 Heinonen OP, Slone D, Shapiro S. Birth defects and drugs in pregnancy. Littleton, Mass: Publishing Sciences Group, 1977

10 Kallen B, Winberg J. A Swedish register of congenital malformations: experience with continuous registration during 2 years with special reference to multiple malformations. Pediatrics 1968; 41: 765–776

11 Leck I. The etiology of human malformations: insights from epidemiology. Teratology 1972; 5: 303–314
12 Leck I, Record RG, McKeown T, Edwards JH. The incidence of malformations in Birmingham, England, 1950–59. Teratology 1968; 1: 263–280
13 Lesi FEA. The significance of congenital defects in developing countries. Medicine Today 1969; 3, No 4: 26–40
14 Morton NE, Chung CS, Mi M-P. Genetics of inter-racial crosses in Hawaii. Basel: Karger, 1967
15 Neel JV. A study of major congenital defects in Japanese infants. Amer J Hum Genet 1958; 10: 398–445
16 Ogbalu MM, Leck I, Hillier VF. The prevalence of malformations at birth in southern Nigeria. Paper presented at the Fifth International Conference on Birth Defects, Montreal, Canada, August 1977
17 Saxén I, Lahti A. Cleft lip and palate in Finland: incidence, secular, seasonal and geographical variations. Teratology 1974; 9: 217–224
18 Smithells RW. Incidence of congenital abnormalities in Liverpool, 1960–1964. Br J Prev Soc Med 1968; 22: 36–37
19 Stevenson AC, Johnston HA, Golding DR, Stewart MIP. World Health Organization Comparative Study of Congenital Malformations: basic tabulations in respect of consecutive post 28-week births recorded in the co-operating centres. Oxford: Medical Research Council Population Genetics Research Unit, 1966
20 Welch J, Hunter AGW. An epidemiological study of facial clefting in Manitoba. J Med Genet 1980; 17: 127–132
21 Lowry RB, Trimble BK. Incidence rates for cleft lip and palate in British Columbia 1952–71 for North American Indian, Japanese, Chinese and total populations: secular trends over twenty years. Teratology 1977; 16: 277–284
22 Niswander JD, Adams MS. Oral clefts in the American Indian. US Publ Hlth Reps 1967; 82: 807–812
23 Kurisu K, Niswander JD, Johnston MC, Mazaheri M. Facial morphology as an indicator of genetic predisposition to cleft lip and palate. Amer J Hum Genet 1974; 26: 702–714
24 Smithells RW. Environmental teratogens of man. Br Med Bull 1976; 32: 27–33
25 Leck I. Correlations of malformation frequency with environmental and genetic attributes in man. In: Wilson JG, Fraser FC; eds. Handbook of teratology, Vol 3 (Comparative, maternal and epidemiological aspects). New York: Plenum, 1977: 243–324
26 Carter CO. Genetics of common disorders. Br Med Bull 1969; 25: 52–57
27 Fujino H, Tanaka K, Sanui Y. Genetic study of cleft-lips and cleft-palates based upon 2828 Japanese cases. Kyushu J Med Sci 1963; 14: 317–331
28 Carter CO, Evans K, Coffey R, Roberts JAF, Buck A, Roberts MF. A three generation study of cleft lip with or without cleft palate. J Med Genet 1982; 19: 246–261
29 Bear JC. A genetic study of facial clefting in Northern England. Clin Genet 1976; 9: 277–284
30 Carter CO, Evans K, Coffey R, Roberts JAF, Buck A, Roberts MF. A family study of isolated cleft palate. J Med Genet 1982; 19: 329–331
31 Leck I. Spina bifida and anencephaly: fewer patients, more problems. Br Med J. 1983; 286: 1679–1680
32 Ferguson-Smith MA. The reduction of anencephalic and spina bifida births by maternal serum alphafetoprotein screening. Br Med Bull 1983; 39: 365–372
33 Suwanwela C. Geographical distribution of fronto-ethmoidal encephalomeningocele. Br J Prev Soc Med 1972; 26: 193–198
34 Elwood JM, Elwood JH. Epidemiology of anencephalus and spina bifida. Oxford: Oxford University Press, 1980.
35 Sever LE. An epidemiologic study of neural tube defects in Los Angeles County II. Etiologic factors in an area with low prevalence at birth. Teratology 1982; 25: 323–334
36 Granroth G, Hakama M, Saxén L. Defects of the central nervous system in Finland: I. Variations in time and space, sex distribution, and parental age. Br J Prev Soc Med 1977; 31: 164–170

37 Elwood JH, Nevin NC. Factors associated with anencephalus and spina bifida in Belfast. Br J Prev Soc Med 1973; 27: 73–80
38 Leck I. Epidemiological clues to the causation of neural tube defects. In: Dobbing J, ed. Prevention of spina bifida and other neural tube defects. London: Academic Press, 1983: 155–182
39 Rogers SC, Weatherall JAC. Anencephalus, spina bifida and congenital hydrocephalus: England and Wales 1964–1972 (Studies on Medical and Population Studies No 32). London: Her Majesty's Stationery Office, 1976
40 Center for Disease Control. Congenital malformations: surveillance report, January–December 1975. Atlanta: Center for Disease Control, 1976
41 Greenberg F, James LM, Oakley GP. Estimates of birth prevalence rates of spina bifida in the United States from computer-generated maps. Amer J Obstet Gynecol 1983; 145: 570–578
42 Buckley MR, Erten O. The epidemiology of anencephaly and spina bifida in Izmir, Turkey, in the light of recent epidemiological theories. J Epidemiol Comm Hlth 1979; 33: 186–190
43 Hashem N, Sever J. Neural tube defects among Egyptians. Amer J Hum Genet 1982; 34: 154A
44 Damyanov I, Dutz W. Anencephaly in Shiraz, Iran. Lancet 1971; i: 82
45 Verma IC. High frequency of neural-tube defects in north India (letter). Lancet 1978; i: 879–880
46 Naggan L. Anencephaly and spina bifida in Israel. Pediatrics 1971; 47: 577–586
47 Naggan L, MacMahon B. Ethnic differences in the prevalence of anencephaly and spina bifida in Boston, Massachusetts. New Engl J Med 1967; 277: 1119–1123
48 Horowitz I, McDonald AD. Anencephaly and spina bifida in the province of Quebec. Canad Med Ass J 1969; 100: 748–755
49 Elwood JH. Major central nervous system malformations notified in Northern Ireland 1964–1968. Develop Med Child Neurol 1972; 14: 731–739
50 Richards IDG, Roberts CJ, Lloyd S. Area differences in prevalence of neural tube malformations in South Wales. A study of possible demographic determinants. Br J. Prev Soc Med 1972; 26: 89–93
51 Fedrick J. Anencephalus in Scotland 1961–72. Br J Prev Soc Med 1976; 30: 132–137
52 Carter CO, Evans K. Spina bifida and anencephalus in Greater London. J Med Genet 1973; 10: 209–234
53 Edwards JH. Congenital malformations of the central nervous system in Scotland. Br J Prev Soc Med 1958; 12: 115–130
54 Imaizumi Y. Statistical analysis on anencephaly, spina bifida and congenital hydrocephaly in Japan. Jap J Hum Genet 1974; 19: 115–135
55 Verstege JCW. Anencephalie in Nederland 1951–1968. The Hague: Centraal Bureau voor de Statistiek, Staatsuitgeverij, 1971
56 Wilson TS. A study of congenital malformations of the central nervous system among Glasgow births 1964–1968. Hlth Bull (Edinb) 1971; 29: 79–87
57 Elwood JH, Elwood JM. Investigation of area differences in the prevalence at birth of anencephalus in Belfast. Internat J Epidemiol 1984; 13: 45–52
58 Myrianthopoulos NC, Chung CS. Congenital malformations in singletons: epidemiologic survey. (Birth Defects Original Article Series 10, No 11.) New York: Stratton, 1974
59 Knox EG. Twins and neural tube defects. Br J Prev Soc Med 1974; 28: 73–80
60 Scragg RKR, Dorsch MM, McMichael AJ, Baghurst PA. Birth defects and household water supply. Epidemiological studies in the Mount Gambier region of South Australia. Med J Aust 1982; ii: 577–579
61 Knox EG. Anencephalus and dietary intakes. Br J Prev Soc Med 1972; 26: 219–223
62 Dobbing J, ed. Prevention of spina bifida and other neural tube defects. London: Academic Press, 1983

British Medical Bulletin (1984) Vol. 40, No. 4, pp. 396–400

THE EPIDEMIOLOGY OF PAGET'S DISEASE OF BONE

D J P BARKER PhD MD FRCP

*MRC Environmental Epidemiology Unit
University of Southampton*

In Paget's disease (osteitis deformans) there is rapid bone remodelling and formation of bone that is structurally abnormal. This causes pain, fractures, and deformity. The aetiology of the disease is unknown. James Paget's original description was of an elderly man.[1] Subsequent clinical, autopsy,[2] and radiological[3] case series have confirmed that the disease is more prevalent among men than women. It is commonest in elderly people although many young patients have been described, symptoms sometimes beginning in the early twenties. Fig. 1 shows the frequency of the disease, occurring as either the principal abnormality or, more often, as an incidental one, in a series of 13 000 abdominal radiographs taken from the stored films within a group of British hospitals. In both sexes the prevalence increases progressively with age. Since spontaneous resolution of the radiological changes is not known to occur, this progressive increase in prevalence reflects the accumulation of cases in the population due to continuing incidence into old age. The pattern of incidence with age has not yet been documented.

Familial Occurrence

There have been many reports of Paget's disease affecting more than one member of a family, including its occurrence in successive generations. Pedigree studies of the distribution of the disease in selected families have led to the conclusion that it is an autosomal dominant disorder.[4] The epidemiological findings which will be described do not support the idea that there is such a clearly defined genetic influence in aetiology. However, studies of the prevalence of the disease among relatives of cases demonstrate a tendency to familial aggregation.[5] Further analyses of the distribution within families, based on representative samples of cases and taking account of subclinical disease, may give useful clues.

1   Time Trends

Paget's disease has been described in various ancient skeletal remains. Perhaps the best authenticated is an Anglo-Saxon skeleton, dated around 950 AD, which was dug up at Jarrow Monastery and is still accessible to examination.[6]

a   Secular Trends

Such evidence as there is on secular trends points to a current decline in frequency of the disease.[7] This evidence derives from deaths in which Paget's disease is given as the underlying cause. (In around 70% of such deaths a patient with Paget's disease dies of cardiac failure or bronchopneumonia.) Table I shows the marked recent decline in deaths in Britain attributed to Paget's disease during the twenty year period 1951–70. The crude average annual mortality rates in England and Wales fell from 3.7 per million in 1951–55 to 3.2 in 1966–70; in Scotland they fell from 2.9 to 1.4. If mortality is analysed in relation to year of birth, it is apparent that successive generations, or cohorts, have had progressively lower death rates from Paget's disease at any particular age over 55 years. Fig. 2 shows age-specific death rates in England and Wales for cohorts of males and females born at around the same time. There is a marked rise in the death rates with increasing age. The cohorts born during the 1880s have the highest death rates. Successive cohorts born thereafter show progressively lower death rates. Analysis of mortality from Paget's disease among whites in the USA reveals a similar pattern of decline, although the USA age-specific death rates are lower.[8]

Paget's disease is rarely fatal and mortality statistics are a manifestly imperfect indicator of incidence. Nevertheless, these findings are supported by secular trends in mortality from primary bone tumours.[7] The rise in mortality from primary bone tumours which occurs over the age of 40 is largely due to osteosarcoma associated with Paget's disease.[9] Knowledge of secular trends in this mortality is based on analyses of bone tumour deaths as coded under the International Classification of Disease (code number 170, eighth revision). This coding includes primary tumours of cartilage and periosteum as well as bone, although osteosarcoma is the commonest type. It also includes secondary bone tumours misclassified as primary; and a review of the accuracy of diagnosis in deaths in 1951–53 coded under this number showed that in only 55% was there acceptable evidence of a primary bone tumour.[9] Data on time trends in bone-tumour mortality must therefore be interpreted with caution. However, unless there is a simultaneous

FIG. 1. Radiological prevalence of Paget's disease according to age and sex

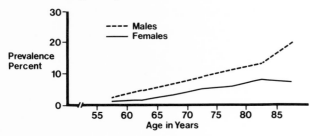

TABLE I. Average annual death rates per million in Britain attributed to Paget's disease

	1951–55	1956–60	1961–65	1966–70
England and Wales	3.7 (826)	3.6 (800)	3.4 (802)	3.2 (771)
Scotland	2.9 (75)	2.4 (62)	2.2 (56)	1.4 (36)

Numbers of deaths are given in parentheses

FIG. 2. Cohort mortality from Paget's disease in England and Wales in five-year periods, 1951–75

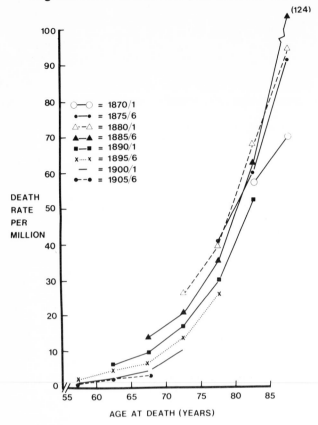

○—○ = 1870/1
●—● = 1875/6
△–△ = 1880/1
▲—▲ = 1885/6
■—■ = 1890/1
x···x = 1895/6
— = 1900/1
●--● = 1905/6

DEATH RATE PER MILLION

AGE AT DEATH (YEARS)

and opposing change in the frequency of the other tumour types, a decline in Paget's disease should be associated with a decline in mortality from malignant bone tumours in middle-aged and elderly people. Such a decline has indeed occurred (Table II). The average annual mortality rates among people aged 55 years and over in England and Wales fell from 48.2 per million in 1951–55 to 28.2 in 1966–70; in Scotland during the same period they fell from 82.4 to 33.7. There was a similar decline in the USA.[8] In both Britain and the USA, successive generations born from around 1870 onwards showed a steep and progressive decline in death rates at any particular age over 35 years.

If these mortality data for Paget's disease and bone tumours are accepted as an indicator of the incidence of Paget's disease, then an inference is that exposure to some aetiological influence has gradually diminished in successive generations.

TABLE II. Average annual death rates per million in Britain from malignant tumours of bone among persons aged 55 years and over

	1951–55	1956–60	1961–65	1966–70
England and Wales	48.2 (2326)	39.7 (2068)	32.6 (1833)	28.2 (1690)
Scotland	82.4 (418)	57.6 (311)	41.2 (236)	33.7 (204)

Numbers of deaths are given in parentheses

b *Cyclic Trends*

Analysis of the ages of 386 patients belonging to a patients' association in Britain, who were born from 1888 to 1924, showed cyclic fluctuations in year of birth.[5] The periodicity of these fluctuations was around three years. Although this was not statistically significant, the lack of significance may be due to small numbers and these observations are being extended.

2 Geography

Although isolated case reports have come from many parts of the world, clinical observations suggest that the disease is common only in Europe, North America, Australia, and New Zealand.[10]

a *Prevalence in Europe*

In a survey in Western Europe the prevalence of the disease was mapped from replies to a postal questionnaire completed by 1416 radiologists in 13 countries.[11] The questionnaire inquired about the frequency with which Paget's disease was seen, as either the principal abnormality or, more often, as an incidental one. There were seven possible responses (once a week or more, once every two weeks, once a month, once every two months, once every six months, once a year, less than once a year). The questionnaire was validated by replies from radiologists in Britain, where the radiological prevalence had already been measured (as will be described) and in Norway, where there was evidence of a low prevalence.[12] The survey excluded replies from radiologists who spent less than half their time in general work.

This is a crude technique. The frequency with which a radiologist sees radiographs with signs of Paget's disease will be influenced by factors other than the prevalence of the disease, such as his or her work load. Nevertheless, replies from radiologists within any one town were generally similar, and from town to town within any one country the medians of the frequencies with which the radiologists reported seeing the disease were surprisingly consistent. A map of these median values across Europe showed a clear pattern. The disease was most common in Britain, where the medians for 61 out of 62 towns were once a week or once a fortnight. In France the frequency was less, with most values being once a month or once every two months. From there the frequencies declined to the south, east and north-east. The disease was rarely reported in Scandinavia, the medians being once a year or less.

More precise data on the geographical distribution came from a series of radiological surveys measuring the prevalence of clinical and subclinical disease.[11,13] Samples of abdominal radiographs of people aged 55 and over were taken from stored films within the radiological departments of general hospitals. Selected films showed the pelvis, sacrum, lumbar spine, and femoral heads—sites that are affected in 95% of people with Paget's disease. Whenever possible, 1000 radiographs were drawn for each town studied with equal numbers for men and women. A research assistant classified them into three groups: positive, having unequivocal signs of the disease, doubtful, and negative. A consultant radiologist examined all positive and equivocal radiographs and a 10% sample of negative ones. The same radiologist took part in every survey. Initially he devised standardized criteria for the radiological diagnosis of the disease by reference to standard texts and consultation with colleagues. Subsequently a study of the trace element content of Pagetoid bone provided the opportunity to test the validity of these diagnostic criteria. Bone biopsy specimens were taken at necropsy from the iliac blades of 21 subjects in whom post-mortem pelvic radiographs had shown the disease in some part of the iliac blade. In 19 out of 21 subjects the biopsy showed histological signs of the disease. (The patchy distribution of the pathological changes in Paget's disease is one possible explanation for the lack of concordance between the radiological and histological appearances in the other two cases.) The repeatability of his survey observations has been formally tested on three occasions when he has examined radiographs while being kept unaware of his previous report. It exceeds 99%.

This technique is only usable because, in the majority of patients, Paget's disease is symptomless and radiographs have been taken because of other, unrelated disorders. Although the frequency of the disease among patients attending for routine radiological investigations is a biased estimate of the true frequency in the population, analyses of the data suggest that the geographical differences discovered will not be greatly influenced by these biases. The differences do not depend on varying levels of clinical suspicion of Paget's disease among doctors referring patients for skeletal radiographs. Within Britain the same geographical variations are seen both in skeletal radiographs and in others, namely those taken during intravenous pyelography, barium studies, and plain abdominal examinations: a study of radiology request forms in England showed that, in patients with radiological evidence of Paget's disease, this diagnosis is rarely stated on the form.

The results of radiological surveys carried out in 15 European towns are shown in Fig. 3. The towns were selected to encompass the range of frequencies of the disease as elicited by the postal questionnaire, the geographical extent of Europe, and areas of various types such as urban, rural, or heavily industrial. The prevalence for Britain is the mean for 31 towns surveyed.[13] This British survey showed that the prevalences were higher in skeletal radiographs (which comprised about 20% of all radiographs) than in others, the age-standardized rates being 6.3% and 4.6% respectively. This was not unexpected since most patients referred for skeletal radiographs presumably have skeletal symptoms, such as back ache, which in some instances will be caused by Paget's

FIG. 3. Age- and sex-standardized prevalences (%) of Paget's disease among hospital patients aged 55 years and over in 15 European towns, and in Britain (see text)

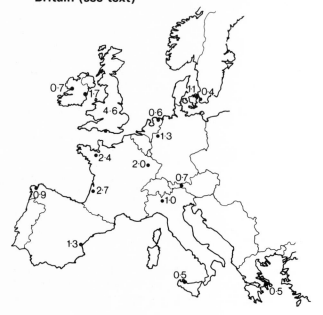

disease. The prevalence recorded in a town will therefore be influenced by the proportion of radiographs which are skeletal. This will depend on the kind of specialist units whose radiographs are being sampled (many European hospitals not having centralized radiograph archives) and on referral practices and indications for radiography among patients with skeletal symptoms. To eliminate this potential source of bias, skeletal radiographs were not used in the European survey.

In Fig. 3 the prevalence rates are directly standardized to allow comparisons corrected for the differing age distributions of the subjects in the various towns. The standardization procedure used five-year age distributions from 55 to 90 years of age and over. In this and all other surveys using the same technique, the combined survey sample of 14 British towns initially studied was used as the standard.

The results corroborate those of the postal questionnaire. Outside Britain the highest prevalences were in the three French towns, Bordeaux (2.7%), Rennes (2.4%), and Nancy (2.0%). These prevalences were lower than the overall prevalence of 4.6% in Britain but were comparable with the lowest values recorded in individual towns (2.7% in Carlisle and 2.3% in Aberdeen in radiographs which included about 20% of skeletal films). In the remaining European towns, the prevalences ranged from 1.7% in Dublin, and 1.3% in Valencia (Spain) and Essen (West Germany), to 0.5% in Palermo (Sicily) and Athens and 0.4% in Malmo (Sweden). As would be expected, the prevalences among men were higher than those among women, except in four towns where the numbers of cases were small. A recent radiological study in Hamburg, W. Germany, using a similar technique to that of the European survey, recorded a prevalence of 1.1% (J D Ringe, personal communication) which is similar to the rate for Essen.

Corroboration of the very low rates in Sweden comes from a previous survey using the same technique, where the prevalence was 0.3%. Radiological and clinical data from Norway[12] and Finland (R Pelkonen, personal communication) clearly indicate the rarity of the disease. The low prevalence in Dublin (1.7%), situated so close to Britain, is remarkable, as is the rarity of the disease in western Ireland (0.7% in Galway).

b *Prevalence in Britain*

The age–sex-standardized prevalences in 31 British towns are shown in Fig. 4 which is based on examination of 29 000 radiographs. Rates above 6.0% occur only in a cluster of six Lancashire towns—Lancaster (8.3%), Preston (7.5%), Bolton (7.1%), Wigan (6.8%), Burnley (6.5%), and Blackburn (6.3%). Outside this small area of high prevalence, the rates fall sharply, with the bordering towns having prevalences of around the average for all towns. Of special interest is the sharp drop that is seen between towns lying within and just outside the area. For example, Wigan and Warrington are only 10 miles apart but the prevalences are 6.8% and 4.2% respectively. There is no evidence of any other focus of high prevalence in the country. Standardization to allow for the differing proportion of skeletal radiographs has little effect on the ranking of towns according to prevalence; indeed, the difference between the six Lancashire towns with a high prevalence and the remainder is somewhat enhanced by this standardization.

c *Prevalence in North America, Australia and New Zealand*

The prevalences in Europe may be compared with those in America, Australia, and New Zealand—the only other countries where the disease is known to occur frequently. In the USA, radiological surveys were carried out in two cities, New York and

FIG. 4. Age- and sex-standardized prevalences (%) of Paget's disease among hospital patients aged 55 years and over in 31 British towns

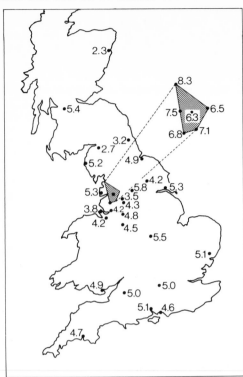

TABLE IV. Prevalence of Paget's disease in Perth, Australia among hospital patients aged 55 years and over, by place of birth and place of residence

Place of birth	Place of residence	No. of radiographs	Age-standardized prevalence %		
			Men	Women	Both sexes
Australia	Australia	1203	3.5	2.8	3.2 (40)
UK	Australia	942	5.7	2.3	4.0 (48)
UK	UK	29054*	6.2*	3.9*	5.0* (1516)

Figures in parentheses are numbers of cases
* Data from survey shown in Fig. 4

observations on immigrants in Perth, Western Australia.[17] Table IV shows the age-standardized prevalence by place of birth and place of residence, and includes the data for UK-born patients living in the UK shown in Fig. 4. Native-born Australians had a lower prevalence (3.2%) than UK-born patients who emigrated to Australia (4.0%), who in turn had lower rates than those who remained in the UK (5.0%). This trend was followed by men; but among women rates for native-born Australians were higher than those for immigrants (2.8% compared with 2.3%). Prevalence rates for women are, however, less reliable than those for men as they are based on smaller numbers. These observations on radiological prevalence are supported by the finding that in Western Australia hospital discharge rates for patients with Paget's disease as the principal diagnosis are 10% higher among UK-born migrants than among its native population.

In Dunedin, whose population largely comprises New Zealanders of European origin, a radiological survey was carried out using the same technique as in the other radiological surveys, but with a different radiologist.[18] Although diagnostic criteria could therefore have differed, the recorded prevalence of 4.4% (5.4% in men and 3.4% in women) supports anecdotal evidence that Paget's disease is more common in New Zealand than in any other country excepting Britain.

3 Discussion

Epidemiological studies on Paget's disease, in particular description of its remarkable geographical distribution, do not of themselves lead to specific aetiological hypothesis. For example, the area of high prevalence in Lancashire has no exclusive cultural, industrial, geological, or climatic characteristics which distinguish it from surrounding areas of England. Nor is there any ready explanation for the comparative rarity of the disease in such places as Scandinavia or Ireland. Although the world distribution of the disease, and knowledge of its occurrence in ancient skeletal remains, compel speculation about a genetically determined disorder disseminated by the migration of peoples, this general idea has yet to be sharpened to the point where it could provide a detailed explanation for the geography of the disease.

A recent analysis of the familial occurrence of the disease concluded that it was consistent with a major environmental influence superimposed on genetic variation in susceptibility to, and perhaps severity of, the disease.[5]

The similar rates of American blacks to those of whites, in contrast to the extreme rarity of the disease in Africa, and the decline in prevalence that accompanies migration from the United Kingdom to Australia (Table IV), point to a dominant role of environmental influences. The rates among Australian immigrants do not fall to the levels of natives of Australia. There are three possible explanations for this. First, immigrants may bring

Atlanta, selected because of an earlier suggestion that the disease is less common in the south.[14, 15] Prevalences were calculated for each of the two major ethnic groups (recorded in hospital records as black or white); other ethnic groups were excluded.

The difference between the two cities (Table III), seen in both sexes and both ethnic groups, indicates a marked variation in prevalence within the USA in which latitude may play some part. New York and Atlanta do not necessarily represent the extremes of this variation. The prevalence among whites in New York (3.9%) is comparable with values recorded in Britain. In Atlanta the prevalence among whites (0.9%) is similar to those in European countries outside Britain and France.

It is of interest that the rates in American blacks (2.6% in New York and 1.2% in Atlanta) are similar to those among whites, for the disease is rarely found among African blacks.[16] This parallels

TABLE III. Prevalence of Paget's disease in two American cities among hospital patients aged 55 years and over, by ethnic group

City	Ethnic group	No. of radiographs	Age-standardized prevalence %		
			Men	Women	Both sexes
New York	Black	950	3.3	2.0	2.6 (24)
New York	White	1082	5.2	2.5	3.9 (43)
Atlanta	Black	1111	1.9	0.6	1.2 (14)
Atlanta	White	1563	0.9	0.8	0.9 (13)

Figures in parentheses are numbers of cases

with them risk factors, related for example to dietary habits or life-style, which persist in their new environment. Secondly, some people who have already developed the disease while living in the UK may be included among the immigrants. Thirdly, there may be a long latent period between initiation of the disease and its first radiological manifestation, so that, progression being to some extent irreversible, migrants carry with them the higher UK risk of developing the disease. It seems likely that the last two explanations apply. Study of the variation in prevalence among immigrants according to the age at migration offers the theoretical possibility of estimating the age at which the initial event in pathogenesis occurs. However, in a case-control study among British migrants in Perth (Australia) there was no difference in the age at migration of cases and age-matched controls.

During the past century many hypotheses about the causation of Paget's disease, for example bacterial infection, a toxin, fluorine poisoning, have arisen and been discarded. Two hypotheses currently command attention. Observations on the localization of Pagetoid bone within the body have suggested a role for mechanical trauma.[19] The pelvic girdle is more frequently involved than the shoulder; the spinal distribution is similar to that seen in vertebral spondylosis; among men there is a pronounced laterality, the right side of the pelvis being more often affected.[20] However, most interest centres on the recent discovery that the nuclei of osteoclast cells in Pagetoid bone contain inclusion bodies whose appearance resembles paramyxovirus nucleocapsides.[21,22] This raises the possibility that the disease is due to infection with a 'slow-virus', which initiates malfunctioning of osteoclast cells—currently thought to be the primary pathological disorder in the disease. Interest is centred on two particular paramyxoviruses, measles virus and respiratory syncitial virus.

The viral hypothesis is unproven. It rests uncertainly on morphology and immunohistology, and laboratory studies are continuing. Confirmation of the periodicity of year of birth of cases would support an infectious aetiology. Cyclic changes in incidence are seen in various childhood infections; measles outbreaks, for example, may occur in three-year cycles. A more pronounced periodicity might be expected from respiratory syncitial virus than from measles since most serious infections due to the former occur in infancy.

Two analytic epidemiological studies have offered little direct support. Environmental indices were studied in the six high-prevalence Lancashire towns and in three Lancashire towns with average prevalence. No correlation was found between the present prevalence of Paget's disease and conditions in the towns during the years 1901–21, the period which covers the childhood of most current cases of the disease. In particular, there was no correlation with overcrowding or infant mortality rates, nor were associations found with the differing frequencies of infectious diseases from town to town, except for an unexpected correlation with notification rates for enteric fever (unpublished data). Studies in Lancaster (the town with the highest recorded prevalence) and Sienna, Italy (a low-prevalence town) are comparing the frequency of factors associated with air-borne infection, for example social class and family size, in cases and controls. To date no differences have emerged (F M Detheridge, unpublished data).

If viral infection is a cause of Paget's disease, the virus must be capable of considerable penetration within populations, for the disease affects up to 8% of people aged 55 and over in British towns. By contrast, its penetration, in so far as this is indicated by the prevalence of the disease, is poor in adjacent populations, notably Ireland and Scandinavia, and in densely populated northern European areas such as Essen in Germany. There is no parallel with any other human viral illness and it seems necessary to postulate the existence of one or more as yet unknown cofactors. Vitamin D deficiency in childhood has been suggested as a possible factor, on the basis of a broad geographical association between the current distribution of Paget's disease and that of rickets at the beginning of the century, and as an explanation for the apparent decline in incidence of the disease. The evidence, however, is no more than suggestive.

Although Paget's disease is often asymptomatic, its high prevalence makes it an important cause of morbidity in the elderly. It is estimated that some 150 000 people in Britain require treatment for it. Research into its causes is poised. In the laboratory all is hypothesis; in epidemiology and clinical research all is description. Should the work of virologists and experimental pathologists progress to a more certain stage then the development of their findings in parallel with analytical epidemiology would be an exciting task.

REFERENCES

1 Paget Sir J. On a form of chronic inflammation of bones (osteitis deformans). Med Chir Trans (Lond) 1877; 60: 37–64

2 Schmorl G. Ueber osteitis deformans Paget. Arch Path Anat 1932; 283: 694–751

3 Pygott F. Paget's disease of bone: the radiological incidence. Lancet 1957; 2: 1170–1171

4 McKusick VA. Mendelian inheritance in man. Catalogs of autosomal dominant, autosomal recessive and X-linked phenotypes 5th ed. Baltimore: John Hopkins University Press, 1978: 294–295

5 Sofaer JA, Holloway SM, Emery AEH. A family study of Paget's disease of bone. J Epidemiol Community Health 1983; 37: 226–231

6 Wells C, Woodhouse N. Paget's disease in an Anglo-Saxon. Med Hist 1975; 19: 396–400

7 Barker DJP, Gardner MJ. Distribution of Paget's disease in England, Wales and Scotland and a possible relationship with vitamin D deficiency in childhood. Br J Prev Soc Med 1974; 28: 226–232

8 Gardner MJ, Barker DJP. Mortality from malignant tumours of bone and Paget's disease in the United States and in England and Wales. Int J Epidemiol 1978; 7: 121–130

9 MacKenzie A, Court Brown WM, Doll R, Sissons HA. Mortality from primary tumours of bone in England and Wales. Br Med J 1961; 1: 1782–1790

10 Barry HC. Paget's disease of bone. Edinburgh: Livingstone, 1969

11 Detheridge FM, Guyer PB, Barker DJP. European distribution of Paget's disease of bone. Br Med J 1982; 285: 1005–1008

12 Falch JA. Paget's disease in Norway. Lancet 1979; 2: 1022

13 Barker DJP, Chamberlain AT, Guyer PB, Gardner MJ. Paget's disease of bone: the Lancashire focus. Br Med J 1980; 280: 1105–1107

14 Guyer PB, Chamberlain AT. Paget's disease of bone in two American cities. Br Med J 1980; 280: 985

15 Rosenbaum HD, Hanson DJ. Geographic variation in the prevalence of Paget's disease of bone. Radiology 1969; 92: 959–963

16 Van Meedervoort E, Richter G. Paget's disease of bone in South African blacks. S Afr Med J 1976; 50: 1897–1899

17 Gardner MJ, Guyer PB, Barker DJP. Radiological prevalence of Paget's disease of bone in British migrants to Australia. Br Med J 1978; 1: 1655–1657

18 Reasbeck JC, Goulding A, Campbell DR, Beale LR, Stewart RDH. Radiological prevalence of Paget's disease in Dunedin, New Zealand. Br Med J 1983; 286: 1937

19 Packard FA, Steele JD, Kirkbride TS. Osteitis deformans. Amer J Med Sci 1901; 122: 552–569

20 Guyer PB, Chamberlain AT, Ackery DM, Rolfe EB. The anatomic distribution of osteitis deformans. Clin Orthop 1981; 156: 141–144

21 Rebel A, Baslé M, Pouplard A, Kouyoumdjian S, Filmon R, Lepatezour A. Viral antigens in osteoclasts from Paget's disease of bone. Lancet 1980; 2: 344–346

22 Singer FR, Mills BG. The etiology of Paget's disease of bone. Clin Orthop 1977; 127: 37–42

British Medical Bulletin (1984) Vol. 40, No. 4, pp. 401–404

URBAN FACTORS IN MENTAL DISORDERS—AN EPIDEMIOLOGICAL APPROACH

M SHEPHERD DM FRCP FRCPsych DPM

Institute of Psychiatry
University of London

1   The psychoses
2   'Minor' psychiatric illness
3   Distress and sub-clinical disorders
4   Conclusion
    References

The process of urbanization has been a major factor in the development of homo sapiens. As in so many spheres of knowledge, Aristotle had the first word when he wrote: 'Men come together in the city to live; they remain there in order to live the good life'. Since then, as Lewis Mumford has documented in his magisterial survey,[1] the city has played a major role in history as the centre of some of man's most civilizing achievements. At all times, however, a delicate balance has existed between the advantages of urban life, with its rich and stimulating environment, and the cost exacted in terms of poverty, unnatural living conditions and adverse environmental pressures. Summing up a substantial body of opinion, one 20th century observer has concluded that to live according to nature, 'we should pass a considerable time in cities for they are the glory of human nature, but they should never contain more than 200000 inhabitants; it is our artificial enslavement to the large city, too enormous for human dignity, which is responsible for half our sickness and misery'.[2] This paper examines the scientific overtones of this assertion in respect of mental disorder.

The coincident arrival of industrialization and modern medicine in the early 19th century led to several attempts to build on the Rousseau-esque notions of a simple life in natural surroundings, paving the way for the view of an environmental concept of health based on favourable social as well as individual conditions. A sanitary ideal was developed by many social reformers who believed in hygiene as a way of life. Identifying dirt, poverty and overcrowding as causes of disease they naturally focused attention on the city. In Germany these ideas were developed prominently by Max von Pettenkoffer in his lectures on 'The Health of a City' that contain an account of the measures introduced successfully into Munich, which included even the planting of trees and flowers because of their supposedly aesthetic effects on the mental health of the population.

In Victorian England the sanitary movement also led to such measures as the formation of the Health and Town Association and the Public Health Act. Its essence is perhaps most vividly exemplified by the famous address delivered by Benjamin Ward Richardson to the Health Section of the Social Science Association in 1875. Aiming 'to show a working community in which death ... is kept as nearly as possible in its proper or natural place in the scheme of life', Richardson presented an idealized view of a community in terms of health issues and, significantly, he concluded that social control of the environment was the key to prevention, an objective which took precedence over curative treatment.

Utopian though it may now seem, it was the spirit of the early sanitarians which paved the way for the laying of the foundations of urban sociology. And it was from the work of men like Booth, Weber, Tönnies, Park and Simmel, all pioneers of the sociological discipline, that there emerged an intense preoccupation with fact-finding and quantification. Not the least significant result of these endeavours was the realization that the definition of a city is itself an issue. The demographers were quick to stress the importance of numbers, density and heterogeneity, but these factors alone do not indicate that the urban ecosystem is a complex physical, biological and psychosocial admixture which includes such diverse elements as climate, noise level, crowding, pollution, occupational specialization and a constant adaptive struggle with stimulus overload.[3] Many studies have now demonstrated that the marked variation between the populations of urban aggregates or societies represents the resultant of a wide variety of factors. For the purpose of scientific inquiry, epidemiology, the quantitative study of health in populations, is the method *par excellence* of studying the pathological aspects of that variation, as I propose to illustrate.

Effects of Urbanization on Health

The simplest demographic level is that of medical geography. In the United Kingdom the routine collection of national statistics had made it possible to compare both mortality and morbidity rates by residential districts. The results demonstrate that urban dwellers are considerably less healthy than their country cousins, with the exception of the risk for traffic-accidents.[4]

The use of such crude indices for mental disorder, however, is unfortunately limited by problems of ascertainment and of definition. Mental disorders are traditionally sub-divided into the two broad categories embodied in the International Classification of Disease, namely the psychoses on the one hand and the neuroses and personality disorders on the other, although the distinction between them is not as sharp as has been maintained. In addition, a third category of distress and sub-clinical reactions has to be included. For convenience, each may be considered in turn.

1   The Psychoses

However they may be defined, the psychotic illnesses are more severe, more socially disruptive and more likely to lead to institutional care than other forms of mental disorder. During the 19th century they were seen by several social commentators as diseases of 'civilization' and were located in large cities. As late as 1903 William Alanson White could write: 'The savage in his simplicity does not know what it is to suffer from the cares and worries which are the daily portion of the European, and it is little wonder that the latter, beset by all manner of disappointments and vexations, should more frequently break down in mind than his less gifted brother'.[5]

The compilation of morbidity statistics derived from mental hospitals opened the door to quantitative investigations like that of Goldhamer and Marshall who were able to show in their monograph, 'Psychosis and Civilisation', that industrialization had not apparently influenced the first admission rates to the Massachusetts mental hospitals for the hundred years after 1840.[6] Here, it should be emphasized, they were testing indirectly the hypothesis that the strains and stresses associated with increasing industrialization centred in cities would lead to an increase in insanity. With a wider range of mental hospitals, more direct comparisons have become possible. Most of them record a larger urban than rural rate of first admissions, but the influence of nosocomial factors may well influence these figures which, further, take no account of those cases which fail to enter institutions. Accordingly, more sophisticated modern investigators have adopted an ecological approach based on detailed surveys of whole communities and areas, chosen for their contrasting characteristics whenever possible.

One of the best-documented and most relevant of these studies was conducted by Eaton and Weil who studied the community of Hutterites, a Protestant sect in the United States of America who live in colonies organized to ensure a pastoral, law-abiding style of life far removed from the cut and thrust of urban existence.[7] Eaton and Weil's conclusions are as follows: 'Our findings do not confirm the thesis that a simple and relatively uncomplicated way of life provides virtual immunity from mental disorders ... Psychoses and other forms of mental disorder were found to occur with regularity in the Hutterite population. Their existence in so secure and stable a social order suggests that there are genetic, organic and constitutional elements which predispose a few individuals to mental breakdown in any social system, no matter how protective and well-protected it may be ... a mental health Utopia is probably impossible'. At the same time they noted that the Hutterites engaged in very little anti-social activity and that their children were rarely disturbed emotionally, a point to which I shall return.

But the possible associations of urban life and mental illness cannot be confined to relatively crude contrasts of this type. The modern town or city is composed of heterogeneous sub-communities and these lend themselves to intra-urban comparison. The model for this type of inquiry was established in Chicago, the major American centre of urban sociology, where Faris and Dunham carried out their classical pre-war study, 'Mental Disorders in

FIG. 1. Areas of residence (shaded areas) in the city of Chicago with high first-admission rates to hospital for schizophrenia in persons aged 15–19 years by 1930 census tract

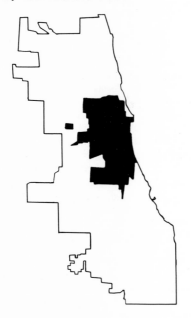

FIG. 2. Areas of residence (shaded areas) in the city of Chicago with high first admission rates to hospital for manic-depressive psychoses in persons aged 15–64 years by 1930 census tract

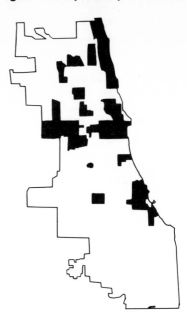

Urban Areas',[8] based on an analysis of first admission rates to hospital from different areas of the metropolis. Their key finding arose from the distribution maps concerning schizophrenia and manic-depressive psychosis which showed that while the pattern formed by the distribution of the manic-depressive psychoses was essentially random, the schizophrenics were concentrated in the poorest, most disorganized areas of the city (Figs. 1 & 2). The results led to the concept of 'insanity areas', comparable to Clifford Shaw's 'delinquency areas', and generated a number of questions, the most significant of which concerned the rival claims of the 'breeder' and 'drift' theorists in relation to schizophrenia. Though this debate now seems to have been decided in favour of the 'drift' or 'social selection' hypothesis it has stimulated a host of careful studies of the social and familial correlates of schizophrenia in different cities and different forms of urban life, all of them based on epidemiological and ecological methods of study.[9] Perhaps the most suggestive result of this work to date has been the notion that the outcome of schizophrenic illnesses is better in developing than in developed countries, a difference reflecting the more stressful impact of the westernized urban environment on the course of the condition.[10]

2 'Minor' Psychiatric Illness

The application of the epidemiological approach to the study of the 'minor' psychiatric disorders faces two problems from the outset. In the first place, only a small proportion of these conditions lead to contact with an institution, so that the use of administrative hospital statistics cannot be employed in their enumeration. Secondly, their identification, assessment and classification all pose a host of unresolved problems, many of which have been illuminated by the information obtained from the general practitioners who assume responsibility for the care of the majority of these patients. In the United Kingdom with its comprehensive health service, it becomes possible to study the primary-care population and the results have shown that psychiatric morbidity constitutes a major segment of the presenting conditions.[11] A National Morbidity Survey, furthermore, has shown marked urban–rural differences (Table I)[12] but here it is necessary to take account of variations in illness behaviour and diagnostic practices among general practitioners as well as possible variations in the patterns of disease. There is also a clear difference in the consultation rates for peptic ulcer, a condition sometimes regarded as stress-induced.

It must be acknowledged that the value of surveys of this type, however carefully conducted, is limited by their static, cross-sectional data. A more dynamic study has been mounted by Muñoz and his colleagues in the Spanish community living in the Baztan valley of Navarra.[13] The population of 8750 inhabits three areas whose socio-demographic features could be characterized as 'urban', 'rural' and 'isolated', according to their respective lifestyles. In this area migration from the less to the more urbanized district is an ongoing process, and a representative sample of subjects was studied in all three areas by means of a two-stage approach—an initial screening with a standardized questionnaire of established reliability, followed by detailed interviews. The key findings demonstrate a positive association between place of residence and neurotic illness, the rates diminishing from 'urban' via 'rural' to 'isolated' areas. The raised urban morbidity, it should be further noted, was significantly associated with males and females characterized as single, aged 15–24 years, unskilled and with poor social and education levels. Support is therefore provided for an association of these phenomena with the process of urbanization which raises the question of whether 'selection' or 'stress'—the equivalents of 'drift' and 'breeder'—may be responsible.

This issue has been examined in greater detail by Rutter and his colleagues in their comparison of the mental health of schoolchildren in the rural Isle of Wight and an Inner London borough.[14] Using a two-stage approach, these workers demonstrated a highly significant excess of neurotic and conduct disorders in the urban areas (Fig. 3). They were also able to relate four factors causally to these differences both between and within the areas: these are family discord, parental deviance, social disadvantage and school characteristics. In several respects their findings confirm the background features identified by West as important correlates of delinquent behaviour: low family income, large family size, parental criminality, low intelligence, and poor parental behaviour.[15] These factors make up a sub-culture in which other anti-

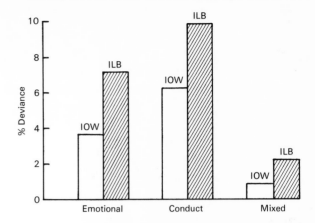

FIG. 3. Percent of schoolchildren with neurotic or conduct disorders (deviance) in the Isle of Wight (IOW) and an Inner London Borough (ILB), 1975

social forms of conduct—e.g. drug-taking, attempted suicide, theft—also occur in the late adolescent and early adult years,[16] and which contrast sharply with the patterns of Hutterite life. Precisely what constitutes these categories of behaviour has still to be determined, but the evidence to date suggest that physical factors like genetic predisposition, coincident physical morbidity and malnutrition play a relatively minor role compared with psychosocial influences.

3 Distress and Sub-Clinical Disorders

The definition and identification of these disorders touches on the borderland between illness and deviant behaviour which lends itself to micro-epidemiological inquiry, in which various environmental influences are studied independently. A few examples may be taken to illustrate the method. In one of our own studies, the site of inquiry was a single London borough within which the patterns of child guidance and delinquency rates were mapped within the smaller, more homogeneous, areas defined by election wards (Fig. 4).[17] Detailed statistical analyses based on socio-demographic features of the districts and the social characteristics of the schools pointed to a complex set of relationships. The best predictor of child-guidance referral proved to be the probation-rate of the school, followed by the proportion of persons living in shared households, the proportion of foreign-born residents and the rate of migration.

To render this type of analysis clinically useful, however, it is necessary to examine personal responses as well as group associations. Thus, while earlier clinical studies of urban living conditions have suggested that residents of high-rise flats, and especially the mothers of young children, are particularly prone to psychiatric disorder,[18] more recent epidemiological work with control groups has indicated the importance of vulnerable individuals, though there is undoubtedly a high degree of expressed dissatisfaction among the young mothers which may serve as the precursor of a depressive reaction.[19]

A comparable state of affairs emerged from our own study of the effects on mental health of another largely urban hazard, namely aircraft noise.[20] Here the areas of the city were sub-divided geographically by noise levels and a survey of some 6000 people was conducted to render comparisons possible. In the event, noise was found to be associated not with overt mental disorder but with

TABLE I. Urban–rural differences in general-practitioner consultation rates
(from 1st National Morbidity Survey, England and Wales[12])

Diagnosis	Consultations per 1000 per year				
	Conurbations	Other towns populations			Rural districts
		> 100000	50000–100000	< 50000	
Psychoneurotic disorders	32	32	25	27	23
Peptic ulcer	15	18	15	14	10
All causes	610	593	607	582	567

From Logan and Cushion 1958

FIG. 4. Numbers of children per 10 000 referred to child guidance clinics by school and election ward within a London Borough, 1962–1966

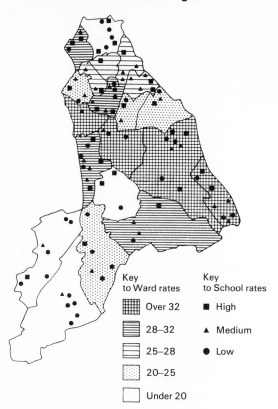

Key to Ward rates

▦ Over 32

▤ 28–32

▤ 25–28

⣿ 20–25

☐ Under 20

Key to School rates

■ High

▲ Medium

● Low

the so-called 'annoyance' of the population, a state of subjective discomfort associated with such symptoms as nervousness, headaches, insomnia, tiredness and irritability. To establish the causal links between annoyance and mental disorder, it proved necessary also to take account of noise sensitivity, a psychophysio-logical factor which varies markedly between members of the general population and was significantly related to both covert psychiatric morbidity and annoyance. With regard to one noxious urban factor, therefore, epidemiological investigation has succeeded in demonstrating that mental disorder is related to predisposition and reactivity as well as to direct causation, depending less on the intensity of any single factor than on the confluence of noxious factors on 'vulnerable' or 'high-risk' members of the population. If the quality of life becomes unbearable there is a transition from annoyance and dissatisfaction to dysthymic states and then to a frankly psychiatric symptom-pattern.

4 Conclusion

So much for this brief overview of the epidemiological approach to psychiatric morbidity in the urban milieu. Clearly the list of potential noxae can be widely extended to include a host of other pollutants but in all cases the objective is the same: to identify adverse factors in the environment and demonstrate their effect on mental health. But what then should be done? In asking this question we are proposing, implicitly or explicitly, that environmental changes may be desirable and by so doing we leave the protected harbour of medical and scientific inquiry for the choppy waters of social administration. The theory of public health is rooted in epidemiology, but its practice depends on political action. In the sphere of physical illness, the pattern has been established for the control of infectious diseases and is now being adapted to tackle such major issues as lead pollution, accident prevention, smoking and other disorders related to lifestyle. So far, relatively little direct action has been taken because of the risks of mental disease but it is worth noting that the United States Appeals Court has ruled that electricity can no longer be generated by the reactor at the Three Mile Island Site in Pennsylvania until it has been shown that the mental health of the population will not suffer as a consequence.[21] The implications of this decision for social policy may be profound, not least because it signifies an awareness of the impact of an environmental pollutant on psychological well-being. As such, it underlines the practical as well as the theoretical significance of the epidemiological approach to mental disorders.

REFERENCES

1 Mumford L. The city in history. Its origin, its transformations and its prospects. Harmondsworth: Penguin Books, 1961
2 Connolly CV. [Palinurus, pseud.] The unquiet grave. A word cycle. London: Arrow Books, 1961
3 Milgram S. The experience of living in cities. Science 1970; 167: 1461–1468
4 Office of Population Censuses and Surveys. The Registrar General's Statistical Review of England and Wales for the year 1971. London: HMSO, 1973
5 White WA. The geographical distribution of insanity in the United States. J Nerv Ment Dis 1903; 30: 257–279
6 Goldhamer H, Marshall A. Psychosis and civilization. Glencoe, Illinois: Free Press, 1953
7 Eaton JW, Weil RJ. Culture and mental disorders: a comparative study of the Hutterites and other populations. Glencoe, Illinois: Free Press, 1955
8 Faris REL, Dunham HW. Mental disorders in urban areas: an ecological study of schizophrenia and other psychoses. 2nd edition. New York: Hafner Publishing, 1960
9 Levy L, Rowitz L. The ecology of mental disorder. New York: Behavioral Publications, 1973
10 World Health Organization. Schizophrenia: an international follow-up study. Chichester: Wiley, 1979
11 Shepherd M, Cooper B, Brown AC, Kalton G. Psychiatric illness in general practice. 2nd edition. Oxford: Oxford University Press, 1982

12 General Register Office. Morbidity Statistics from General Practice, Vol. 1 (General) by Logan WPD, Cushion AA. (Studies on Medical and Population Subjects, No. 14). London: HMSO, 1958
13 Vázquez Barquero JL, Muñoz PE, Madog Jaúregui V. The influence of the process of urbanization on the prevalence of neurosis: a community survey. Acta Psychiat Scand 1982; 65: 161–170
14 Rutter M. The city and the child. Am J Orthopsychiatry 1981; 51: 610–625
15 West DJ. Present conduct and future delinquency. First report of the Cambridge study in delinquent behaviour. London: Heinemann, 1969
16 Mills IH, Eden MAM. Social disturbances affecting young people in modern society. In: Harrison GA, Gibson JB, eds. Man in urban environments. Oxford: Oxford University Press, 1977
17 Gath D, Cooper, B, Gattoni F & Rockett D. Child guidance and delinquency in a London borough. (Institute of Psychiatry Maudsley Monograph 24). Oxford: Oxford University Press, 1977
18 Moore NC. Psychiatric illness and living in flats. Br J Psychiatry 1974, 125: 500–507
19 Brown GW, Harris T. Social origins of depression: a study of psychiatric disorder in women. London: Tavistock, 1978
20 Tarnopolsky A, Morton-Williams J. Aircraft noise and prevalence of psychiatric disorders. Research report. London: Social & Community Planning Research, 1980 (P. 460)
21 Editorial: Can change damage your mental health? Nature, 1982; 295: 177

Notes on Contributors

DR E D ACHESON has been Chief Medical Officer at the Department of Health and Social Security since January 1984. Previously, he was Professor of Clinical Epidemiology at the University of Southampton and Honorary Consultant Physician at the Royal South Hants Hospital (1968–83); Foundation Dean of the Faculty of Medicine of Southampton University (1968–78) and Director of the Medical Research Council Unit in Environmental Epidemiology (1979–83). His research interests have been in epidemiology with a particular interest in the environmental and occupational fields. He has been a member of various advisory committees to Government and the MRC, and a member of the Royal Commission on Environmental Pollution between 1979–83. Between 1980–81, he was Chairman of the DHSS Working Group on Primary Health Care in Inner London.

DR A M ADELSTEIN was Chief Medical Statistician at the Office of Population Censuses and Surveys from 1967 to 1981, after which he was Visiting Professor at the London School of Hygiene and Tropical Medicine. His earlier career included practice in industrial medicine and a senior lectureship in epidemiology at the University of Manchester. He is currently working on the epidemiology of various cancers, for example, rates of cancer in immigrants, and in persons who were born to mothers with virus infections during pregnancy. His publications include: 'Accident proneness' (J R Stat Soc 1952; CXV; Part III); with G B Hill, 'Cohort mortality from carcinoma of the cervix' (Lancet 1967; ii: 605–606); and, with W H W Inman, 'Rise and fall of asthma mortality in England and Wales in relation to use of pressurised aerosols' (Lancet 1969; ii: 279–285). In 1983 Dr Adelstein was awarded the Bisset Hawkins Medal by the Royal College of Physicians.

DR B K ARMSTRONG is Director of the National Health and Medical Research Council of Australia's Research Unit in Epidemiology and Preventive Medicine in the University of Western Australia. He is a fellow of the Royal Australasian College of Physicians and received his DPhil degree from the University of Oxford after three year's work with Sir Richard Doll on the epidemiology of cancer in the urinary tract. In Australia, he has continued research in the epidemiology of cancer and cardiovascular disease and has made recent contributions in the environmental epidemiology of malignant melanoma and the role of diet in the aetiology and control of hypertension.

PROFESSOR D J P BARKER is Director of the Medical Research Council's Environmental Epidemiology Unit, Professor of Clinical Epidemiology at the University of Southampton, and a Consultant Physician at the Royal South Hants Hospital. After qualifying at Guy's Hospital, he was Research Fellow in Social Medicine and then Lecturer in Medicine at the University of Birmingham. In 1969 he went to Uganda on a grant from the Medical Research Council to investigate the transmission of Myco ulcerans infection. Returning to England in 1972, he joined the staff of the new medical school at Southampton. He has studied the geographical distribution of disease within Britain in order to explore suspected causes, in particular nutritional and occupational. He is the author of two textbooks of epidemiology.

L BULUSU is currently a statistician in the Medical Statistics Division of the Office of Population Censuses and Surveys, London. After qualifying in statistics, he first worked as a lecturer in statistics and then as a member of the scientific staff of the Medical Research Council. His past work was associated with calcium and phosphate metabolism, bone formation/resorption and density with special reference to osteoporosis, and

clinical trials. His current work is in the field of mortality statistics, related to geography, immigration and seasonal variation. He is joint author with M M Marmot & A M Adelstein of Immigrant mortality in England and Wales, 1970–78.

MR DENIS BURKITT worked from 1946–1964 in Uganda as a government surgeon and as a member of the Surgical Department at the Makerere University Medical School after serving for five years as a surgeon in the Army. In 1964 he joined the external scientific staff of the Medical Research Council, returning to England to continue work with the MRC two years later. Leaving the MRC in 1976, he was appointed Honorary Senior Research Fellow in the Unit of Geographical Pathology at St. Thomas' Hospital Medical School. His past scientific work included the recognition of Burkitt's lymphoma as a specific clinical entity. He also helped to pioneer the chemotherapy of this disease. Subsequently he became involved in epidemiological studies of the diseases now recognized to be characteristic of modern Western culture. He has been awarded The Gold Medal of the British Medical Association, The Paul Ehrlick-Ludwig Darmstaedter Gold Medal (Germany), and an honorary Fellowship of Trinity College Dublin.

DR DAVID COGGON is a member of clinical scientific staff at the Medical Research Council's Environmental Epidemiology Unit, University of Southampton. He graduated from the University of Oxford in 1976 and, after a period of training in general medicine, took up his current post in 1980. His main research interest is the epidemiology of cancers related to occupation (e.g., D Coggon & E D Acheson. 'Do phenoxy herbicides cause cancer in man?' Lancet 1982; i: 1057–1095.

NICHOLAS E DAY is a graduate of Oxford University. His major interests are cancer epidemiology and the development of statistical methods and models for use in this field. After graduating in mathematics, he obtained a PhD in statistics at Aberdeen University. Three years as a research fellow at the Institute of Advanced Studies at the Australian National University preceded his move, in 1969, to the International Agency for Research on Cancer in Lyon, whee he is currently head of the Unit of Biostatistics and Field Studies. Three major publications are: Statistical methods in cancer research, Vol. I— The analysis of case-control studies (IARC Scientific Publications No. 32); Cancer in Singapore (IARC Scientific Publications No. 47); and Second cancer in relation to radiation treatment for cervical cancer (IARC Scientific Publications No. 52); for all of which he is co-author and editor.

PROFESSOR SIR RICHARD DOLL has been engaged in epidemiological and clinical research since 1945. He succeeded Sir Austin Bradford Hill as director of the Medical Research Council's Statistical Unit in 1961, was Regius Professor of Medicine at the University of Oxford from 1969–79, and the first Warden of Green College, Oxford, from 1979–83. He is now an honorary consultant in the Imperial Cancer Research Fund's Cancer Epidemiology and Clinical Trials Unit, which he had previously directed since its foundation. His early work with Sir Austin first demonstrated the causal relationship between cigarette smoking and lung cancer. Later work showed the importance of asbestos and other occupational chemicals in producing the same disease, the quantitative relationship between leukaemia and exposure to ionizing radiations (with the late Professor Michael Court Brown), and the long term effects of the use of oral contraceptives (with Professor Martin Vessey). He was elected a Fellow of the Royal Society in 1966 and has received awards for his work from many organizations, including the United Nations, and academic bodies in the United States, Canada, France, and Italy, as well as Britain.

DR JEAN-MARIE EKOE qualified in medicine in the Faculty of Medicine, University of Lausanne in 1976,

and had held posts in several Swiss Hospital Centres. In 1980, he became Chief Resident in the Diabetes Unit of the University Cantonal Hospital, Geneva, where he acquired training and research interests in diabetes and its management. In October 1983, he competed successfully for the newly founded Kelly M West Epidemiology Research Fellowship, a joint World Health Organisation/International Diabetes Federation venture funded by Eli Lilly. In the Division of Non-Communicable Diseases of WHO, he has undertaken the task of collating information on the prevalence manifestations and impact on health of diabetes globally and has a particular interest in diabetes in the developing world.

PROFESSOR JOHN FOX has been Professor of Social Statistics at City University since 1980. After completing a PhD in statistics at Imperial College, on a project sponsored by the Medical Research Council, he spent four years planning, conducting and analysing epidemiological studies for the Employment Medical Advisory Service. Of particular interest at this time was work on the 'healthy worker effect' (with P F Collier, 'Low mortality rates in industrial cohort studies due to selection for work and survival in the industry', Br J Prev Soc Med 30: 225–230). A background in occupational health epidemiology was of major importance to his next post in the Office of Population Censuses and Surveys where he was responsible for preparing the most recent decennial supplement on occupational mortality (Occupational mortality 1970–72, Series DS no. 1, HMSO, 1978). For the past six years he has been working on the OPCS Longitudinal Study (with P O Goldblatt, Sociodemographic mortality differentials; OPCS longitudinal study 1971–75, Series LS no. 1, HMSO, 1982) and has recently brought together, in the Social Statistics Research Unit at City, a number of researchers who are looking at migration, cancer incidence and survival, bereavement and mortality using this source.

DR MARTIN GARDNER graduated as a mathematician and later received a PhD degree in statistics from the University of London. He worked for the Medical Research Council for a number of years, before becoming Senior Lecturer in Medical Statistics at the University of Southampton on the setting up of the new medical school. He was later appointed Reader in Medical Statistics before moving to the new MRC Environmental Epidemiology Unit also at Southampton. His interests have long been in the geographical patterns of disease, and he has recently published with other authors, the Atlas of cancer mortality in England and Wales, 1968–78. He also published on time trends in cancer mortality (with C Osmond, E D Acheson & A M Adelstein, Trends in cancer mortality, analyses by period of birth and death, 1951–80, England and Wales. OPCS Series DH1, No. 11.) and asbestos and health (with E D Acheson, The control limit for asbestos. HMSO 1983).

DR P O GOLDBLATT is a statistician in the Medical Statistics Division of the Office of Population Censuses and Surveys ()PCS). He completed his degrees in mathematics and statistics at the University of Manchester. His doctoral research was on Bayesian methods in population sampling. This was carried out at Manchester and at the Indian Statistical Institute, Calcutta. From 1975–77 he worked on an SSRC project on subjective probability assessment. Since joining OPCS in 1977, he has worked on a variety of medical research projects (for example, with P Fraser & C Chilvers, 'Census-based mortality study of fertiliser manufacturers' BJIM; 39: 323–329; with J H Fuller, J Elford & A M Adelstein, 'Diabetes mortality: new light on an underestimated public health problem' Diabetologia; 24: 336–341; and with A J Fox, Longitudinal study: sociodemographic mortality differentials, Series LS no. 1 HMSO 1982).

PROFESSOR M S R HUTT is Professor of Geographical Pathology in the Histopathology Department of St Thomas's Hospital Medical School, London. He graduated in medicine at the University of London and subsequently trained in pathology. In 1957 he was appointed consultant in clinical pathology to the Louis Jenner Laboratories in St Thomas' Hospital, and in 1962 became the second Professor of Pathology at Makerere University College in Kampala, Uganda. In 1970 he returned to the United Kingdom to take up his present post. While in Uganda he became interested in the epidemiological and geographical aspects of disease and has published widely on these topics, particularly in the field of cancer, renal and heart disease. His publications include *Medicine in a tropical environment*, edited with A G Shaper & J Kibukamusoke; and *Cardiovascular disease in the tropics*, edited with A G Shaper & Z Fejfar. He is Chairman of the Editorial Board of *Tropical Doctor* and on the Council of the Royal Society of Tropical Medicine and Hygiene.

DR D R JONES is a senior research fellow in the Social Statistics Research Unit at The City University in London. After obtaining undergraduate and higher degrees in mathematics, he worked briefly in town planning research. Thereafter he was a research fellow in the National Health Service, principally concerned with statistical modelling of its patterns of resources (with S Masterman, 'NHS resources: scales of variations', *Br J Prev Soc Med* 1976; 30: 244–250). Following a move to the Institute of Cancer Research in Sutton, he developed an interest in the methodolody of clinical trials and epidemiological studies which he continued to pursue when appointed Senior Lecturer in Medical Statistics at Westminster Medical School, London (with J Whitehead, 'The analysis of sequential clinical trials', *Biometrika* 1979; 443–452; with L Rushton, 'Simultaneous inference in epidemiological studies' *Int J Epidemiol* 1982; 11: 276–282). In 1982 he joined the Social Statistics Research Unit, where his current interests include anaysis of patterns of mortality and widowhood in the OPCS Longitudinal Study by socio-demographic and enviromental variables.

PROFESSOR HARRY KEEN qualified in medicine at St. Mary's Hospital in 1948, where he spent several years in the Medical Unit with the late Professor Sir George Pickering and subsequently Professor W S Peart. During this period, he started a study of the family links between diabetes and hypertension and this laid the basis for his continuing interest in the epidemiology and genetics of these diseases. Following a research fellowship in diabetes at NIH, Bethesda, he returned to the Department of Medicine, Guy's Hospital, London, in 1961. There, he has continued studies of diabetes, combining laboratory investigation with clinical studies and epidemiologically based investigation of population samples. The retinal and renal complications of diabetes have become a major research interest, inspired a book, *The complications of diabetes* (jointly with Professor R J Jarrett), and are the main lines of work in the Unit for Metabolic Medicine at Guy's Hospital.

IAN LECK has been Professor of Community Medicine in the University of Manchester since 1979. He is also Honorary specialist in Community Medicine, Central Manchester Health District. He first came to Manchester in 1971 as Reader in Social and Preventive Medicine and Director of the Regional Cancer Epidemiology Unit, where he was particularly involved in studying the epidemiology of childhood neoplasms and bladder cancer and in developing quality control methods for cancer registration and anticoagulent therapy. He has reviewed aspects of the epidemiology of malformations in several books including *Handbook of teratology*, Vol. 3, pp. 243–324 (edited by J G Wilson & F C Fraser, 1977) and *Obstetrical epidemiology* pp. 263–318 (edited by S L Barron & A M Thomson, 1983) and in two earlier numbers of the Bulletin (*Br Med Bull* 1974; 30: 158–163; and 1976; 32: 45–52).

DR M G MARMOT is Senior Lecturer in Epidemiology at the London School of Hygiene and Tropical Medicine, and Honorary Consultant in the Cardiac Department, University College Hospital, London. He trained in medicine at the University of Sydney, Australia. In 1971 he went to the University of California, Berkeley, for postgraduate work in epidemiology including a PhD degree. While there, he worked on studies of heart disease among men of Japanese ancestry living in Japan, Hawaii and California. His interest in blood pressure and cardiovascular disease took him to Panama, New Zealand and the Philippines. After lecturing in epidemiology at Berkeley he moved to the London School of Hygiene and Tropical Medicine where his interests have included social influences on cardiovascular disease, a study of disease in immigrants, and now international studies of electrolyte excretion and blood pressure.

MRS P J COOK-MOZAFFARI is a member of the external staff of the Medical Research Council attached to the Department of Community Medicine and General Practice in the University of Oxford. After initial training as a geographer, she did postgraduate work in epidemiology and statistics in Oxford and then worked as a research associate in the Cancer Registry in Birmingham fro 1964 to 1966. She subsequently joined the MRC Statistical Research Unit in London and has been an employee of the MRC ever since, in London until 1974 and then in Oxford. Between 1969 and 1976 she also worked for extended periods as a consultant for the International Agency for Research on Cancer (WHO) on projects in Africa and Iran. Work has centred on the establishment of cancer registries and assessment of the regional distribution of cancer in Africa, on detailed studies of the aetiology of cancer and the oesophagus; and on the use of British mortality and incidence data to study small-scale variations in cancer frequency.

HUGH TUNSTALL PEDOE is Director and Professor of the Cardiovascular Epidemiology Unit, Ninewells Hospital and Medical School, Dundee, and Honorary Consultant Cardiologist and Specialist in Community Medicine, Tayside Health Board. He qualified in medicine in 1964, obtaining his MD degree there in 1978. He is a Fellow of the Royal College of Physicians and a Fellow of the Faculty of Community Medicine.

DR M C PIKE has, since October 1983, been the director of the Imperial Cancer Research Fund's Cancer Epidemiology and Clinical Trials Unit at the Radcliffe Infirmary, Oxford. Dr Pike received his initial mathematical training at Witwatersrand University in Johannesburg. He subsequently trained as a mathematical statistician at Cambridge University and at the University of Aberdeen where he obtained his PhD in 1962. He joined Professor Sir Richard Doll's MRC Statistical Research Unit in London in 1963 and moved with Professor Doll to Oxford in 1969. Between 1966 and 1969 he worked for some two years at Makerere Medical School in Uganda. From 1973 to 1983 Dr Pike was Professor of Preventive Medicine at the University of Southern California Medical School in Los Angeles. Dr Pike's current interests concern the aetiology of hormone-related cancers, in particular breast cancer and testicular cancer.

DR SCHALK VAN RENSBURG initially spent 13 years researching the pathophysiology of the reproductive system, making basic contributions to the causes of parturition initiation and the endocrinology of habitual abortion. In 1969 he joined the newly established South African Medical Research Council, soon to head the Division of Nutritional Pathology, until becoming Assistant Director in the Institute for Nutritional Diseases in 1982. Etiological investigations on diseases peculiar to remote parts of rural Africa, including some

possible mycotoxicoses and both liver and oesophageal cancer, are still receiving attention. Some 80 publications include 'Primary liver cancer rate and aflatoxin intake in a high cancer area'. (*S Afr Med J* 1974; 48: 2508a–2509d) and 'Epidemiologic and dietary evidence for a specific nutritional predisposition to oesophageal cancer' (*JNCI* 1981; 67: 243–251).

DR RONALD K ROSS is an associate professor of preventive medicine at University of Southern California School of Medicine in Los Angeles. Dr Ross's current research interests concern the aetiology of hormone-related cancers and the risks and benefits of hormone replacement therapy. His published works include: R K Ross, A Paganini-Hill, T M Mack, M Arthur & B E Henderson, 'Menopausal estrogen therapy and protection from heart disease death' (*Lancet* 1981; i: 858–860); R K Ross, A P Hill, V R Gerkins et al. 'A case-control study of menopausal estrogen therapy and breast cancer' (*JAMA* 1980; 243: 1635–1639); B E Henderson, R K Ross, M C Pike & J T Casagrande, 'Endogenous hormones as a major factor in human cancer (*Cancer Res* 1982; 42: 3232–3234); and A Paganini-Hill, R K Ross, V R Gerkins, B E Henderson, M Arthur & T M Mack, 'A case-control study of menopausal estrogen therapy and hip fractures' (*Ann Int Med* 1981; 95: 28–31).

PROFESSOR A G SHAPER has been Professor of Clinical Epidemiology at the Royal Free Hospital School of Medicine, University of London since 1975. Before this he was a member of the Scientific Staff of the MRC Social Medicine Unit at the London School of Hygiene and Tropical Medicine. He was WHO Professor of Cardiovascular Research at Makerere University, Uganda until 1970, having been successively a Lecturer, Senior Lecturer and Reader in Medicine there from 1957. His main interests lie in the field of cardiovascular disease with particular reference to the role of nutrition, to geographical variations and to risk factors in ischaemic heart disease and hypertension. Since 1975 he has directed the Regional Heart Study which is concerned with regional variations in cardiovascular disease in Great Britain and with the aetiology of ischaemic heart disease and hypertension.

PROFESSOR MICHAEL SHEPHERD has held the chair of Epidemiological Psychiatry at the Institute of Psychiatry, University of London, since 1967. He is also Honorary Consultant to the Bethlem Royal and Maudsley Hospitals and to King's College Hospital, and is Honorary Director of the General Practice Research Unit. In addition to his research into various aspects of the epidemiology of mental disorders, he has contributed to the fields of clinical psychiatry, psychopharmacology, medical education and medical history. His current research programme is centred on the causes, identification and treatment of mental illness in the community. His publications number some 200 papers and 15 books, two of them volumes of collected papers, and include *The psychosocial matrix of psychiatry* (1983) and, with B Cooper, A C Brown & G W Kalton, *Psychiatric illness in general practice* 2nd edition (1981). Professor Shepherd is general editor of the 5-volume *Handbook of psychiatry* (1983–1984) and the founder-editor of *Psychological Medicine*. He received the Donald Reid medal for epidemiology in 1982 and the Rema Lapouse award of the American Public Health Association in 1983.

WILLIAM CAIRNS SMITH qualified in medicine in Aberdeen in 1974. In 1982 he obtained his MPH degree in Dundee and became a Member of the Faculty of Community Medicine. From 1977 to 1980, he was Medical Superintendent of General and Leprosy Hospitals, India. He is currently an epidemiologist in the Cardiovascular Epidemiology Unit at Ninewells Hospital and Medical School, Dundee, and Honorary Specialist in Community Medicine, Tayside Health Board.

INDEX

Computer typeset by SB Datagraphics. Printed in Great Britain by Spottiswoode Ballantyne Printers Ltd.

The value of epidemiological studies and the large amount of information which they provide are clearly demonstrated in the papers contained in this volume.

Whilst the majority of chapters concern specific diseases or disease groups, examples of widely applicable methodologies are also discussed. The importance of collaboration between epidemiologists and their laboratory and clinical colleagues is emphasised. Not only does this volume report on established issues but it also provides ideas and direction for future research and investigation.

The contents of this book are identical to the October, 1984 issue of the British Medical Bulletin (Volume 40, Number 4) and are made available in this format for non-subscribers.

ISBN 0 443 03085 5